Cardiovascular Surgery

Rui Manuel de Sousa Sequeira
Antunes de Almeida
Fabio Biscegli Jatene
Editors

Nathalia Ribeiro Pinho de Sousa
Gabriel Romero Liguori
Marcus Rodrigo Monteiro
Leila Nogueira Barros
Associate Editors

Cardiovascular Surgery

A Clinical Casebook

Springer

Editors
Rui Manuel de Sousa Sequeira Antunes de Almeida
Department of Cardiology and Cardiovascular Surgery
University Center Assis Gurgacz Foundation
Cascavel, PR
Brazil

Fabio Biscegli Jatene
Department of Cardiovascular Surgery
University of São Paulo Medical School
São Paulo, SP
Brazil

Associate Editors
Nathalia Ribeiro Pinho de Sousa
Faculdade de Medicina da Universidade Federal do Ceará
Fortaleza, CE
Brasil

Marcus Rodrigo Monteiro
Universidade Federal de São Paulo
Escola Paulista de Medicina
Residente de Cirurgia Geral SUS SP
São Paulo, SP
Brazil

Gabriel Romero Liguori
Instituto do Coração (InCor)
Hospital das Clínicas HCFMUSP
Faculdade de Medicina
Universidade de São Paulo
São Paulo, SP
Brazil

Leila Nogueira Barros
Faculdade de Ciências Médicas da Santa Casa de São Paulo
Residente de Cirurgia Cardiovascular da Santa Casa de São Paulo
São Paulo, SP
Brazil

ISBN 978-3-319-57083-9 ISBN 978-3-319-57084-6 (eBook)
https://doi.org/10.1007/978-3-319-57084-6

Library of Congress Control Number: 2018961581

This Springer imprint is published by the registered company Springer Nature Switzerland AG
The registered company address is: Gewerbestrasse 11, 6330 Cham, Switzerland

Foreword

It was a pleasure and privilege to write the preface to this book, *Cardiovascular Surgery: A Clinical Casebook*. A great number of books on cardiovascular surgery are written every year, both here in Brazil and internationally. Some of these publications deal with a special field or subspecialty. Each one plays an important role in updating the literature and educating new trainees. The main limitation of all books is the time period required to prepare the text for publication, when new advances will undoubtedly appear in a rapidly developing specialty such as cardiovascular surgery.

This book has a number of features that make it special—and therefore make me happy to comment on it here. First, the text was prepared by graduate medical students in English, thus fulfilling the recommendation that all medical students have proficiency in this particular language. Furthermore, the authors come from different medical schools and were supervised by an editorial board of professionals from different academic institutions.

Secondly, the book focuses on clinical cases, with additional questions and answers based on a particular case. There is also discussion of the subjects related to the case and literature references. This format is of utmost practical importance for students and trainees in cardiovascular surgery. For decades, our specialty has become progressively more complex and is incorporating more technology into its practice. Transcatheter and minimally invasive procedures have introduced even more complexity into the procedures of cardiovascular surgery.

This field can be highly challenging for medical students and residents. Educational programs and participation in cardiovascular surgery societies can help in the training of future specialists. However, the current 5-year minimum duration for residency is longer than that of other specialties. Furthermore, there is a greater need for human and financial resources at the institutions where these younger colleagues can practice their specialty after training. These factors may discourage potential candidates from entering the field of cardiovascular surgery. However, a number of initiatives can help to increase students' interest in pursuing a career as a cardiovascular surgeon and are fundamental to the future of the specialty, including the academic leagues of cardiovascular surgery, the participation of students in congresses of the specialty, and this book, which has been mainly prepared by students.

Finally, I want to congratulate the medical students who prepared the cases and participated in other aspects of the chapters in this book. I also congratulate the supervisors who supported this initiative and contributed to the quality of the publication.

Noedir A. G. Stolf
Emeritus and Senior Professor
University of São Paulo Medical School
São Paulo, SP, Brazil

Preface

The book *Cardiovascular Surgery—A Clinical Casebook* is a great team effort from a group of medical students who are interested in cardiovascular surgery. Born from the wish to contribute to the development of graduating medical students and residents in this specialty, this book was a massive undertaking by students that belong to academic leagues in cardiology and cardiovascular surgery, as well as the Department of Academic Leagues of the Brazilian Society of Cardiovascular Surgery.

The initial dream for this book was to publish 20 chapters from different national leagues, but the final publication ended up having 40 chapters. The book is divided into 12 sections that are of great importance to this field: aortic disease, arrhythmias, cardiac tumors, coronary insufficiency, congenital heart disease, endovascular therapies, heart failure, heart transplantation, mechanical circulatory support, pericardial disease, pulmonary embolism, and valvular heart disease.

Each section discusses one or more clinical cases using a common format, which includes the clinical presentation, diagnosis, assessment, and treatment. After the clinical case presentation, the authors of each chapter answer some questions related to any challenging points, positions that are not well defined in current practice, and any controversies in a way that allows the reader to follow a straight line of clinical judgment. All 40 clinical cases are especially relevant because they are common cases that were chosen by the cardiac surgeon to orientate the students. The chapters are richly illustrated with figures from common imaging examinations and the surgery itself.

This book can be read from front to back or in no particular order. It should be consulted when you have a similar clinical case and have to make clinical or surgical decisions. Furthermore, it will allow you to see if your clinical judgment and conduct is similar to or different from those of the chapter's authors.

This is a unique book for two reasons. First, it was written and edited by students, under the supervision of cardiovascular surgeons. Furthermore, it is a work of the medical students of the Brazilian Society of Cardiovascular Surgery; however, it was not written in their native language so that a large number of global students would also have the opportunity to read it.

Professor Noedir Stolf was invited to write the Introduction because of his great contributions to cardiac surgery and medical education. He is a true believer in the formation of young people in this specialty and is a mentor to a great number of residents. We personally think that early exposure to cardiovascular surgery during medical school, in addition to a true mentor relationship, are the primary factors that influence a medical school graduate to embrace this specialty.

On behalf of all authors, we hope that you enjoy reading this book, are able to review the concepts and ideas on all the cases present herein, and learn from what is described and the manner in which the patients were treated.

Rui M. S. Almeida
Paraná Western State University
Medical School Dean University Center FAG
Cascavel, PR, Brazil

Contents

Part IV Coronary Insufficiency

Contributors

Leonardo Jadyr Silva Rodrigues Alves Unified School of Brasília (UNICEUB), Brasília, DF, Brazil

Rafael Ramos Amaral Unified School of Brasília (UNICEUB), Brasília, DF, Brazil

Vitor Abaurre Amaral School of Sciences of Santa Casa de Misericórdia de Vitória (EMESCAM), Vitória, ES, Brazil

Gabriel Donato Amorim School of Sciences of Santa Casa de Misericórdia de Vitória (EMESCAM), Vitória, ES, Brazil

Heloísa Guedes Andrade Assis Gurgacz Foundation University (FAG), Cascavel, PR, Brazil

Luciano Castiglioni Andriato University Center of Espírito Santo (UNESC), Colatina, ES, Brazil

Emanuel Sampaio Araújo Federal University of Ceará (UFC), Sobral, CE, Brazil

Anderson Dias Arruda Federal University of Ceará (UFC), Sobral, CE, Brazil

Fernando Antibas Atik Cardiology Institute of Federal District (ICDF), Brasília, DF, Brazil

Débora Cristina Haack Bassani Santa Cruz do Sul University (UNISC), Santa Cruz do Sul, RS, Brazil

Leandro Pedro Goloni Bertollo Faculty of Medicine of University of São Paulo (FMUSP), São Paulo, SP, Brazil

Elisa Cao Bicalho School of Sciences of Santa Casa de Misericórdia de Vitória (EMESCAM), Vitória, ES, Brazil

Valquiria Pelisser Campagnucci Santa Casa de São Paulo School of Medical Sciences (FCMSCSP), São Paulo, SP, Brazil

Luiz Fernando Caneo Faculty of Medicine of University of São Paulo (FMUSP), São Paulo, SP, Brazil

Marcos Antonio Cantero Federal University of Grande Dourados (UFGD), Dourados, MS, Brazil

Lucas Alves Bessa Cardoso Federal University of Viçosa (UFV), Viçosa, MG, Brazil

João Vitor Ferreira Carvalho Federal University of Grande Dourados (UFGD), Dourados, MS, Brazil

Marisa Wanderley Casado Federal University of Paraíba (UFPB), João Pessoa, PB, Brazil

Eduardo Gregório Chamlian Federal University of São Paulo (UNIFESP), São Paulo, SP, Brazil

Graziela Chequer Minas Gerais Federal University (UFMG), Belo Horizonte, MG, Brazil

Eugênio Antônio Mascarenhas Colonnezy Federal University of Bahia (UFBA), Salvador, BA, Brazil

Dhaisa Thaina Souza Conceição Federal University of Bahia (UFBA), Salvador, BA, Brazil

Anderson Berni Cristofari Santa Cruz do Sul University (UNISC), Santa Cruz do Sul, RS, Brazil

Vanessa Dias D'Avila Sperandio School of Sciences of Santa Casa de Misericórdia de Vitória (EMESCAM), Vitória, ES, Brazil

Fernando Augusto Alves da Costa Anhembi Morumbi University (UAM), São Paulo, SP, Brazil

Claudio Ribeiro da Cunha Cardiology Institute of Federal District (ICDF), Brasília, DF, Brazil

Felipe Bruno Santos da Cunha Unified School of Brasília (UNICEUB), Brasília, DF, Brazil

Assiane Gabriela Anceles da Rocha Catholic University of Pernambuco (UNICAP), Recife, PE, Brazil

Amanda Késsia da Silva Sales Federal University of Ceará (UFC), Sobral, CE, Brazil

Rayane da Silva Souza Federal University of Paraíba (UFPB), João Pessoa, PB, Brazil

Luciana Baltazar da Silveira de Araujo Federal University of Bahia (UFBA), Salvador, BA, Brazil

Daniel Tomasi Keppen Sequeira de Almeida Assis Gurgacz Foundation University (FAG), Cascavel, PR, Brazil

Filipe T. K. S. Almeida Assis Gurgacz Foundation University (FAG), Cascavel, PR, Brazil

Rui M. S. Almeida Assis Gurgacz Foundation University (FAG), Cascavel, PR, Brazil

Mamede Francisco Johnson de Aquino Filho Federal University of Ceará (UFC), Sobral, CE, Brazil

Nilton Freire de Assis Neto Anhembi Morumbi University (UAM), São Paulo, SP, Brazil

Rômulo Martins de Camargo Federal University of São Paulo (UNIFESP), São Paulo, SP, Brazil

Guilherme Henrique Ribeiro de Carvalho Faculty of Medicine of University of São Paulo (FMUSP), São Paulo, SP, Brazil

Laryssa Alves de Farias Catholic University of Pernambuco (UNICAP), Recife, PE, Brazil

Orival de Freitas Filho Faculty of Medicine of University of São Paulo (FMUSP), São Paulo, SP, Brazil

Daniel Bartholo de Hyppolito Santa Casa of Sao Paulo School of Medical Sciences (FCMSCSP), São Paulo, SP, Brazil

Eduardo Teles de Lima Lopes Federal University of Viçosa (UFV), Viçosa, MG, Brazil

José Antônio de Lima Neto Federal University of Ceará (UFC), Sobral, CE, Brazil

Thainá de Lima Quinteiro Federal University of Bahia (UFBA), Salvador, BA, Brazil

Maria Tereza de Magalhães Andrade Federal University of Bahia (UFBA), Salvador, BA, Brazil

André Gorle de Miranda Chaves Minas Gerais Federal University (UFMG), Belo Horizonte, MG, Brazil

Eugênio Patrício de Oliveira Federal University of Paraíba (UFPB), João Pessoa, PB, Brazil

Felipe Bezerra Martins de Oliveira Cardiology Institute of Federal District (ICDF), Brasília, DF, Brazil

Jéssica Silva de Paula Minas Gerais Federal University (UFMG), Belo Horizonte, MG, Brazil

Bárbara Liss de Sousa Freire Federal University of Ceará (UFC), Sobral, CE, Brazil

Helmgton José Brito de Souza Unified School of Brasília (UNICEUB), Brasília, DF, Brazil

Jéssica Krieger de Souza Federal University of Grande Dourados (UFGD), Dourados, MS, Brazil

Gilberto Loiola De Vasconcelos Federal University of Ceará (UFC), Sobral, CE, Brazil

Camila Lopes do Amaral Federal University of Ceará (UFC), Sobral, CE, Brazil

Thiago do Amaral Cavalcante Unified School of Brasília (UNICEUB), Brasília, DF, Brazil

Carla Mayara Forte dos Santos Federal University of Ceará (UFC), Sobral, CE, Brazil

Caroline Kelli Domingues dos Santos State University of Western Paraná (UNIOESTE), Cascavel, PR, Brazil

Tailana Paiva Dourado Federal University of Bahia (UFBA), Salvador, BA, Brazil

Ana Carolina Gonçalves e Silva Cardiology Institute of Federal District (ICDF), Brasília, DF, Brazil

Mateus Fagundes Assis Gurgacz Foundation University (FAG), Cascavel, PR, Brazil

Nathalia Spandl Falqueto School of Sciences of Santa Casa de Misericórdia de Vitória (EMESCAM), Vitória, ES, Brazil

André Maurício Souza Fernandes Federal University of Bahia (UFBA), Salvador, BA, Brazil

Marcus Vinícius Silva Ferreira Cardiology Institute of Federal District (ICDF), Brasília, DF, Brazil

Heraldo Guedis Lobo Filho Federal University of Ceará (UFC), Fortaleza, CE, Brazil

José Glauco Lobo Filho Federal University of Ceará (UFC), Fortaleza, CE, Brazil

Maikon Augusto Vogado Aranda Florenciano Federal University of Grande Dourados (UFGD), Dourados, MS, Brazil

Evandro Luis Queiroz Flores Assis Gurgacz Foundation University (FAG), Cascavel, PR, Brazil

Laura Gomes Flores Assis Gurgacz Foundation University (FAG), Cascavel, PR, Brazil

Mariana Vano Galvão Almeida França Anhembi Morumbi University (UAM), São Paulo, SP, Brazil

Patrícia Freitag Assis Gurgacz Foundation University (FAG), Cascavel, PR, Brazil

Leonardo Cristiano Frigini University Center of Espírito Santo (UNESC), Colatina, ES, Brazil

Edmo Atique Gabriel Grandes Lagos Faculty (UNILAGO), São José do Rio Preto, SP, Brazil

Fabio Antonio Gaiotto Faculty of Medicine of University of São Paulo (FMUSP), São Paulo, SP, Brazil

Letícia Lanzarin Gehm Santa Cruz do Sul University (UNISC), Santa Cruz do Sul, RS, Brazil

João Carlos Guaragna Pontifical Catholic University of Rio Grande do Sul (PUC- RS), Porto Alegre, RS, Brazil

Basem Juma Abdalla Abdel Hamid Santa Cruz do Sul University (UNISC), Santa Cruz do Sul, RS, Brazil

Augusto Emilio Hinterholz Santa Cruz do Sul University (UNISC), Santa Cruz do Sul, RS, Brazil

Yuri Justi Jardim Faculty of Medicine of University of São Paulo (FMUSP), São Paulo, SP, Brazil

Fabio Biscegli Jatene Faculty of Medicine of University of São Paulo (FMUSP), São Paulo, SP, Brazil

Armindo Jreige Júnior Cardiology Institute of Federal District (ICDF), Brasília, DF, Brazil

Nelson Américo Hossne Junior Federal University of São Paulo (UNIFESP), São Paulo, SP, Brazil

Roque Aras Junior Federal University of Bahia (UFBA), Salvador, BA, Brazil

Flávia Cristina Kufner Assis Gurgacz Foundation University (FAG), Cascavel, PR, Brazil

Francisco Coelho Lamachia Santa Cruz do Sul University (UNISC), Santa Cruz do Sul, RS, Brazil

Caroline Cleophas Lobo Leite Federal University of Ceará (UFC), Fortaleza, CE, Brazil

Isadora Simão Almeida Liberato Anhembi Morumbi University (UAM), São Paulo, SP, Brazil

Melchior Luiz Lima School of Sciences of Santa Casa de Misericórdia de Vitória (EMESCAM), Vitória, ES, Brazil

Rodolpho Poeys Lima Federal University of Viçosa (UFV), Viçosa, MG, Brazil

Jackson Brandão Lopes Federal University of Bahia (UFBA), Salvador, BA, Brazil

Henrique Louzan Machado Unified School of Brasília (UNICEUB), Brasília, DF, Brazil

Sergio Rodrigues Maranha University Center of Espírito Santo (UNESC), Colatina, ES, Brazil

Rízia Kérem Gonçalves Martiniano University Center of Espírito Santo (UNESC), Colatina, ES, Brazil

Fernanda Schuh Martins Santa Cruz do Sul University (UNISC), Santa Cruz do Sul, RS, Brazil

Rodrigo Mendes Federal University of São Paulo (UNIFESP), São Paulo, SP, Brazil

Jéssica Nathiele Meotti Assis Gurgacz Foundation University (FAG), Cascavel, PR, Brazil

Gabriel Lorente Mitsumoto Santa Casa de São Paulo School of Medical Sciences (FCMSCSP), São Paulo, SP, Brazil

Rodrigo Mont'Alverne Guimarães Federal University of Ceará (UFC), Sobral, CE, Brazil

Daniela Moraes Santa Cruz do Sul University (UNISC), Santa Cruz do Sul, RS, Brazil

Leonardo Jadyr Silva Rodrigues Alves Unified School of Brasília (UNICEUB), Brasília, DF, Brazil

Daiane Thaysa Brito Nakamura Federal University of Bahia (UFBA), Salvador, BA, Brazil

Filipe Alves Nery University Center of Espírito Santo (UNESC), Colatina, ES, Brazil

Joaquim David Carneiro Neto Federal University of Ceará (UFC), Sobral, CE, Brazil

Saulo Victor Benevides Nunes Federal University of Ceará (UFC), Sobral, CE, Brazil

Gabrielle Santos Oliveira Cardiology Institute of Federal District (ICDF), Brasília, DF, Brazil

Letícia Oliveira Grandes Lagos Faculty (UNILAGO), São José do Rio Preto, SP, Brazil

Fabiano André Pereira Federal University of São Paulo (UNIFESP), São Paulo, SP, Brazil

Matheus Ramos Dal Piaz School of Sciences of Santa Casa de Misericórdia de Vitória (EMESCAM), Vitória, ES, Brazil

Matheus Duarte Pimentel Federal University of Ceará (UFC), Fortaleza, CE, Brazil

Luiz Antonio Rivetti Presidente do Instituto de Pesquisa e Inovação Tecnológica da Santa Casa de São Paulo, São Paulo, SP, Brazil

Bruno da Costa Rocha Federal University of Bahia (UFBA), Salvador, Salvador, Brazil

Lissa Canedo Rocha School of Sciences of Santa Casa de Misericórdia de Vitória (EMESCAM), Vitória, ES, Brazil

Yasmine Lailla Vasconcelos Rodrigues Federal University of Ceará (UFC), Sobral, CE, Brazil

Carlos Henrique Romancini State University of Western Paraná (UNIOESTE), Cascavel, PR, Brazil

Gabriel Prado Saad Minas Gerais Federal University (UFMG), Belo Horizonte, MG, Brazil

Eduardo Keller Saadi Pontifical Catholic University of Rio Grande do Sul (PUC- RS), Porto Alegre, RS, Brazil

Marina Petersen Saadi Pontifical Catholic University of Rio Grande do Sul (PUC- RS), Porto Alegre, RS, Brazil

Rodrigo Petersen Saadi Pontifical Catholic University of Rio Grande do Sul (PUC- RS), Porto Alegre, RS, Brazil

Pedro Rafael Salerno Catholic University of Pernambuco (UNICAP), Recife, PE, Brazil

Manuela Xavier Cajado Sampaio Salvador University (UNIFACS), Salvador, BA, Brazil

Larissa Lucas Schloicka Cardiology Institute of Federal District (ICDF), Brasília, DF, Brazil

Fábio Selig Assis Gurgacz Foundation University (FAG), Cascavel, PR, Brazil

Adriana Fernandes Silva Assis Gurgacz Foundation University (FAG), Cascavel, PR, Brazil

Felipe Machado Silva Santa Casa de Sao Paulo School of Medical Sciences (FCMSCSP), São Paulo, SP, Brazil

Joely Nataly Silva Federal University of Ceará (UFC), Fortaleza, CE, Brazil

Pedro Guimarães Silva Federal University of Bahia (UFBA), Salvador, BA, Brazil

Carolina Kuchenbecker Soares Minas Gerais Federal University (UFMG), Belo Horizonte, MG, Brazil

Diogo Assis Souza Unified School of Brasília (UNICEUB), Brasília, DF, Brazil

Gabriel Pelegrineti Targueta Federal University of Paraíba (UFPB), João Pessoa, PB, Brazil

Henry Eiji Toma Santa Casa de Sao Paulo School of Medical Sciences (FCMSCSP), São Paulo, SP, Brazil

Amanda Dorighetto Tomazelli School of Sciences of Santa Casa de Misericórdia de Vitória (EMESCAM), Vitória, ES, Brazil

Cassiana Tomazoni Assis Gurgacz Foundation University (FAG), Cascavel, PR, Brazil

Camila Rocha Vieira Torres Federal University of Paraíba (UFPB), João Pessoa, PB, Brazil

Priscilla Gomes Tosta School of Sciences of Santa Casa de Misericórdia de Vitória (EMESCAM), Vitória, ES, Brazil

Anna Luiza Amâncio Vidal Federal University of Viçosa (UFV), Viçosa, MG, Brazil

Luana Luiza Vieira Assis Gurgacz Foundation University (FAG), Cascavel, PR, Brazil

Vanessa Lopes Vieira Faculty of Medicine of University of São Paulo (FMUSP), São Paulo, SP, Brazil

Raphaella von Sohsten Calabria Lima Catholic University of Pernambuco (UNICAP), Recife, PE, Brazil

Antonio Eduardo Zerati Faculty of Medicine of University of São Paulo (FMUSP), São Paulo, SP, Brazil

Nágila Simon Ziebell Santa Cruz do Sul University (UNISC), Santa Cruz do Sul, RS, Brazil

Part I
Aorta Disease

Aortic Dissection Associated with Ischemic Stroke

Rízia Kérem Gonçalves Martiniano, Filipe Alves Nery, Luciano Castiglioni Andriato, Sergio Rodrigues Maranha, and Leonardo Cristiano Frigini

Clinical Presentation

O.C.S., a 60-year-old male patient, a smoker, with a medical history of hypertension under control using captopril 25 mg, once a day. He was admitted to the emergency room on the first day with symptoms of cold sweats and angina after falling from a ladder. Because of the severity of his case, O.C.S was admitted to the Hospital Silvio Avidos (HSA), located in Colatina/ES, showing a decreased level of consciousness, hemiplegia of the left inferior limb, and a deviation of the labial commissure of mouth. Therefore, some preliminary clinical tests were performed and he was transferred 2 days later to Hospital Maternidade São José (HMSJ), also in Colatina, for better therapeutic approaches.

Because of the serious condition the patient was in, he was admitted to the Intensive Care Unit of the HMSJ,

R. K. G. Martiniano (✉) · F. A. Nery · L. C. Andriato
S. R. Maranha · L. C. Frigini
University Center of Espírito Santo (UNESC), Colatina, ES, Brazil

R. M. S. Almeida, F. B. Jatene (eds.), *Cardiovascular Surgery*,
https://doi.org/10.1007/978-3-319-57084-6_1

hemodynamically stable, pale (1+/4+), hydrated, and with an axillary temperature of 37.7 °C. In the neurological examination, the patient scored 12 points on the Glasgow Coma Scale, the pupils were mitotic and reactive to light stimulus, there was a deviation from the face to the right and hemiparesis of the left side of the body with predominance in the area of the thigh. In the cardiovascular system, the rhythm was regular, twice with normal heart sounds, but with a systolic murmur in the aortic focus. The heart rate was at 82 beats per minute, invasive blood pressure of 177 × 61 mmHg, average arterial blood pressure of 89 mmHg and he also had preserved capillary perfusion. On physical examination of the respiratory tract, the patient had vesicular breathing sounds with diffuse rhonchi, oxygen saturation of 100%, and a respiratory rate of 20 breaths per minute. There were no changes in the abdomen and lower limbs. In the genitourinary system, the diuresis was 25 ml, concentrated in a collecting bag. The patient's glycemic index was 98 mg/dl. There was no exteriorized bleeding. At the time, antibiotics were not used.

Diagnosis, Assessment, and Treatment

Before admission, investigative examinations such as computed tomography (CT) of the skull (Fig. 1) were carried out at Hospital Silvio Avidos. CT showed an area of a recent ischemic event in the territory of the right middle cerebral artery and deletion of other grooves cortical of the right brain hemispheres suggesting edema; a transthoracic echocardiogram (TTE) demonstrated mild dilatation of the aortic arch, with an image suggesting a dissection flap; on CT angiography of the abdominal and thoracic aorta (Fig. 2) dilatation of the ascending segment of the aorta was identified (measuring 5.6 × 5.5 cm in diameter), showing a blade of dissection that extends at this aortic segment to the arch, observing the extension of the dissection to the brachiocephalic trunk and left subclavian artery, with signs of partial thrombosis, including no

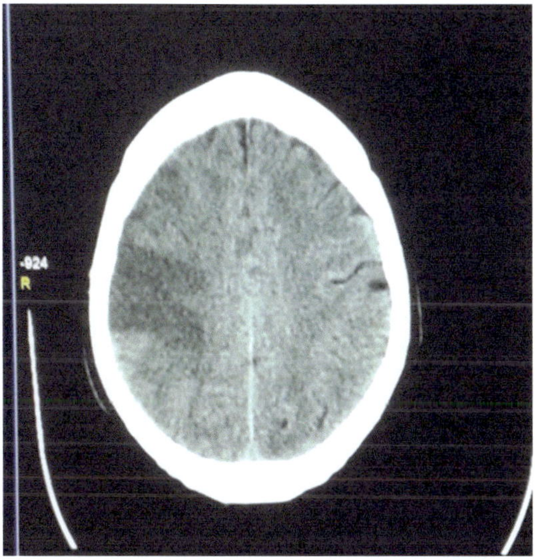

FIGURE 1 Computed tomography of the skull showing the stroke

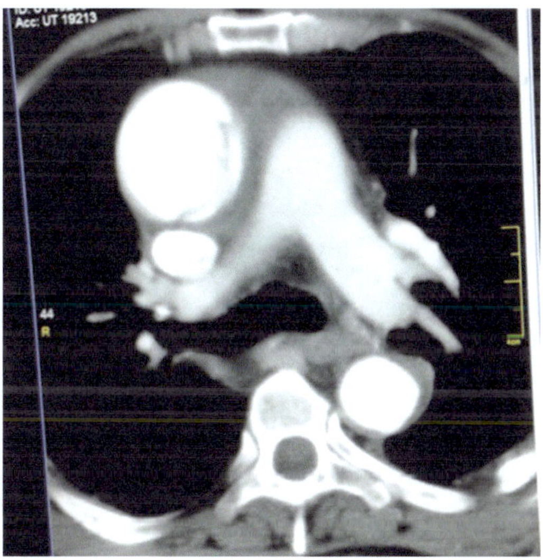

FIGURE 2 Computed tomographic angiography of the chest showing aortic dissection

opacification of portions of the right common carotid artery characterized. For that reason, the management involved maintaining a zero diet with basal serum with glucose and potassium, strict control of the blood pressure and heart rate (HR), another electrocardiogram (ECG), X-ray and biochemistry at admission, intense neurological monitoring because of the risk that the symptoms would worsen; and assessed the real benefit of the surgical procedure owing to the extent of the ischemic stroke. With this, the patient's family was informed about the severity of the condition, the sequelae, and the high probability of death, including during the perioperative period, regardless of the treatment chosen, whether conservative or surgical.

After discussing the risks with the family, on the same day of the patient's admission to HMSJ, surgery of exchange of the ascending aorta, correction of its arch, and stent graft in the descending aorta was performed. The procedure, which began in the late afternoon, lasted approximately 8 h. Cardiopulmonary bypass (CPB) had been performed by 145 min, with two concentrates of erythrocytes, and diuresis of 900 mL. After the operation, the patient needed a blood transfusion of 20 IU of platelets because the index was about 60,000 per mm^3. After the procedure, the patient recovered in the ICU, where he stayed for 16 days of intensive support and physiotherapy. Within this period, a tracheostomy and gastrostomy were required on the 7th day after surgery.

The patient has evolved well, but was transferred to the high-dependence unit at HMSJ 15 days after surgery, where he received clinical support and continued under the care of physiotherapists and speech therapists. After clinical improvement, he was discharged.

There were no complications involving the cardiac procedure. However, the patient remained with sequelae such as paresis of the left lower limb (LLL) and plegia of the upper limb (MSE) and remains in outpatient follow-up because of the ischemic stroke. On returning for the follow-up visit, there was an improvement of strength in the lower left limb.

Questions

1. What are the main causes of cerebral vascular accident?

The cerebral vascular accident (CVA) is caused by various pathological conditions. The etiology may be classified into three main mechanisms: cardioembolism, atherosclerosis of the great artery, and occlusion of the small vessels, among others. Aortic dissection is one possible cause of ischemic stroke.

2. What are the main causes of aortic dissection?

Hypertension and atherosclerosis occur in 75% of cases. Marfan syndrome is the etiological agent in approximately 10% of cases. There may be other changes in connective tissue as the Ehler–Danlos syndrome, Behçet's, and others. Coarctation of the aorta, bicuspid aortic valve, congenital aortic stenosis and other less frequent causes, such as pregnancy, blunt chest trauma, ascending aortic cannulation for a cardiopulmonary bypass, may also be responsible for aortic dissection.

3. What tests assist in the diagnosis of aortic dissection?

Transthoracic echocardiography (TTE); transesophageal echocardiography (TEE); magnetic resonance imaging (MRI); conventional computed tomography; and aortography. All these tests present a diagnostic sensitivity of 65–100% and a specificity of 85–100%. In addition, coronary angiography; helical computed tomography; chest X-ray; and electrocardiography are used.

4. What is the pathophysiology of the disease aortic dissection?

The aorta is made of collagen, elastin, and muscle cells that contribute to the structural integrity, vascular tone, and distensibility respectively. As we age, the degenerative changes damage the elastic tissue and cause the loss of smooth muscle. The disease may be related to the artery intima of a major break when the pressure of the pulsatile blood flow induces arterial longitudinal separation of layers. The vasa vasorum break with the start of intramural hemorrhage is also suggested to be the initial event, with subsequent disruption of the formation of the intima and dissection. Most of these dissections propagate forward, which leads to poor distal perfusion syndromes, but can sometimes result in retrograde dysfunction and cause the aortic valve or acute myocardial infarction because of the involvement of the right coronary artery. Increased pressure within the false lumen induces relaxation and the collapse of the true light, reducing the caliber and distal hypoperfusion.

5. What are the main signs and symptoms presented in cases of ischemic stroke related to aortic dissection?

It is indicated by the intense pain, in the form of heartburn in a type A dissection and in the back in a type B dissection (according to the Stanford classification). Syncope, dyspnea, and hemoptysis may occur. Patients tend to have hypertension and possibly arterial hypotension.

6. What are some of the risk factors for aortic dissection?

Hypertension, age greater than 50 years, smoking, dyslipidemia, cocaine, amphetamine, connective tissue disorders (Marfan syndrome, Loeys–Dietz, Turner, Ehlers–Danlos syndrome, among others), vascular inflammation, trauma deceleration (car accident), and iatrogenic factors.

7. How is the Stanford classification used?

The Stanford classification distinguishes two types: type A, which involves the ascending aorta, is more frequent, severe, and requires urgent surgical treatment; and type B, which affects only the descending aorta.

8. What is the appropriate approach in cases of combined aortic dissection and stroke?

When we suspect the diagnosis of aortic dissection, we must, after the clinical examination, ask for chest X-rays, which may show a widening of the superior mediastinum, at the expense of the dilatation of the ascending aorta in contrast with the normal diameter of the abdominal aorta. If dissection is suspected, evaluation should be supplemented with an aortoiliac arteriography, except if clinical symptoms of hypotension and hypovolemic shock are presented. In these cases, the aortoiliac arteriography is always performed using the retrograde catheterization technique, usually demonstrating a false lumen; we see only a reduction in the caliber of the artery.

Once the arteriographic diagnosis of ascending dissection of the aorta is confirmed, and there are no clinical contraindications, almost all patients are treated by surgery. The surgical technique consists of the resection of the compromised aortic segment and its replacement with a Dacron graft. If necessary, exchange of the aortic valve is carried out at the same time. The surgical risk is about 20%.

Review of the Addressed Disease or Treatment

According to the European Society of Cardiology's definition, aortic dissection is a break of the middle tunica caused by intramural bleeding, which causes separation of the layers of the aorta and the formation of a true lumen and a false lumen with or without communication. In most the cases, an intimal tear is the trigger, resulting in a track of blood in a dissection area with the middle tunica. This whole process is followed by an aortic break if the adventitia is involved or reentry into the aortic lumen if a second intima occurs. The dissection has two main classifications: DeBakey and Stanford. DeBakey classifies the anatomical topography and Stanford classifies the extent of the dissection. DeBakey type I has its origin in the ascending aorta and propagates to a descending aorta; type II only affects the ascending aorta, and type III has its origin in the descending aorta. Stanford type A is when the ascending aorta is involved in the lesion and type B occurs far from the left subclavian artery. In addition, dissections that occur only in the aortic arch are classified as type non-A.

The dissection of the aorta is not a frequent lesion, but has a high mortality rate. The main predisposing factor is chronic arterial hypertension, followed by others such as obesity, smoking and connective tissue diseases. Usually, the patient feels a sudden, high-intensity chest, abdominal or interscapular pain. There may also be other neurological symptoms as a consequence, such as persistent or transient ischemic stroke (CVA), spinal cord ischemia, ischemic neuropathy, and hypoxic encephalopathy.

Ischemic stroke (CVA) is the most frequent neurological symptom and affects 6–32% of patients with aortic dissection. It is caused by many pathological conditions. The etiology can be categorized into three mechanisms: cardioembolism, atherosclerosis of large arteries, and occlusion of small vessels, and others (unusual or indeterminate etiology). Aortic dissection is not a major but is a possible cause of ischemic stroke. In this case, it may cause abrupt occlusion or narrowing of the proximal extracranial carotid artery or vertebral artery branches from the aorta causing CVA. The prevalence of the involvement of supra-aortic branches in aortic dissection was reported to be 29% by postmortem investigation or 43% by imaging or intraoperative visualization. In particular, carotid (81%) and right-sided arteries (69%) are frequently affected.

There are two possible mechanisms for ischemic stroke secondary to aortic dissection. In the first one, dissection obstructs the blood flow through the true lumen of branched arteries, thereby reducing cerebral perfusion and eventually causing damage to brain tissue. In the second one, in the case of true lumen reentry, the thrombus is transferred to the distal portion of the arteries and causes thromboembolism. In patients with CVA with aortic dissection, the supra-aortic arteries were involved in 62.5%, whereas others suffered from ischemic stroke without extension of the dissection toward the supra-aortic vessels, indicating that stroke is caused by an embolic mechanism.

Most patients with aortic dissection present with sudden chest pain and this typical or distinctive pain is indicative of aortic dissection. However, painless dissection may occur. The frequency of painless aortic dissection is 6–15%. In the case of aortic dissection complicated by ischemic stroke, the presentation of pain may be less frequent. Chest pain at the beginning may not be seen in patients with dysfunction of consciousness or aphasia because of the difficulty involved in inquiring about the initial symptoms. In addition, syncope occurs in 6–19% of patients with aortic dissection, and this may also hinder recognition of the condition. The findings may have several implications for patients with aortic dissection and stroke. In addition to the chest or back pain that precedes the stroke, a study by Bossone et al. (2016), and others suggests that a high degree of suspicion should also be raised for type A aortic dissection in stroke patients with syncope hypotension, pulse deficit, and aortic regurgitation. In patients with these symptoms, early imaging would allow the diagnosis of dissection if present to help prevent inadvertent use of fibrinolytic therapy, which could lead to fatal outcomes in this cohort, as thrombolysis can cause critical adverse effects such as cardiac tamponade or hemothorax.

To diagnose underlying aortic dissection in patients with early-stage ischemic stroke, chest or back pain at the beginning should be confirmed with the possibility of this disease in mind. A careful physical examination is also needed to check the pulse or blood pressure differentials and aortic regurgitation. A chest X-ray should be routinely performed to assess mediastinal or aortic enlargement. In addition, carotid ultrasound imaging is indispensable in identifying arterial dissection because the non-invasive test can be performed at the bedside without loss of time.

The diagnosis of aortic dissection is confirmed by CT, MRI, TTE, TEE, or aortography. The sensitivity of these diagnostic tests is 65–100% and the specificity is 85–100%.

Bossone et al. (2016) found that an urgent surgical repair is necessary for aortic dissection because conservative management is associated with a high incidence of early mortality. However, some studies suggest that immediate surgical repair of dissection in the presence of CVA might carry a prohibitive risk associated with hemorrhagic aggravation of an ischemic stroke after reperfusion following cardiopulmonary bypass and complete anticoagulation.

Bibliography

1. Castrillo SM, Rodeño BO, Sanz EA, Salaices MG. Ictus isquémico secundario a disección aórtica: un reto diagnóstico. Neurología. 2016;79:192–4.
2. Kamouchi M. Editorial: aortic dissection as a possible underlying cause of acute ischemic stroke. Offl J Jpn Circ Soc. 2015;79:1–2.
3. Dietrich W, Erbguth FJ, Gaul C. Neurological symptoms in aortic dissection: a challenge for neurologists. Cerebrovas Dis. 2008;26:1–8.
4. Zárate M. Disección Aórtica Tipo A: Reto Quirúrgico. Revista Colombiana de Cardiología. 2013;20(5):331–3.
5. Alvarado C, Arias CA, Barragán R, Guzmán F, Vargas F. Síndromes aórticos agudos. Revista Colombiana de Cardiología. 2013;20(2):114–21.
6. Erbel R, et. al. 2014. 2014 ESC guidelines on the diagnosis and treatment of aortic diseases [Online] 35. Available: http://eurheartj.oxfordjournals.org/content/ehj/35/41/2873.full.pdf [Accessed 23 Jan 2017].
7. Bossone E, et al. Stroke and Outcomes in Patients With Acute Type A Aortic Dissection. Am Heart Assoc J. 2013;128 (suppl 1):S175–9.

Bentall-De Bono Technique in the Ascending Aorta Aneurysm, Aortic Regurgitation, and Coronary Reimplantation

Filipe T. K. S. Almeida, Luana Luiza Vieira, Adriana Fernandes Silva, Evandro Luis Queiroz Flores, and Rui M. S. Almeida

Clinical Presentation

J.C.H. a 53-year-old male patient, caucasian race, retired, married and catholic. The patient reported recent dyspnea during moderate effort and had been diagnosed with hypertension 10 years ago, making use of medication. The cardiovascular physical test identified a regurgitation systolic murmur (3+/6+) audible in the aortic focus, preserved B1 and hypophonic B2, and palpable ictus displaced inferiorly to the left.

F. T. K. S. Almeida (✉) · L. L. Vieira · A. F. Silva · E. L. Q. Flores
Assis Gurgacz Foundation University (FAG), Cascavel, PR, Brazil

R. M. S. Almeida
Department of Cardiology and Cardiovascular Surgery,
University Center Assis Gurgacz Foundation, Cascavel, PR, Brazil

R. M. S. Almeida, F. B. Jatene (eds.), *Cardiovascular Surgery*,
https://doi.org/10.1007/978-3-319-57084-6_2

Diagnosis, Assessment, and Treatment

Additional tests: The electrocardiogram showed sinus rhythm, heart rate of 70 bpm, and overloading of the left atrium and ventricle. The 2-D echocardiogram showed a severe aortic valve insufficiency, due to non-coaptation of the aortic valve leaflets, with a mild thickening, a LV diastolic dysfunction with an altered relaxation pattern, enlarged left chambers, an ascending aortic aneurysm, with an aortic ascending transverse diameter of 65 mm, in its middle third and 61 mm at the level of the sinus of Valsalva and aortic arch diameter of 31 mm, a left ventricular hypertrophy and an ejection fraction of 50%. Cardiac catheterization found an elevation of Pd2 in the left ventricle. The aortography showed an aneurysm of the ascending aorta (Fig. 1b). The aortography showed an aneurysm in the ascending aorta. The left ventriculography shows dilated left ventricle with hypertrophy and end-systolic volume increase, due to diffuse hypokinesia (2+/4+). CT angiography of the thoracic aorta showed an aneurysm affecting the entire length of the ascending thoracic aorta and dilation of the tubular segment and aortic root, with a transverse diam-

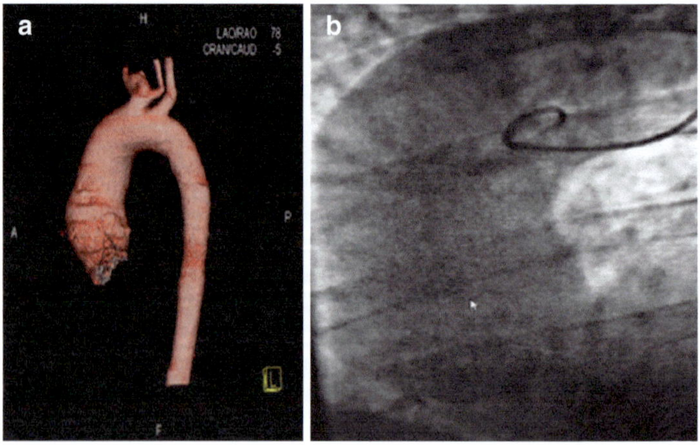

Figure 1 (**a**) CT angiography of the thoracic aorta, showing an aortic aneurysm. (**b**) Ascending aortic aortography also showing an aortic aneurysm

eter of 65 mm in the middle third of the tubular portion and 61 mm in the level of sinus Valsalva (Fig. 1a). The aortic diameter before the emergence of the innominate artery was estimated at 38 mm and the diameter in the middle third of the aortic arch 33 mm. The isthmus and the descending thoracic aorta have diameters within the normal range, estimated at 30 and 29 mm, respectively.

Diagnosis: Aneurysm of the ascending aorta and aortic valve insufficiency.

Treatment: Surgical treatment with Bentall-De Bono technique and aortic valve and ascending aorta replacement with the anastomosis of the coronary buttons. On-pump surgery was performed and the cardioplegic solution used to protect the heart with Custodiol®.

The patient recovered well from the surgery, and after 2 months, the tests showed no abnormalities. The echocardio-

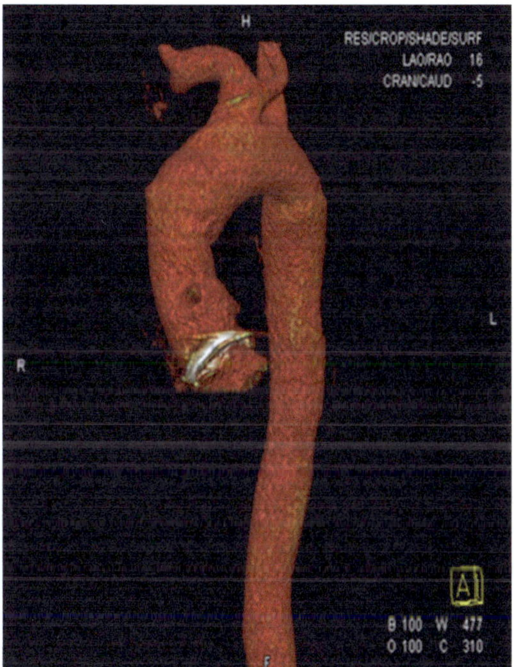

FIGURE 2 CT angiography of the thoracic aorta after treatment

gram shows the maintenance of normal left ventricular ejection fraction values. The preoperative 58.5 mm's valve area was replaced by the diameter of St. Jude's valvar tube No. 29, with 30 mm, as seen in CT (Fig. 2). As a follow-up, it recommends the monitoring of this patient by a cardiologist in the first 6 months and annually thereafter. If asymptomatic we perform echocardiography, CT, and prothrombin time tests.

The use of the Bentall-De Bono technique has had lower mortality rates. Studies show a percentage of 87.17% survival in patients followed up for 10 years [6].

Questions

1. What are the epidemiological and pathophysiological features of aortic aneurysms and aortic insufficiency?

It is understood as pathological, the diameter of the ascending aorta where the aortic dilatation is greater than 50% predicted for age and body surface of the patient. This results from the progressive weakening or defect in the layers of the aortic wall [10]. An aortic regurgitation (AR), in turn, is characterized by the backflow of blood from the aorta to the left ventricle (LV) through the aortic valve during diastole. The presence of a congenital bicuspid aortic valve is considered the more likely cause of this condition; however, in elderly patients, the most frequent cause is calcification of the leaflets and in developing countries, there is a relationship with rheumatic heart disease. In addition, aortic regurgitation results from primary diseases, causing dilation of the ascending aorta or sinus of Valsalva [5].

The regurgitated blood increases the final diastolic volume and wall tension in the left ventricle, causing a progressive compensatory myocardial hypertrophy. The natural evolution of this heart condition is characterized, in most cases, by a lack of symptoms and a normal LV ejection fraction for years. Diseases that affect the valve ring or ascending aorta and cause simultaneous AR, such as Marfan and Ehlers-Danlos syndromes, ankylosing spondylitis, syphilitic aortitis, and hypertension, should be also considered. In these situations, the AR is a consequence of the ostium dilatation, followed by coaptation failure of the leaflets [7].

2. From the symptomatology of the disease, which additional tests should be performed?

Some additional tests should jointly assist in clarifying the diagnostic hypotheses and possibly confirm the diagnosis. Among them, there is a chest X-ray and the echocardiography for AR. The gold standard for the investigation of the ascending aortic aneurysm is computed tomography (CT) with iodinated contrast; it is used for diagnosis, monitoring, and surgical planning. Magnetic resonance imaging (MRI) is a high-accuracy test, whose advantage is the nonuse of contrast and radiation and, however, presents long-time acquisition of images, which impairs their use in emergencies.

When we suspect an aortic aneurysm, the chest X-ray is important at the beginning of the evaluation process, because it can identify abnormalities such as calcification and aortic dilation. To measure the increased diameter, a 2-D echocardiography is used. The transesophageal echocardiogram can be used as a supplement due to the high-accuracy rate for the ascending aorta, sometimes confirming the initial diagnostic. The CT is useful to visually reconstruct different dimensional planes, providing a better visualization of an important structure. This exam also complements the understanding of anatomical structures with a sensitivity of 98–100%. MRI is highly sensitive as CT and allows to assess the left ventricular function and the involvement of aortic branches. The aortic angiography, in turn, fell into disuse because it is more invasive and less specific than CT, but it is important for the evaluation of the coronary arteries.

The AR investigation by chest radiograph shows anatomical changes such as calcification and cardiomegaly with left ventricular dilatation expense. Echocardiography can give information about morphological features of the valve, assessing the number of brochures, the fusion of the cusps, the calcification, and the failure of coaptation. It is considered especially useful in measuring the diastolic and systolic diameter, ejection fraction, and degree of reflux in conjunction with aortography and MR [4].

3. What is the classification of the patient as the aortic regurgitation?

Aortic regurgitation can be divided into four categories measured by anatomy and valve hemodynamics and the presence of symptoms. Internships vary among patients at risk for aortic insufficiency (stage A), with progressive AR medium-moderate asymptomatic (stage B), with asymptomatic severe AR (stage C), and with symptomatic AR (D stage) [4, 5].

The patient showed a small calcification in a leaflet of the aortic valve, ascending aortic aneurysm, left ventricular ejection fraction of 50% with the presence of dilation, and symptoms of dyspnea and angina. So, the patient was classified as severe AR, stage D.

4. About the therapeutic approach, what types of treatments this patient could be submitted?

The recommended treatment of AR is the surgery, for valve replacement in cases of symptomatic patients at rest or after exercise testing. The valve replacement is also indicated for patients with lower left ventricular ejection fraction or equal to 50%, although asymptomatic, or those who have other comorbidities that require surgical intervention.Until surgery can be performed, the use of vasodilators is recommended, such as nifedipine, captopril, and enalapril, which act reducing the diastolic blood pressure and, consequently, the aortic regurgitation. The patient had an aortic aneurysm, with a diameter greater than 60 mm, which implies a surgical recommendation grade A, mainly due to the risk of rupture and/or dissection that increases 2–30% in similar cases [4, 5].

Clinical treatment is controversial, mainly by the use of beta-blockers, even reducing the impact of blood on the walls of the aneurysmal aorta; it can cause side effects by decreasing the elasticity of the same. Thus, the clinical management involves the regulation of risk factors for rupture of an aneurysm, such as hypertension, dyslipidemia, and evaluation of correlated genetic diseases [10].

5. How is the surgical procedure done?

The Bentall-De Bono technique - a median transsternal thoracotomy is performed, followed by the opening of the

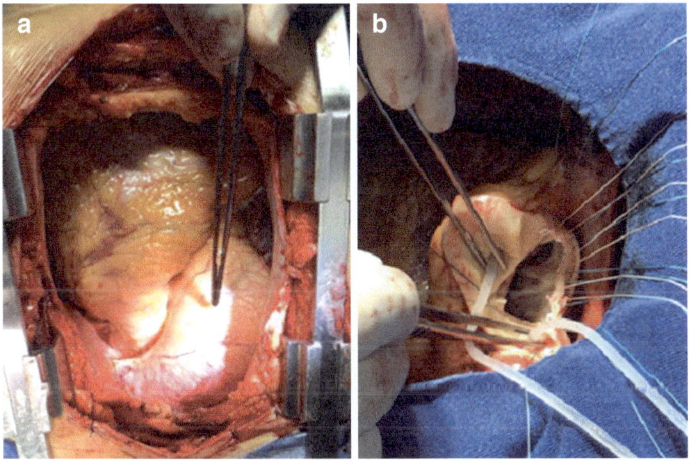

FIGURE 3 (**a**) The ascending aortic aneurysm in comparison with an anatomical forceps. (**b**) The aortic valve, post section, and the buttons of the coronary arteries

pericardial sac; the ascending aortic aneurysm and dilated left ventricle, was viewed (Fig. 3a). The patient is placed in extracorporeal circulation and hypothermia at 32 °C is achieved. The aorta is clamped, opened and its structures visualized; the aneurysmal portion of the ascending aorta and the aortic cusps are excised, after separating the coronary ostiums, and replaced by a valvar tube with a mechanical valve; both coronary buttons are anastomosed to the tube(Fig. 3b).

All anastomosis are performed by means of continuous suture; hemostatic sealant is used. Deairing manouvers are performed, during reheating and the aortic clamp is opened, and gradually the patirent is withdraw from the extracorporeal circulation. A drain is placed in the anterior mediastinum as weel as of two temporary epicardial pacemaker wires, in the right ventricle and right atrial appendage. A complete review of hemostasis is performed. Partial closure of the pericardial sac, sternum and underlying plans, complets the surgery [1].

6. How is the coronary arteries' anastomosis technique done? What is its relevance?

With the patient in cardiopulmonary bypass and hypothermia, and after removing the calcified aortic valve, the coronary arteries are removed while maintaining a generous portion of the aortic wall, called button. This structure is useful for the coronary implant since it avoids bending and unwanted tissue tension. After the valved tube placement, the coronary's ostium is implanted directly on the prosthesis. When the diameter of an aneurysm is very significant, laterally away from the ostium, it is advisable to use the second graft between this and the prosthesis. Such behavior prevents tension on the anastomosis, which is usually the most frequent point of bleeding after repair. After that, holes are made in the graft on the opposite sides of the arteries' ostium, and an adequate amount of the graft must be left out between the prosthesis' suture ring and the new way to the coronary artery. After that, the anastomosis of the left coronary artery is initially made, all the suture loops around the bottom edge of the coronary ostium are placed before pulling, so the area comes close to graft accurately. Cartwheel stitches are made around the coronary artery ostium. The right coronary anastomosis is made after complete anastomosis of the left coronary artery [2, 3].

The procedures that reconstruct the coronary ostium using homologous or autologous tissues are susceptible to intimal hyperplasia, thrombosis, or calcification. Furthermore, the new ostium location after implantation allows easy catheterization in future interventional procedures [2, 3].

7. What are the most common types of complication of the Bentall-De Bono procedure?

In the short term, the most common complications of the Bentall-De Bono technique include bleeding due to the positioning and fixation of the prosthesis or valved tube, which can result in cardiac tamponade. In addition, a complete heart block and arrhythmias may occur by an injury to the cardiac conduction system. The thrombus formation can also happen with the withdrawal of the stenotic valve structures, mainly causing neurological injuries by embolism and stroke by occlusion.

The prolonged use of cardiopulmonary bypass should be considered as a factor that increases the incidence of inflammatory reactions and is directly related to the prevalence of these [3, 8].

8. Did we find any abnormalities in the ascending aortic wall?

During surgery, there was a tear in the tunica intima, of the ascending aortic wall, with approximately 4 cm in length and 10 cm distally from the aortic valve. The lesion showed signs of fibrosis, which probably prevented the development of a dissection (Fig. 4). It is understood that it began as a spontaneous aortic dissection due to the rupture of the tunica intima and the commitment of the tunica media, without tearing it. There is almost no connection between patients with aortic regurgitation, ascending aortic aneurysm, and a loss of elastic

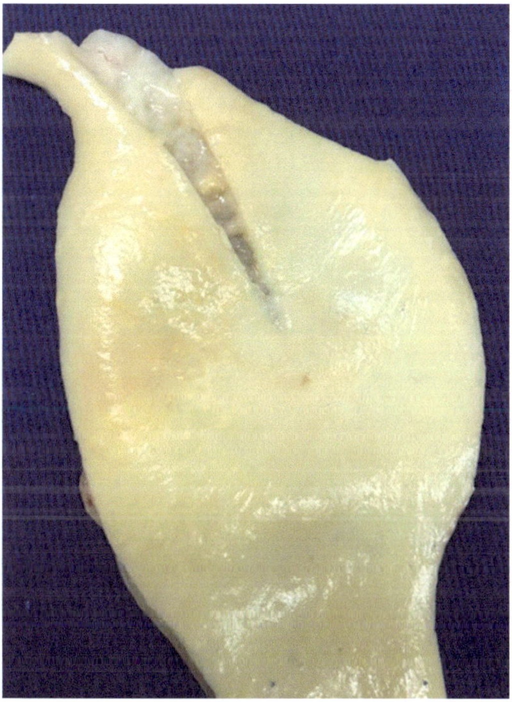

FIGURE 4 Lesion in the wall of the ascending aorta

fibers. Generally, in cases of Marfan syndrome, it is expected that a preexisting injury is responsible for starting the laceration and degeneration of the tunica media. However, this patient did not have specific comorbidities that could cause histological alterations. Although the patient was hypertensive, the presence of hypertension is not a confirmed cause for the appearance of spontaneous dissection, but it may promote the progression of the medial hematoma. Thus, antihypertensive medications can effectively limit a developing dissection, justifying its use for tissue healing [6, 7].

Review About the Addressed Disease or Treatment

Suffering from valvular and vascular comorbidities, the treatment recommended by the AHA/ACC's guidelines is the surgery for valve replacement and aortic tube placement. These guidelines indicate the surgical option to correct the aortic insufficiency due to the symptoms of the patient during the moderate effort, ejection fraction lower or equal to 50%, and vascular comorbidities. Having an aortic diameter greater than 60 mm, the same procedure is indicated to treat an aneurysm. Thus, the option of performing the Bentall-De Bono surgery and valve tube implantation was in consonance with international recommendations.

The high survival rate of the technique, approximately 87% in 10 years, and the long life span of the mechanical aortic prosthesis were convincing factors to the patient.

The surgery was successful, reducing the aortic diameter to 30 mm and obtaining normal values for left ventricular ejection fraction. During surgery, a laceration was found in the tunica intima of the ascending aorta with approximately 4 cm in length and with signs of fibrosis, indicating a possible early dissection.

It is recommended for this patient initially semiannual follow-up and annual after the symptoms cease.

Bibliography

1. Bentall H, De Bono A. A technique for complete replacement of the ascending aorta. Thorax. 1968;23:338–9.
2. Bongiovani HL, Haddad JL. Re-implant of the right coronary artery: a surgical technique for treatment of ostial lesion. Rev Bras Cir Cardiovasc. 2002;17(4):352–4.
3. Kouchoukos NT, et al. (2013). Cardiac surgery. vol. 1(4). Philadelphia: Elsevier Saunders.
4. Liguori GR, et al. Manual acadêmico de cirurgia cardiovascular SBCCV/DBLACCV. São Paulo: Atheneu; 2014.
5. Nishimura RA, et al. Guideline for the management of patients with valvular heart disease: executive summary. J Am Coll Cardiol. 2014;63(22):2438–88.
6. Roberts, W. C. et al. (2010). Comparison of the structure of the aortic valve and ascending aorta in adults having aortic valve replacement for aortic stenosis versus for pure aortic regurgitation and resection of the ascending aorta for aneurysm. Circulation [online]. 123(8). Available at: http://circ.ahajournals.org/content/123/8/896 [Accessed 12 Aug 2016].
7. Paola AAV, et al. Cardiologia: Livro Texto da Sociedade Brasileira de Cardiologia. Manole: Burueri; 2012.
8. Paparellaa D, Yaua TM, Young E. Cardiopulmonary bypass induced inflammation: pathophysiology and treatment. Eur J Cardiothorac Surg. 2002;21:232–44.
9. Silva VF, et al. Bentall and Bono surgery for correction of valve ascending aortic disease: long-term results. Rev Bras Cir Cardiovasc. 2008;23:256–61.
10. Townswend CM. Tratado de Cirurgia: as bases biológicas da prática cirúrgica moderna. 6th ed. Rio de Janeiro: Guanabara Koogan, 2003.

Correction of Interrupted Aortic Arch in an Adult: Ascending-to-Descending Aorta Bypass

Dhaisa Thaina Souza Conceição, Daiane Thaysa Brito Nakamura, Tailana Paiva Dourado, Jackson Brandão Lopes, and Bruno da Costa Rocha

Clinical Presentation

A 24-year-old woman presented with hypertension since she was 17 years old. Her past medical history included asthmatic bronchitis, presenting 3–4 episodes per year, and a Cesarean section 3 years ago. She denied allergies to medicines and foods. The medications in use were losartan (50 mg 2 times a day) and hydrochlorothiazide (25 mg 1 time a day).

Physical examination revealed:

General appearance: a female who is awake and alert and who appears healthy and looks her stated age

D. T. S. Conceiçao (✉) · D. T. B. Nakamura · T. P. Dourado
J. B. Lopes · B. da Costa Rocha
Federal University of Bahia (UFBA), Salvador, BA, Brazil

R. M. S. Almeida, F. B. Jatene (eds.), *Cardiovascular Surgery*,
https://doi.org/10.1007/978-3-319-57084-6_3

Vitals: RF 18 ipm, 220 × 120 mmHg arterial pressure in both right and left superior members; systolic pressure of 120 mmHg in left inferior member; radial pulse palpation 81 bpm, regular; oxygen saturation level of 97% in moment of exam

Head: normocephalic; eyes, ears, nose, throat, and mouth without changes

Neck: without JVD at 45° and other abnormalities in the trachea, thyroid, or suprasternal notch

Cardiovascular: precordium without lifts or heaves – PMI not visible; PMI – palpable in fifth ICS, MCL; S1 and S2 heard, without extra sounds and murmurs

Thorax and lungs: without abnormalities in inspection; resonant at percussion; auscultation clear, with vesicular breath sounds normal

Abdomen: plan, without scars and striae; palpation superficial and deep without tenderness and masses; liver edge not palpable

Extremities: lymph nodes not palpable; normal in color and texture, without cyanosis, clubbing, and deformities

Neurologic: awake and alert; oriented to person, place, and time; without other abnormalities

Diagnosis, Assessment, and Treatment

She was submitted to magnetic resonance imaging (MRI), which showed left ventricle function of 70%, ascending aorta measuring 28.1 × 31.9 mm in diameter, the proximal aortic arch of 20 × 18 mm, descending aorta of 18 × 16.6 mm, the distal aortic arch of 11.7 × 11.3 mm, and interrupted aorta at isthmus level. Echocardiogram showed left ventricular diameter of 89 × 25 mm, ventricular septum of 8 mm, and left ventricular ejection fraction (LVEF) of 63%. Cranial CT scan showed dilated vessels without aneurysms. The patient was submitted to pneumology evaluation and counseling before surgery.

Surgery description: The operative strategy was the correction of aortic arch interruption performing an ascending-to-descending aorta bypass. The surgery started with a medium sternotomy, mainly because of the intense collateral arteries developed for adults' survival. Both superior and inferior vena cava and ascending aorta were cannulated for bypass circulation. After the cardioplegic arrest, the apex was dislocated superiorly. At this time, the surgeon could open the posterior pericardium and dissect the descending thoracic aorta above the diaphragm insertion. A partial clamping of the descending aorta was made, intense collateral arteries surrounding surgical field were ligated with hemoclip 200 or 300, and the descending aorta was clamped. An end-to-side anastomosis with Goretex 18 mm graft was performed; continuous suture using a 6-0 polypropylene and biological glue was applied. Partial clamping time was 22 min. A proximal end-to-side anastomosis was made in the ascending aorta above the Valsalva aortic sinus, and the graft was settled anteriorly to the inferior vena cava. The bypass circulation time was 120 min.

Postoperative setting: The patient was sent to ICU using low doses of adrenaline and milrinone. During 48 h in ICU, the patient had no adverse events and was discharged from the hospital on the sixth postoperative day. At the time of writing, she was at the eighth postoperative month and presented asymptomatic with a good tolerance to exertion. Physical examination revealed weight of 81 kg, arterial pressure of 130 × 80 mmHg at the left superior member, 140 × 90 mmHg at the right superior member, and systolic above 160 mmHg at the right inferior member. Echocardiogram showed normal flow through the graft without gradients. MRI (Figs. 1, 2, and 3) showed LVEF of 77%, left ventricular mass of 251 g, graft diameter of 19 × 19 mm, and great collateral arteries in regression (Fig. 4). She was using losartan 25 mg two times a day and aspirin. The doctor indicated physical activity, a healthy lifestyle, and endocrinological counseling.

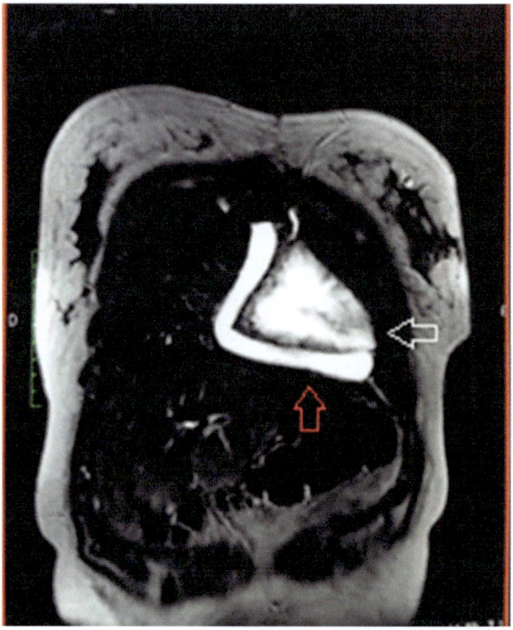

Figure 1 MRI after the ascending-to-descending bypass shows the graft (*red arrow*) descending next to the right margin of the heart, anteriorly to the IVC, and then making a curve on the apex (*white arrow*)

Questions

1. What is the diagnosis?

This is a patient with a type A aortic arch interruption. The interrupted aortic arch (IAA) is a rare congenital cardiac malformation which causes a completely impervious area in the aorta. IAA can be divided into three types, based on the location of the interruption: type A, the second most common, refers to interruptions located distal to the left subclavian artery; type B, the most common, is located between the left common carotid and the left subclavian artery; and type C is located between the innominate and left common carotid arteries. Most cases are associated with other cardiac

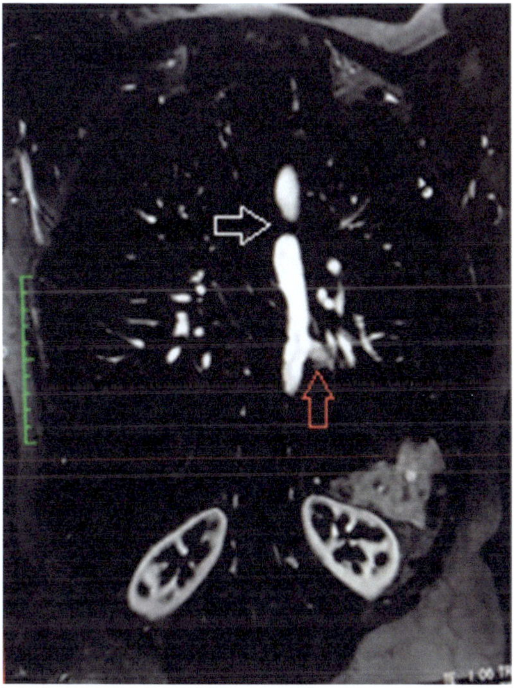

FIGURE 2 MRI shows the aortic arch interruption at the aortic isthmus level (*white arrow*) and the end-to-side anastomosis between the Goretex graft and descending thoracic aorta (*red arrow*)

abnormalities, such as ventricular septal defect or subaortic obstruction of the outflow tract, and the isolated form is very uncommon [4]. Symptoms usually start at the moment of birth, and they progress fast, requiring neonatal emergency surgery. If not identified and treated, half of the patients will die in the following 10 days [8].

2. What is the importance of measuring the blood pressure in the four members in clinical practice?

In this case, an uncommon isolated and asymptomatic IAA was found in the patient's adulthood. However, the diagnosis could have been made earlier, if pressure measurement of all four limbs were made, and an early diagnosis could reduce

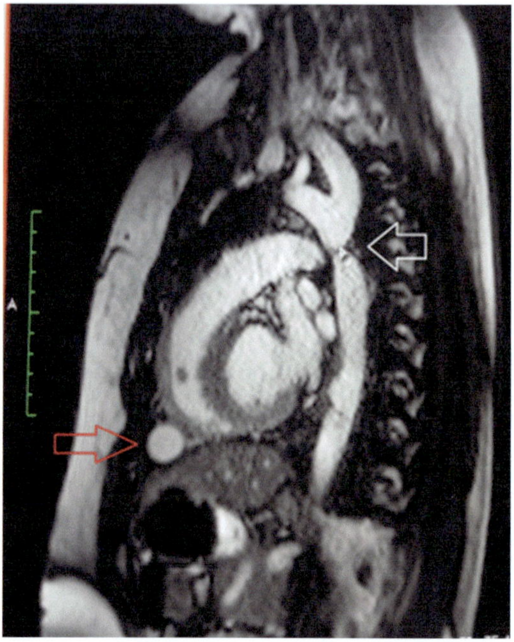

FIGURE 3 Sagittal view of MRI shows the aortic arch interruption (*white arrow*) and the graft (*red arrow*) on the diaphragmatic surface of the heart

surgical risks and improve the prognosis of this disease. In addition, we would like to stress that IAA could also happen between the innominate and left common carotid arteries, which would cause a difference in blood pressure of the superior members.

Blood pressure gradient could also indicate other abnormalities, such as aortic coarctations, which are associated with heart failure, aneurysm or aortic dissection, stroke, and coronary artery disease. Other disorders that could cause an adult patient to present with blood pressure gradient include arterial obstructive disease (atherosclerosis or thromboembolism), previous surgical ligation, aortic dissection, and supra-valvar aortic stenosis.

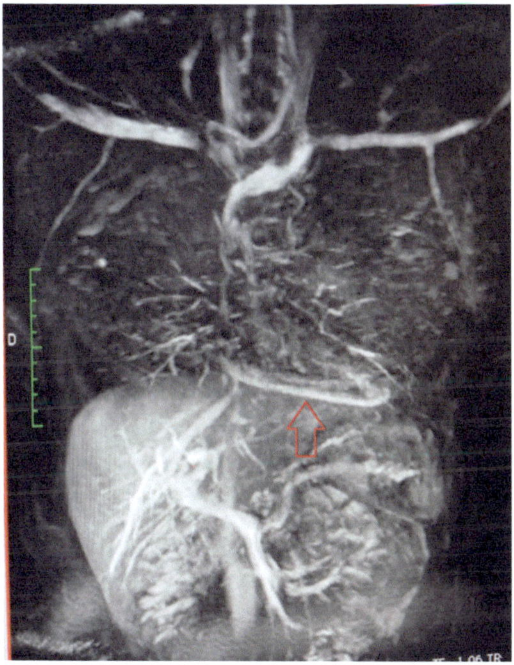

FIGURE 4 This view of the MRI highlights multiple collateral arteries developed during patient's life. They persisted even 8 months after surgery. The great graft flow (*red arrow*) can be observed

3. What complementary exams can be used for IAA diagnosis?

In those cases, imaging studies can be especially useful. Exams such as chest radiography, aortography, echocardiography, and magnetic resonance imaging could be applied.

4. Why was this patient submitted to cranial CT angiography?

Cases of IAA can be associated with multiple cardiovascular abnormalities. It is necessary to investigate carotid and intracranial vessels to exclude the possibility of arteriovenous abnormalities, and angiography, magnetic resonance imaging (MRI), or computed tomography (CT) scan will be useful both for the evaluation of the aorta and the Willis polygon

[2]. Patients under suspicion of coronary disease must be submitted to coronary angiography.

5. What is surgery indicated in this case?

The surgery indication should be analyzed in each individual case. In IAA, the correction strategy is usually invasive, and some surgery techniques can be found in literature: resection and end-to-end anastomosis, angioplasty with placement of polytetrafluoroethylene (PTFE) patch, graft placement (Dacron), and aortoplasty with subclavian flap. In this case, chosen was graft placement with PTFE graft once it is at the patient who had an IAA diagnosed in adulthood and had already developed signs of heart function compromise due to the disease.

6. How to choose the best surgical approach?

In the literature, there are still discussions about the best approach. We preferred the median thoracotomy to avoid multiple collaterals from supra-aortic vessels passing through intercostal spaces surrounding connective tissue along the thoracic aorta. Those are friable and might lead to major bleeding during dissection.

7. Why wasn't the graft positioned next to the sternum?

The graft was anastomosed and positioned in a way that it made a curve around the heart's apex, toward to the diaphragmatic surface of the heart. This choice was considered safer because it prevents graft rupture if a future surgery is ever needed. Rupturing a graft of that diameter could lead to fatal bleeding.

8. What is the Aristotle basic complexity score (ABC) of this patient?

Aristotle score is a comprehensive risk score used to analyze detailed information about the complexity of congenital heart surgery. They were considered possible risk factors for each procedure and assigned scores based on the risk of mortality, morbidity, and surgical difficulty expected. The minimum values of surgical risk range from 0.5 to 15.0, then specific values are added for each morbidity condition, and finally, an amount of up to 5 points can be added due to factors such as anatomical variations, age, and associated procedures. In the case of our patient, her Aristotle score was 7.8.

9. How important is the use of beta-blockers in the postoperative period?

One of the most frequent complications in the postoperative period is persistent hypertension. Postoperative hypertension is defined as systolic blood pressure >140 mmHg and/or diastolic blood pressure >90 mmHg in two consecutive measurements. Pressure elevations in the postoperative period are related to pain, anesthesia time, hypoxia, hypothermia, fluid overload, hypercapnia, and physical or emotional stress, especially in patients who had a history of hypertension.

The use of beta-blocker reduces hospitalization length time and improves left ventricular function and left ventricular remodeling once our patient had an important left ventricular hypertrophy (LV 14 mm) and blood pressure control. Drug treatment with antihypertensive drugs is indicated. Beta-blockers, angiotensin-converting enzyme (ACE) inhibitors, and angiotensin receptor blockers are the most appropriate, even if there may be a need for a therapy with a combination of drugs.

Review About the Addressed Disease or Treatment

Interrupted aortic arch (IAA) is an extremely rare congenital heart disease, with estimated incidence of three per million live births [5], and it accounts for less than 1% of all congenital heart disease [3]. It's defined as a complete discontinuation between the aortic arch and the descending aorta, because of an error during embryonic development, once the aortic arch segments are derived from different components. In 1959, Celoria and Patton developed a very useful classification [7]:

Type A: this type occurs at the level of the isthmus, which is a constriction of the aorta immediately distal to the left subclavian artery at the point of attachment of the *ductus arteriosus*.

Type B: the interruption occurs between the left common carotid artery and the left subclavian artery.

Type C: IAA located between the innominate artery take-off and the left common carotid.

In children, type B is the most prevalent (53–69%) [3, 7], followed by type A (43%) and type C (4%) [3]. After the ductal closure, most of the children become acidotic and anuric, and the ischemic injury of many organs may result in death if the IAA wasn't corrected. However, a few children manage to survive, and IAA can be diagnosed in adults.

There are 37 published cases in the last 40 years describing adults with IAA [3]. In adults, the type A appears to be the most prevalent (79%), followed by types B (16%) and C (3%) [3]. One of the reasons for this change would be that the IAA is the "end point" of a coarctation of the aorta [3, 5]. Other hypotheses include the fact that the type A appears to develop collaterals more easily and types B and C would have disparate upper extremities pressures, which were more often diagnosed at the childhood and adolescence [3]. Associated abnormalities are common, including bicuspid aortic valve, ventricular septal defects, patent ductus arteriosus, mitral stenosis, and persistent left superior vena cava [5].

The most common symptoms presented by these patients were hypertension refractory to medical management (70%), claudication (13%), congestive heart failure (6%), and aortic insufficiency (10%) [3]. Patients with refractory hypertension, presenting a large pressure difference between upper and lower extremities and diminished pulses at the lower extremities, should be investigated for IAA. The anatomic diagnosis can be made using echocardiography, providing information about the site and length of the interruption, the diameter of the aortic annulus, and the diameter of the ascending aorta and if there are associated anomalies. Chest x-ray, cardiac catheterization, percutaneous angiography, and magnetic resonance angiography can be used.

The IAA management in adults is mainly surgical. The sternotomy is the most indicated approach; however, either the sternotomy or thoracotomy seems to be reasonable depending on the size and location of the collaterals [3]. The end-to-end anastomosis has a limited use in adults, as the length of the interruption or stenosis can be quite long. The placement of interposition grafts is often used in an older population. If the patient needs another procedure, an extra-anatomic graft can be used. The ascending-to-descending bypass graft can be indicated for patients who need another cardiac repair, complicated aortic disease, or aortic arch hypoplasia [5]. If the patient had a known coarctation as a child, a percutaneous wire perforation of the septum with dilation and stent placement within the aorta can be performed [3].

The surgery can be made without cardiopulmonary bypass, once the collateral flow is sufficient, but it can be used if the distal aortic pressure fell below 50 mmHg [5]. The cardiopulmonary bypass and the extra-anatomic graft can also be used in older patients since the thin walls of the collaterals present a higher risk of bleeding [5].

Recoarctation and stenosis of the graft can occur with time, and a catheter-based intervention is a possibility. Hypertension can persist after IAA correction, especially if the defect was corrected after the childhood. These patients have a higher risk for an aneurysm or pseudoaneurysm formation and dissection, and they also should be screened for intracranial aneurysms at the circle of Willis [5].

Bibliography

1. Cooley DA. Techniques in cardiac surgery. 2nd ed. Philadelphia: WB Saunders Company; 1984.
2. Croti AU, Mattos SS, Pinto VC Jr, Aiello VD, Moreira VM. Cardiology and pediatric cardiac surgery. 2nd ed. São Paulo: Roca; 2012.
3. Gordon EA, Person T, Kavarana M, Ikonomidis JS. Interrupted aortic arch in the adult. J Card Surg. 2011;26:405–9.
4. Jacobs ML, Chin AJ, Rychik J, Steven JM, Nicolson SC, Norwood WI. Interrupted aortic arch: impact of subaortic stenosis on management and outcome. Circulation. 1995;92:128–31.

5. John AS, Schaff HV, Drew T, Warnes CA, Ammash N. Adult presentation of interrupted aortic arch: case presentation and a review of the medical literature. Congenit Heart Dis. 2011;6:269–75.
6. Lacour-Gayet F, Clarke D, Jacobs J, Gaynor W, Hamilton L, Jacobs M, Maruszewski B, Pozzi M, Spray T, Tchervenkov C, Mavroudis C, Committee A. The Aristotle score for congenital heart surgery. Semin Thorac Cardiovasc Surg Pediatr Card Surg Annu. 2004;7:185–91.
7. Mavroudis C, Backer CL. Pediatric cardiac surgery. West Sussex: Wiley-Blackwell, Ltd; 2013.
8. Reardon MJ, Cooley DA, Hallman GL. Interrupted aortic arch: brief review and summary of an eighteen-year experience. Tex Heart Inst J. 1984;11(3):250–9.

Giant Ruptured Sinus of Valsalva Aneurysm

Saulo Victor Benevides Nunes, Anderson Dias Arruda, Yasmine Lailla Vasconcelos Rodrigues, Joaquim David Carneiro Neto, and Camila Lopes do Amaral

Clinical Presentation

Patient EAC, female, 33-year-old, married, brown, peasant, presented dyspnea, palpitations, and edema of the lower limbs for about 15 years, with worsening for approximately 10 months and evolving to dyspnea at rest and paroxysmal nocturnal dyspnea in recent days. The patient had a personal history of hypertension, and she was not a smoker or drinker.

On physical examination, the patient was conscious, oriented, responsive, normal colored, hydrated, and cyanotic, had no fever (36.4 °C) and heated and perfused limbs, and was without edema and with heart rate of 145 bpm, respiratory rate of 20 bpm, oxygen saturation of 96%, and blood pressure of 92 × 60 mmHg. On examination of the respiratory system, the vesicular murmur was present in both hemithorax and no adventitious sounds. Cardiac auscultation was irregular heart rhythm with a holosystolic murmur (5+/6+) continues

S. V. B. Nunes · A. D. Arruda (✉) · Y. L. V. Rodrigues
J. D. C. Neto · C. L. do Amaral
Federal University of Ceará (UFC), Sobral, CE, Brazil

R. M. S. Almeida, F. B. Jatene (eds.), *Cardiovascular Surgery*,
https://doi.org/10.1007/978-3-319-57084-6_4

along the right sternal border. On examination of the abdomen, it showed up flabby, not painful on palpation with important hepatomegaly and fluid sounds.

Diagnosis, Assessment, and Treatment

Laboratory evaluation without significant changes. Electrocardiogram showed high ventricular response, atrial fibrillation rhythm, and the presence of polymorphic ventricular premature beats. Echocardiography showed a significant increase in cardiac chambers and a significant degree of diffuse hypokinesia of the left ventricle FE (Teicholz): 25%. An oval image was observed with pendulous movement swinging the tricuspid valve with a continuity area near the aortic valve and aortic sinuses. At the Doppler, turbulent flow of high speed was observed inside the aorta and right chambers (right coronary aortic sinus berry aneurysm measuring 38 × 43 mm with fistulation signals). An aneurysm was protruded into the right chambers, causing coaptation failure of the tricuspid valve and a significant degree of failure. Aortography confirmed aneurysm of the right coronary sinus with rupture and release of contrast to the right atrium (Figs. 1 and 2).

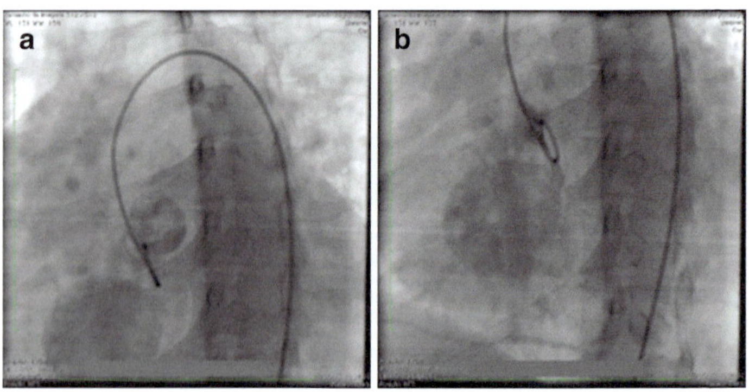

FIGURE 1 Aortography in OE showing (**a**) filling the sinus of Valsalva aneurysm immediately after contrast injection; (**b**) pedunculated image of the aneurysm with communication with the right sinus of Valsalva

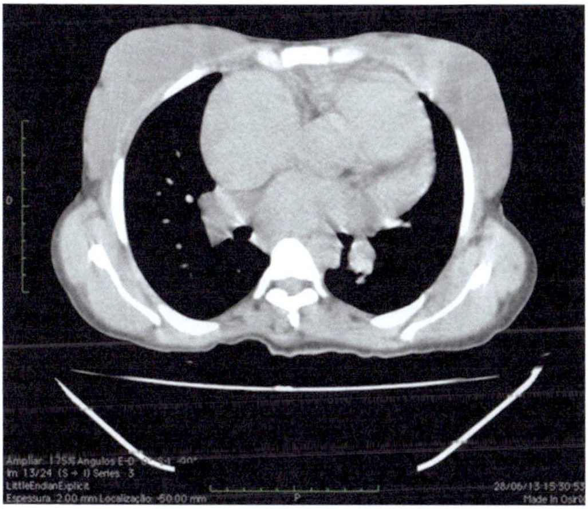

FIGURE 2 Computed tomography of the chest showing the following: projection of the sinus of Valsalva emerging and invading the right atrium; ascending aorta; dilatation of the main pulmonary artery

The patient underwent surgical excision of the aneurysm and reconstruction of the right coronary sinus with a bovine pericardial patch. Cardiopulmonary bypass time was 90 min, and anoxia time was 79 min. The patient recovered uneventfully throughout the intraoperative. She was discharged from the hospital on the eighth postoperative day and evolves, nowadays, with significant improvement of congestive symptoms.

Questions

1. What are the possible etiologies of a sinus of Valsalva aneurysm (SVA)?

Sinus of Valsalva aneurysm (SVA) is an abnormality which may be congenital or acquired. Acquired aneurysms may result from trauma, infections (endocarditis, syphilis, tuberculosis), degenerative diseases (atherosclerosis), systemic inflammatory diseases (Behcet's disease, ankylosing spondylitis), and connective tissue disorders (systemic lupus erythematosus, Marfan syndrome) or even senile-type dilatation in which the three sinuses dilate as a result of the ordinary aging process [1]. The Takayasu arteritis, an inflammatory arteritis affecting large vessels, is an extremely rare cause of this disease, with only one previously reported case.

About the congenital aneurysm, hypotheses suggest that the aneurysm results from the incomplete fusion of the aortopulmonary septum (which forms right coronary aortic sinus) and interventricular septum (which forms the noncoronary sinus), creating a transitional tissue between the fragile sinus and prone to form an aneurysm [1].

2. What is the epidemiology of this aortic disease?

The aneurysmal dilatation of the SV is a rare pathology, constituting about 1% of congenital cardiac anomalies. According to the literature, the ruptured sinus of Valsalva aneurysm is a rare condition, ranging between 0.26% and 3.5% of all types of operations for the treatment of congenital heart diseases. The incidence has been five times higher in Eastern countries than in Western countries, based on Japan and India's numbers. It is more frequent in men than in women, and the vast majority of patients are operated in adulthood. The most common coexisting injuries are ventricular septal defect (VSD) and aortic insufficiency, mainly in Asian patients. VSD is usually related to the ruptured aneurysms in the right sinus of Valsalva which break in the right ventricle (RV) and are usually the supracristal type. Some authors noted VSD of this type in 75% of patients, while others have found 84% of VSD in their cases and 100% of sub-arterial type. In Western patients, the incidence of VSD and aortic insufficiency is lower, not reaching 50%. Often, the diagnosis is made in the third or fourth decade of life after the rupture of the aneurysm into a cardiac cavity (most often the right atrium) [2].

3. What is the clinical presentation of a patient with an SVA?

The clinical condition is variable, and it will depend, in most cases, on the presence or absence of fistula in an aneurysm, as well as the magnitude of the blood flow through the fistula and its location. In the literature, many patients are asymptomatic, and routine medical examination can provide continuous blowing near the location of the fistula, and about 45% of the patients may have angina or cardiac insufficiency symptoms [3].

4. What is the pathophysiology of heart failure in an SVA patient?

The decompensation occurs mainly after the rupture of the aneurysm (more frequent in right chambers). With the rupture or fistula of the aneurysm to the right chambers, there is an increased blood flow in the pulmonary artery and a volume overload to the left chambers. After the loss of compensatory mechanisms, the failure of the left ventricle occurs [4].

5. What are the methods used to diagnose an SVA?

The diagnosis by clinical examination is difficult due to the variety of symptoms that can be manifested. The chest radiography shows unspecific changes to SVA. It can show increased cardiothoracic index, dilation of the aortic button and the left ventricle, and even associated arrhythmias.

The two-dimensional color Doppler echocardiography and transesophageal echocardiography are noninvasive tests, with low risk, that determine the precise anatomy of the sinus of Valsalva and identify associated heart diseases and the effect of them on the heart. Aortography and coronarography can define the structure of the aneurysm and relate it to the coronary anatomy [5].

6. What is the appropriate management of an SVA patient?

The early surgical repair of SVA is the treatment of choice in symptomatic patients and in cases of aneurysm rupture. The optimal management is less clear for asymptomatic not-ruptured aneurysms. The operative risk is low, and the long-term outcome is good. The straight closure can cause or worsen aortic regurgitation by deformation of the aortic annulus and may also be responsible for relapses. Thus, the lock by the graft is recommended even when the hole is small, as was done in this case. Other incisions (atriotomy, ventriculotomy) can be performed when there is rupture of the aneurysm into other cardiac chambers or when there are associated abnormalities [6].

7. What are the main complications of SVA ?

The ruptured SVA, generally symptomatic, have a poor prognosis and may set a catastrophic event; they may present complications related to their break:

(a) Cardiac tamponade, to drain the pericardium
(b) Cardiac insufficiency, when it drains into the heart chambers
(c) Arrhythmias and/or bundle branch block

The unruptured SVA are usually asymptomatic. There are reports of patients diagnosed with SVA after complaining of angina pectoris caused by compression of the coronary artery [5].

8. What is the prognosis for patients with this malformation?

The rupture of the SV is associated with a high mortality, and life expectancy of these patients is less than 4 years, so surgical correction is the recommended treatment. Operative mortality is less than 5%, and the long-term results are excellent (85% of patients were in functional class I in the mean follow-up of 11.1 years). The risk of recurrence is low. In particular cases, the closure of fistulas percutaneously is already an option. Late deaths, as well as reoperations, are usually related to the replacement or repair of the aortic valve [5].

Review About the Addressed Disease or Treatment

Sinus of Valsalva aneurysms (SVA) are rare, and they present a varied symptomatology. This case presents a patient with symptoms of a long-term heart failure and progressive clinical worsening due to late diagnosis.

The early diagnosis can prevent complications such as significant dilation of the cardiac chambers, ejection fraction decrease, and the development of atrial fibrillation. In this case, the patient was admitted for decompensated heart failure, classified in functional class IV (NYHA), and with atrial fibrillation with rapid ventricular response [6]. The initial treatment was the clinical compensation with diuretics and the control of heart rate; therefore, hospitalization in the intensive care unit was necessary [6].

An emergency echocardiogram was conducted, which showed an SVA and significant systolic dysfunction. After clinical stability, the transesophageal examination confirmed an SVA projecting into the right atrium and large turbulent flow into the right chambers (volume overload). In the long run, the fistula or aneurysm's rupture caused the progressive dilatation of the right and left chambers. The right ventricle is the most common fistula site (60–90%) followed by the right atrium.

The sinus of Valsalva aneurysms are classified according to the affected sinus and protrusion or rupture in [5]:

Type I: connection between the right coronary sinus and the outflow tract of the right ventricle, with the pulmonary valve
Type II: connection between the right coronary sinus and the right ventricle in supraventricular crest
Type IIIa: right coronary sinus and right atrium
Type IIIv: posterior region of the right coronary sinus and right ventricle
Type III (a + v): right coronary sinus and both, the atrium and right ventricle
Type IV: no coronary sinus and right atrium

As stated in the literature, the diagnosis is most commonly performed after the rupture of the aneurysm by rapid progression of heart failure. In this case, in the absence of symptoms of other conditions and changes in laboratory tests, congenital etiology was considered the most likely.

There are many complications of SVA, which may be cited as follows:

1. Potential risks of expansion, rupture, heart failure, and sudden death
2. Acute myocardial infarction by coronary artery compression

3. Total atrioventricular block (compression of conducting tissues and atrioventricular node)
4. Right ventricular outflow obstruction
5. Infective endocarditis
6. Pericardial tamponade

In addition to the complications, the SVA can follow other congenital anomalies: VSD (30–60%), bicuspid aortic valve (15–20%), and aortic insufficiency (44–5%). It affects up to 10% of patients with the Marfan syndrome [7].

The initial pharmacological treatment could offset the symptoms of heart failure. The persistence of the left-right shunt maintains a constant volume overload cycle of the heart chambers, and thus, the risk of new decompensation is high. Therefore, the definitive treatment is the correction of the causative agent, in other words surgery with resection of the aneurysmal sac and anatomical reconstruction of the coronary sinus.

The prognosis after surgical treatment is excellent, mainly with a fast and accurate diagnosis. In this case, the diagnosis was made by echocardiography and aortography. Angiotomography with three-dimensional reconstruction has been used because it allows a correlation between the findings of the aneurysm and the coronary anatomy [5].

Bibliography

1. Goldberg MD, Krasnow MD. Sinus of valsalva aneurysms. Clin Cardiol. 1990;13:831–6.
2. Bonatelli Filho L, Rampinelli A, Collaço J. Correção cirúrgica do aneurisma roto do seio de Valsalva: relato de dois casos. Rev Bras Cir Cardiovasc. 1999;14(4):344–7.
3. Gopro AA, Coimbra LF, MVN DS. Fístula da artéria coronária: relato de três casos operados e revisão da literatura. Rev Bras Cir Cardiovasc. 2002;17(13):271–4.
4. Abe T, Komatzu S. Surgical repair and long-term results in ruptured sinus of Valsalva aneurysm. Ann Thorac Surg. 1998;46:520–5.
5. Fiarresga A, Branco LM, Da Silva MN, Feliciano J, Pelicano N, Fernandes RM, Fragata J, Quininha J. Rupture of a congenital

aneurysm of the non-coronary sinus of Valsalva into the right atrium. Rev Port Cardiol. 2006;25(1):79–85.
6. Dias RR, Camurça FD, Leite Filho OA, Stolf NAG. Right sinus of Valsalva aneurysm causing extrinsic coronary compression. Arq Bras Cardiol. 2009;92(6):74–7.
7. Hamid IA, Jothi M, Rajan S, Monro JL, Cherian KM. Transaortic repair of ruptured aneurysm of sinus of Valsalva – fifteen-year experience. J Thorac Cardiovasc Surg. 1994;107(6):1464–8.

Retroesophageal Right Aortic Arch Associated with an Aortic Aneurysm and a Ventricular Septal Defect

Marcus Vinícius Silva Ferreira, Gabrielle Santos Oliveira, Ana Carolina Gonçalves e Silva, Fernando Antibas Atik, and Cláudio Ribeiro da Cunha

Clinical Presentation

A 57-year-old woman with hypertension, dyslipidemia, past history of smoking, past history of tuberculosis, and asymptomatic heart murmur during childhood was admitted due to complaints of shortness of breath on exertion, chest pain upon exertion radiating to the back, and episodes of tachycardia, with a history of a syncope episode 6 months ago after her mother's death and a presyncope 1 month ago associated with a hypertensive crisis. The patient was in the regular use of 25 mg of hydrochlorothiazide and 25 mg of losartan twice a day and 50 mg of atenolol every 8 h. Examination revealed the following: weight, 64 kg; height, 155 cm tall, blood pressure, 188/96 mmHg in the left arm and 175/101 mmHg in the

M. V. S. Ferreira (✉) · G. S. Oliveira · A. C. G. e Silva · F. A. Atik
C. R. da Cunha
Cardiology Institute of Federal District (ICDF), Brasília, DF, Brazil

R. M. S. Almeida, F. B. Jatene (eds.), *Cardiovascular Surgery*,
https://doi.org/10.1007/978-3-319-57084-6_5

right arm; and a systolic heart murmur that was heard all over the cardiac area radiating to the back. The remainder of the examination was normal.

Diagnosis, Assessment, and Treatment

The patient was evaluated after drug optimization and hypertension control, and a chest X-ray and a new echocardiography were performed in our service. The echocardiography showed a perimembranous ventricular septal defect (VSD) partially occluded by a tricuspid tissue, measuring 7 mm in diameter with a left-to-right shunt (pressure gradient of 125 mmHg), Qp:Qs of 1.90, left ventricular ejection fraction of 56%, and a dilated and hypertrophic left ventricle with mild systolic dysfunction. Chest X-ray presented an expanding opacity in the right mediastinum blurring the cardiac area, suggesting a large mass.

A contrast-enhanced computed tomography (CT) angiography was then performed to evaluate the radiographic findings and revealed (Fig. 1):

- A dilated (39 mm) ascending aorta
- A right aortic arch with a retroesophageal elongated and tortuous segment whose branches emerged in the following order: 1. left common carotid artery, 2. right common carotid artery, 3. right subclavian artery, and 4. left subclavian artery (elongated and tortuous)
- A saccular aneurysm with calcified walls on the middle third measuring 92 × 73 mm, partially compressing the right subclavian artery, the innominate veins, and the esophagus

The patient was then submitted to preoperative coronary CT (no obstructive lesions) and to right cardiac catheterization that showed a mild pulmonary hypertension (systolic pulmonary artery pressure (SPAP), 45 mmHg) and mild increase in pulmonary vascular resistance (PVR, 4.1 UW).

Surgical treatment was indicated to correct the aortic arch aneurysm altogether with the VSD. The cardiopulmonary

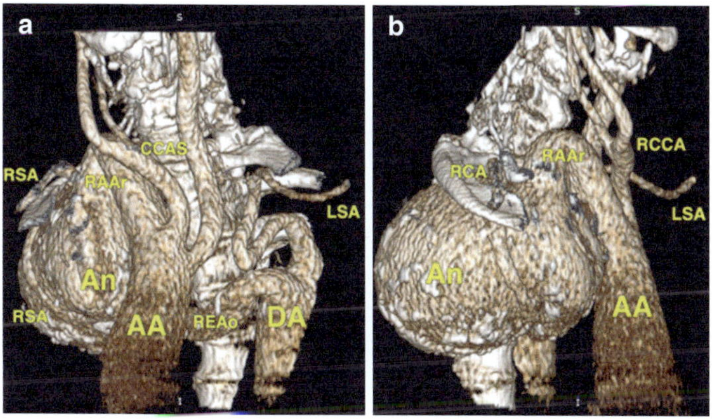

FIGURE 1 Preoperative three-dimensional computed tomography reconstruction of the thoracic aorta showing the retroesophageal right aortic arch and the aneurysm emerging from the arch. (**a**) Frontal view. (**b**) Right side view (AA ascending aorta, DA descending aorta, An aneurysm, RAAr right aortic arch, REAo retroesophageal aorta, CCAS common carotid arteries, RCCA right common carotid artery, RSA right subclavian artery, LSA left subclavian artery)

bypass (CPB) was performed with a double arterial cannula (distal ascending aorta and right femoral artery) and a double venous cannula (superior and inferior vena cava), associated with a 32 °C hypothermia. Cardioplegia was achieved through antegrade (aorta) and retrograde (coronary sinus) cannulation with cold solution (St. Thomas number 2) every 15 min. The aorta was cross-clamped and sectioned after the origin of the carotid arteries, and before the aneurysm, with stitches placed in a two-plane suture at the proximal end with Polypropylene 5.0. Another cross-clamp and section were performed immediately after the aneurysm end and the right subclavian artery origin, with an interposition of an 18-mm Dacron graft sutured with continuous stitches of Polypropylene 5.0, creating an aortic bypass from the ascending aorta to the retroesophageal portion of the aorta (Fig. 3, IG1). The right subclavian artery was sutured in a terminoterminal anastomosis to a 10-mm Dacron tube that was interposed with a

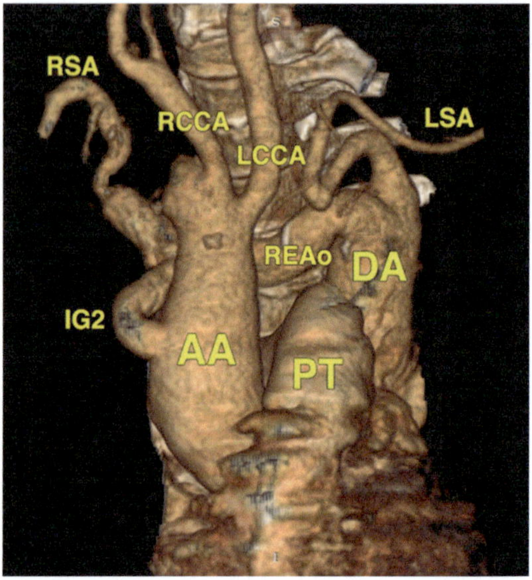

FIGURE 2 Postoperative three-dimensional computed tomography reconstruction of the thoracic aorta (AA ascending aorta, PT pulmonary trunk, REAo retroesophageal aorta, DA descending aorta, RCCA right common carotid artery, LCCA left common carotid artery, RSA right subclavian artery, LSA left subclavian artery, IG2 second interposition graft)

terminolateral suture to the ascending aorta (Figs. 2 and 3, IG2). The ventricular septoplasty was then performed with a double U-stitch suture through a right atriotomy. The patient was rewarmed and successfully weaned from CPB after 122 min and after 76 min of aortic cross-clamping.

After surgery, the patient was admitted to the ICU henodinamically stable under 7 mcg/kg/min of dobutamine and 0.4 mcg/kg/min of nitroprusside, which were totally weaned after 24 h. The patient remained hospitalized in the ICU for a period of 10 days due to respiratory insufficiency requiring reintubation and a right upper lobar pneumonia treated with cefepime for 4 days, changing to polymyxin B, meropenem, and vancomycin for completion, as a complication of transi-

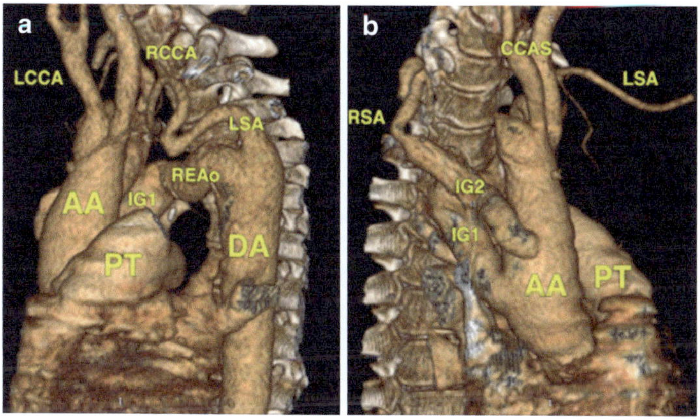

FIGURE 3 Postoperative three-dimensional computed tomography reconstruction of the thoracic aorta (**a**) Left side view. (**b**) Right side view (AA ascending aorta, PT pulmonary trunk, REAo retroesophageal aorta, DA descending aorta, CCAS common carotid arteries, RCCA right common carotid artery, LCCA left common carotid artery, RSA right subclavian artery, LSA left subclavian artery, IG1 first interposition graft, IG2 second interposition graft)

tory diaphragmatic paresis due to neuropraxis of the phrenic nerve and tuberculosis sequelae in the right upper pulmonary lobe. After 29 days' postsurgery, the patient was discharged with mild respiratory distress and improvement of lung auscultation, with no sign of infectious process. On a 1-month follow-up consultation, she presented complete remission of chest pain and improvement of respiratory symptoms.

Questions

1. What are vascular rings?

The term vascular ring was first used to refer to vascular anomalies that encircled the intrathoracic portion of the esophagus and trachea, leading to various degrees of compressions and symptoms depending on the tightness of the ring ([5]: 511). A vascular ring is an aortic arch or pulmonary artery anomaly that presents an abnormal relationship with the esophagus and trachea, often causing compression symptoms (dysphagia and/or respiratory symptoms) ([6]: 1435).

The first vascular ring described was a double aortic arch noted by Hommel in 1737. Bayford reported retroesophageal right subclavian artery in 1794 after performing an autopsy on a woman who had experienced dysphagia for years and died of starvation. Maude Abbott described five cases of double aortic arch in 1932 and made the suggestion that surgical intervention should be undertaken in such cases. Finally, in 1945, Gross used the term vascular ring in the publication that he wrote after performing the first successful division of a double aortic arch. Since that time, numerous reports of successful treatment have occurred, and the forms of aortic arch anomalies causing this problem have been well delineated [3].

2. How is the aortic arch formed during the embryonic period?

The aorta and the supra-aortic vessels originated from several structures during the embryonic development. By the fifth week of embryogenesis, the ascending aorta is formed through the division of the truncus arteriosus by the truncal ridges (posteriorly fusing with the bulbar ridges and forming the aorticopulmonary septum) as it undergoes a 180° spin, originating the ascending aorta and the pulmonary trunk. Almost simultaneously, by the fourth week of gestation, the pharyngeal arch arteries start developing altogether with the pharyngeal arches and will originate the aortic arch, the supra-aortic vessels, the pulmonary arteries, and the ductus arteriosus ([8]: 324).

The pharyngeal arch arteries are composed of six pairs of arteries connecting the aortic sac (dilated segment at the distal end of the truncus arteriosus) to the ipsilateral dorsal aorta. However, these pairs of arteries are not all present at the same time and are formed progressively and simultaneously disappear, leaving by the eighth week the final arterial arrangement. The aortic arch originated from the aortic sac, the left fourth pharyngeal arch artery and the left dorsal aorta, with its left curvature formed through

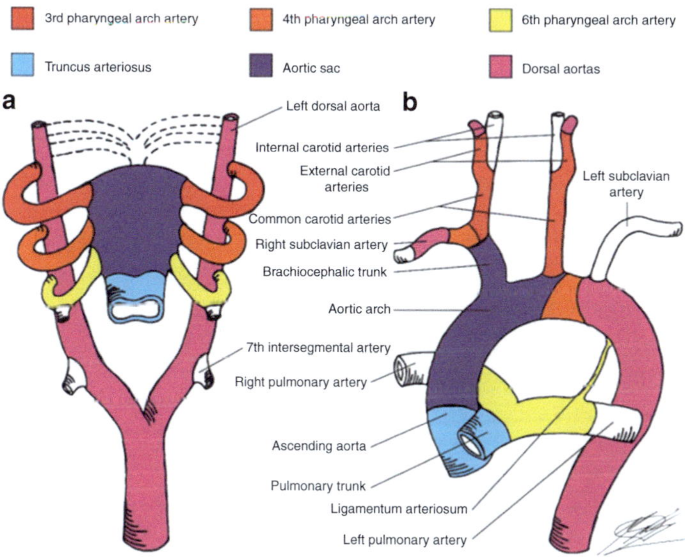

FIGURE 4 Schematic drawings representing the embryonic formation of the adult arterial pattern. (**a**) Pharyngeal arch arteries and dorsal aortas at the sixth week of pregnancy. (**b**) Adult arterial pattern (*Illustrations by Daniel Ferreira and Marcus Ferreira*)

the regression of a segment of the right dorsal aorta (Fig. 4). The left dorsal aorta completes the aorta, originating the descending aorta ([8]: 326).

3. How is a vascular ring formed during the embryonic period?

This congenital malformation originates during the formation of the adult arterial system from the pharyngeal arch arterial system when the arteries that should disappear persist or when arteries that should persist disappear. The failure of the pharyngeal arch arteries to form, fuse, or disappear may lead to a vascular ring formation ([8]: 327). The types of malformation that may occur will be further discussed in the next topic.

4. What types of vascular rings do exist?

There are five major types of vascular rings described in the medical literature ([6]: 1435). They can be further divided into two groups accordingly to the presence or not of a continuous structure encircling the trachea and the esophagus, despite the presence or not of compressive symptoms: complete or incomplete ([5]: 514).

Complete Vascular Rings

- Double aortic arch: This is the most common form of vascular ring and is a result of the failure of the distal part of the right dorsal aorta to disappear, with the persistent fourth pharyngeal arches originating two arches (a left one immediately before the trachea and a right one behind the esophagus) with a single left descending aorta. Usually, only one arch is patent, but if they both are, the right arch is usually larger. These two arches' fusion may lead to compression of the structures trapped inside the ring, causing the associated symptoms.
- Right aortic arch: This type of vascular ring is formed due to the abnormal persistence of the right dorsal aorta, disappearing the left dorsal aorta. The ring is completed by a left ductus or ligamentum arteriosum, but rarely it compromises any structures or promotes symptoms. Usually, the symptomatic forms are accompanied by a Kommerell diverticulum.
- Retroesophageal aortic arch: A rarer and more complicated form of a vascular ring that can be either formed by a right aortic arch with a descending left aorta or by a left aortic arch and descending right aorta. The ring is also completed by a right- or left-sided ligamentum arteriosum and may cause tracheal compression.

Incomplete Vascular Rings

- Anomalous origin of the right subclavian artery: Despite being described in this group, rarely is a vascular ring formed in this anomaly (only in the presence of a right ligamentum arteriosum). The right subclavian artery has an aberrant origin at the distal end of the aortic arch and runs posterior to the esophagus to supply the right upper limb. Symptoms are only present in 5% of patient in adult age due to the rigidity of the vessel passing behind the esophagus.

- Pulmonary artery sling: Here the left pulmonary artery arises from the right pulmonary artery and runs behind the trachea and anteriorly to the esophagus. There might be significant hypoplasia of the bronchial tree, and symptoms are usually related to respiratory tract compression.

5. What are the associated anatomical anomalies that may occur?

The anatomical compression of the airways might contribute to abnormal development of the tracheobronchial tree leading to tracheomalacia (usually in the double aortic arch and right aortic arch) and trachea stenosis (pulmonary artery sling). Other cardiac malformations have been reported, such as ventricular septal defect, tetralogy of Fallot, transposition of the great vessels, truncus arteriosus, coarctation of the aorta, and patent ductus arteriosus ([5]: 517).

Reports on the medical literature also associate vascular rings to numerous different congenital malformations and chromosomic syndromes. Renal agenesis, cross-fused ectopia, horseshoe kidney, tracheoesophageal fistula, hiatus hernia, diaphragmatic eventration, imperforate and ectopic anus, PHACE syndrome, and Down syndrome are some of the previously described ([5]: 515). In a case series reported by McElhinney et al. ([7]: 2115), the association with the deletion of chromosome 22q11 was present in 24% of patients and should be suspected in the presence of other congenital anomalies.

6. How frequent are vascular rings in the general population?

The prevalence of vascular rings is estimated in 0.1–3% of the adult population, and it represents approximately 1% of all cases of congenital heart defects that are surgically corrected ([2]: 975). They occur equally distributed by gender, with no predilection for race or geographical location ([5]: 513). However, the available data comes from old studies, and there are no more current studies that have evaluated its incidence or prevalence, mainly due to its rarity among congenital malformations and its multiple presentations and variations.

7. How do vascular rings clinically present?

The presence, age of onset, and severity of the symptoms depend on the type of vascular ring and on the degree of constriction of the esophagus and trachea. Some patients with incomplete rings may be asymptomatic, and diagnosis may only be made incidentally during the evaluation of chronic heart disease at adult age. Most of the symptomatic cases are identified early in life, with some case being investigated for complaints about dysphagia later in childhood and other cases never to be diagnosed ([6]: 1435).

When present, the most classical symptoms consist mainly of respiratory and digestive symptoms. Respiratory manifestations are present in 70–97% of symptomatic cases and include respiratory distress, cyanosis, chest pain, stridor, wheezing, seal-bark cough, apnea, and recurrent respiratory infections, usually in the first year of life. Later in childhood, with the introduction of solid diet, patients may present feeding problems such as dysphagia, slow feeding, and neck extension while eating. Since the clinical manifestations may also be present in other prevalent diseases of infancy such as asthma and gastroesophageal reflux, misdiagnosis is common and may delay by several years the correct diagnosis ([5]: 515).

8. What imaging studies should be requested upon clinical suspicion?

Clinical suspicion is essential to initiate the investigation of the symptoms; thus imaging studies that usually include chest radiography, bronchoscopy, barium esophagogram, echocardiography, cardiac magnetic resonance imaging, and computed tomography angiography should be requested upon clinical suspicion. Radiography is the first line of investigation with great negative predictive value and may provide evidence of a right- or a left-sided aortic arch (compared to the tracheal position), airway narrowing and bowing, hyperinflation of lung fields, retrotracheal opacity, and posterior indentation of the esophagus on barium esophagogram. Bronchoscopy may differentiate dynamic from static compression of airway and level and extent of compression and discard other conditions and should be provided to all patients prior to surgery ([5]: 515).

Upon suspicious image, other imaging studies are required to confirm the diagnosis and further evaluate the anatomy and compromise of adjacent structures. The echocardiography may identify the laterality of the aortic arch, anomalous branching, and associated cardiac defects. Magnetic resonance imaging and computed tomography angiography are the preferred modes of evaluation of vascular rings and are essential for the determination of the treatment plan. The gold standard for the evaluation of the aorta and its branches is the magnetic resonance imaging, with the disadvantage of requiring deep sedation and general anesthesia in children. Cross-sectional studies can provide detailed anatomic assessment and evaluation of posterior vascular structures, required prior to a surgical approach, especially by video-assisted thoracoscopic techniques ([6]: 1435; [5]: 522).

Prenatal diagnosis is nowadays becoming more common with the widespread use of prenatal ultrasound. Upon suspicion, fetal echocardiography with color Doppler investigation is warranted, and detection of vascular rings should be followed by appropriate counseling at a specialist center to prepare for delivery in the best available conditions ([5]: 522). Prenatal diagnosis of the presence and type of vascular ring can be accurately provided in 68–100% of cases, but should not preclude postnatal confirmation through other imaging studies ([2]: 975).

9. When and how should surgical intervention be performed?

The presence of symptoms and the evaluation anatomy of the malformation are essential for indication surgery ([6]: 1435). Symptomatic cases may require early intervention in order to prevent the effects of prolonged vascular and airway compression (loss of weight, failure to thrive). The surgical approach may vary depending on the type and associated anomalies and may be achieved through open or video assisted thoracoscopic surgery (VATS) ([5]: 522).

Surgical division of the vascular ring is the main procedure performed, but may be unnecessary or insufficient in some cases requiring extra-anatomic reconstructions. Konstantinov and Puga ([4]: 2021) described a 32-year-old patient with right aortic arch, Kommerell diverticulum, and anomalous origin of the left subclavian artery submitted to the division of the left-sided ligamentum arteriosum without improvement, requiring resection of the aortic arch and diverticulum associated with surgical bypass (ascending-descending retrocardiac interposition graft). In another report, Emil de Goma et al. ([1]: 2375) described a patient with right aortic arch causing tracheal compression treated singly with sling wrapped around the ascending aorta and second ribs.

10. What is the prognosis before and after surgery?

Vascular rings when occurring as isolated anomalies may present a benign prognosis, sometimes without repercussion through lifetime. Prolonged symptomatic cases may lead to failure to thrive, low weight during infancy, and even more serious complications due to apneic episodes. However, they are prevented through early surgery that can be performed with low morbidity and mortality ([5]: 522). Tracheal narrowing requiring surgical intervention increases the mortality rate, as does its association with intracardiac malformations ([6]: 1435). Sudden death or further tracheobronchial damage may occur in cases with delayed intervention, reinforcing the need for prompt investigation of all cases ([5]: 522).

Patients respond well to surgery, with significant improvement in symptoms, even in the immediate postoperative. After repair, the patients should be examined for the persistence of respiratory symptoms, since rarely symptoms resolve immediately after surgery, usually persisting for another 6 months. If there are any residual symptoms, some exercise restrictions may apply, as cardiologist follow-up is recommended. Despite that, there will be no restrictions to exercise and no increased susceptibility to the development of arrhythmias or sudden death. Pregnancy may be undertaken without added risk if there is no persistence of significant respiratory obstruction [9].

Review About the Addressed Disease or Treatment

Vascular rings are abnormalities that originated from the impaired regression or persistence of the pharyngeal arteries and dorsal aorta, which leads to an abnormal relationship between the aorta/pulmonary trunk and the esophagus/trachea. The presence of compressive symptoms is further determined by the type of vascular ring formed, especially in the presence of complete vascular rings, and might lead to further malformations of the tracheobronchial tree. Despite these local consequences, other cardiac malformations and chromosomic syndromes have been described altogether and should be part of the initial investigation upon the diagnosis of a vascular ring.

Although unknown by many healthcare providers, vascular rings are estimated to be present in 0.1–3% of the general population, despite the lack of sufficient data due to its rarity. Most of the cases that are diagnosed usually become apparent in early life due to compressive symptoms, but some patients, especially with incomplete rings, might remain asymptomatic through a lifetime and remain undiagnosed. Special attention should be given to patients that present with respiratory and digestive symptoms, such as dyspnea, cyanosis, chest pain, stridor, wheezing, seal-bark cough, apnea, recurrent respiratory infections, and dysphagia, and slow feeding and neck extension while eating in later childhood. Since there are more common causes of these symptoms, vascular rings should not come as the main hypothesis but remain as a differential diagnosis not to be missed in these cases. In other words, clinical suspicion is of the essence to the diagnosis.

Initial investigation of symptomatic cases should include imaging studies, with radiography being used as first-line exam due to its high sensitivity. Upon a suspicious image, further investigation should include other image modalities to confirm the diagnosis, better understand its anatomy, and evaluate adjacent structures compromise. Magnetic resonance imaging (gold standard) and computed tomography angiography are the preferred modes of evaluation due to the details they provide, but echocardiogram, bronchoscopy, and esophagogram may be as well useful. One brief commentary should be made on prenatal diagnosis since due to the widespread use of prenatal ultrasound, more and more cases of cardiac anomalies have been suspected. Upon suspicion, fetal echocardiography with color Doppler investigation is warranted, with further follow-up by a specialist center and postnatal confirmation studies.

Surgical intervention is indicated upon the presence or not of symptoms and the complexity of the anatomy of the malformation, where compression of adjacent structures might require early correction to relief symptoms. Surgical division of the vascular ring may be achieved through open or video-assisted thoracoscopic surgery (VATS), but the surgical strategy may change in the presence of concomitant malformations. Despite the worse prognosis related to the presence of digestive or tracheobronchial compression (failure to thrive and apneic episodes), its correction presents low morbidity and mortality and leads to early relief in symptoms and good long-term prognosis. In cases where symptoms persist after 6 months, however, the therapy should focus on symptomatic relief only, since there are no additional risks or restrictions related to physical activities or pregnancy. In contrast, when vascular rings present as isolated and asymptomatic anomalies, patients might present no repercussion through lifetime and remain undiagnosed.

Bibliography

1. de Gomma EM, Wright CD, Pelikan PC, Leal JE, Karlsberg RP. Surgically corrected right-sided aortic arch. J Am Coll Cardiol. 2011;57(23):2375.
2. Galindo A, Nieto O, Nieto MT, Rodríguez-Martín OM, Herraiz I, Escribano D, Granados MA. Prenatal diagnosis of right aortic arch: associated findings, pregnancy outcome, and clinical significance of vascular rings. Prenat Diagn. 2009;29:975–81.

3. Hardin RE, Brevetti GR, Sanusi M, Bhaskaran D, Burack JR, Genovesi MH, Lowery RC, Rafii S, Bondi E. Treatment of symptomatic vascular rings in the elderly. Tex Heart Inst J. 2005;32(3):411–5.
4. Konstantinov IE, Puga FJ. Surgical treatment of persistent esophageal compression by an unusual form of right aortic arch. Ann Thorac Surg. 2001;72:2121–3.
5. Licari A, Rispoli GA, Mannarino S, Pelizzo G, Marseglia GL. Congenital vascular rings: a clinical challenge for the pediatrician. Pediatr Pulmonol. 2015;50:511–24.
6. Mann DL, Zipes DP, Libby P. Braunwald's heart disease: a textbook of cardiovascular medicine. 10th ed. Philadelphia: Saunders Elsevier; 2015.
7. McElhinney DB, Clark BJ, Weinberg PM, Kenton ML, McDonald-McGinn D, Driscoll DA, Zackai EH, Goldmuntz E. Association of chromosome 22q11 deletion with isolated anomalies of aortic arch laterality and branching. J Am Coll Cardiol. 2001;37(8):2114–9.
8. Moore KL, Persaud TVN, Torchia MG. The developing human: clinically oriented embryology. 9th ed. Philadelphia: Saunders Elsevier; 2013.
9. Suh YJ, Kim GB, Kwon BS, Bae EJ, Noh CI, Lim HG, Kim WH, Lee JR, Kim YJ. clinical course of vascular rings and risk factors associated with mortality. Korean Circ J. 2012;42:252–8.

Aortic Aneurysm

Yuri Justi Jardim and Antonio Eduardo Zerati

Clinical Presentation

NNC, female, 74 years, retired, and born and raised in São Paulo, SP.

Clinical examination: Good general condition. Mucous stained. Hydrated, afebrile, acyanotic, and eupneic. Conscious, vile, and oriented. FC, 70 bpm, and FR, 18 ipm. Temperature, 36.5 °C. No jugular stasis. Nonpalpable ganglia. Thyroid with normal appearance and consistency. Abdominal examination: flat abdomen, with no scars or marks. Aircraft noise present. Cardiology examination: heart with rhythmic sounds, without blows. Ictus not palpable. Palpable and symmetrical carotid and brachial pulses. Normal and symmetrical popliteal, malleolar, and pedicular pulses. No edema or signs of TVP.

Pulmonary exam: Thorax with normal appearance (normal skin, shape, and rhythm). Expansivity and symmetrical thoraco vocal sympathies in all fields. Vesicular murmurs

Y. J. Jardim (✉) · A. E. Zerati
Faculty of Medicine of University of São Paulo (FMUSP), São Paulo, SP, Brazil

R. M. S. Almeida, F. B. Jatene (eds.), *Cardiovascular Surgery*, https://doi.org/10.1007/978-3-319-57084-6_6

present, with clear pulmonary sound. No snoring, wheezing, or crackling. Normal voice listening.

Patient with thoracoabdominal aortic aneurysm diagnosed during the investigation for hepatic hemangioma. Asymptomatic in regard to the aneurysm.

Diagnosis, Assessment, and Treatment

Considering the maximum transverse diameter of the aneurysm of the aorta, the option was the indication for surgical treatment.

As for the technique, because of the high surgical risk posed by patient age and its comorbidities, we chose the endovascular due to its less invasive nature, aimed at minimizing the risk of complications.

Less diseased areas of the aorta, with the nearest normal diameter limits, are the most appropriate to support the proximal and distal ends of the stent. For this concept, in this case, the proximal stent should be positioned at the emergence of the left common carotid artery, covering the ostium of the left subclavian artery. The distal most suitable support, in turn, should be the aorta below the origin of the renal arteries. Thus, with the coverage of this entire segment of the aorta, there is a need for revascularization of the celiac trunk, the superior mesenteric artery, and the renal arteries. Therefore, surgical planning was based on the use of a branched prosthesis to the celiac trunk and fenestrated to the superior mesenteric artery and renal arteries.

Thus, based on angiotomographic study, the project of the customized stent adapted to the anatomical characteristics of the patient was done.

In order to reduce the risk of paraplegia, some measures have been taken. First, we decided to revascularize the left subclavian artery, which would have its ostium covered in an endoprosthesis to maintain pulsatile flow through the left vertebral artery and left internal thoracic, which aid in collateral circulation to the spinal cord through a left subclavian carotid bridge left. Another decision was to perform the procedure two times to reduce the surgical time.

So, initially, we performed carotid-subclavian left bridge with Dacron prosthesis and implantation of the first thoracic endoprosthesis module, covering the ostium of the left subclavian artery to a part of the descending aorta (Fig. 1). After 30 days, we perform the implantation of other two stent modules to the abdominal aorta, placing the last module in the celiac trunk and fenestrating the stent to the superior mesenteric and renal arteries. Coated stents were positioned joining the trunk branch celiac in this arterial branch and also through the fenestrae of the endoprosthesis to the superior mesenteric and renal arteries (Fig. 2). Control arteriography showed perfusion in all visceral branches without contrast leakage ("endoleak"), characterizing the success of the procedure (Fig. 3).

In this second stage, the patient's CSF pressure was continuously monitored for 48 h in order to reduce the risk of paraplegia. In a unique opportunity, within the first 24 h, the CSF pressure reached 14 mmHg, requiring drainage of the cerebrospinal fluid.

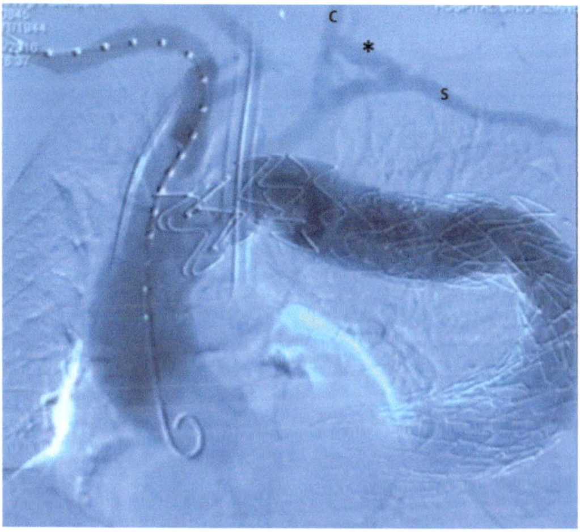

Figure 1 Intraoperative arteriography showing the absence of control proximal endoleak (thoracic aorta) and patency of the subclavian-carotid left bridge. C left carotid artery, S left subclavian artery, (*) subclavian-carotid bypass

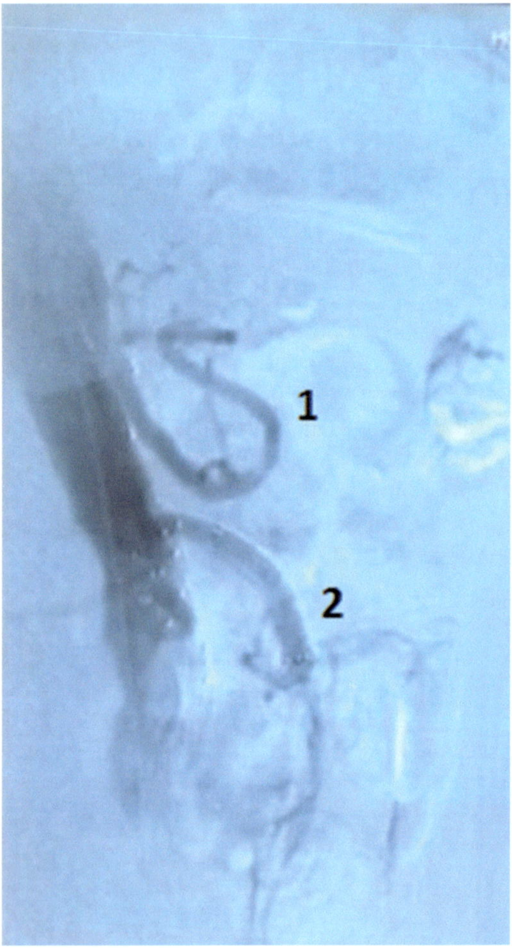

FIGURE 2 Arteriography Intraoperative control profile (abdominal aorta) showing the absence of distal endoleak and patency of the celiac trunk (1) and superior mesenteric artery (2)

The patient had elevated serum creatinine postoperatively, which returned to normal after 2 weeks. There was clinical improvement without any deficits in the lower limb , and the patient was discharged after 21 days.

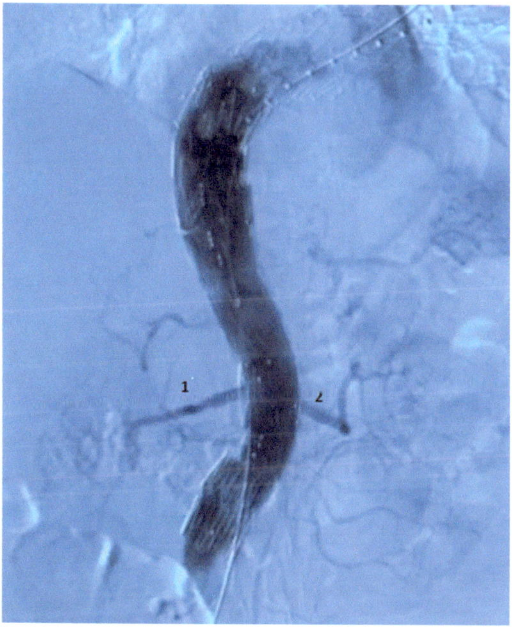

FIGURE 3 Arteriography intraoperative control in the anteroposterior projection (abdominal aorta) showing the absence of distal endoleak and patency of the right renal artery (1) and left (2)

Angiotomographic control after 3 months of the surgery showed complete exclusion of the aneurysm (Fig. 4) and discreet decrease in its maximum transverse diameter (5.6 cm) beyond the patency of all visceral trunks and carotid-subclavian left bridge (Fig. 5).

Questions

1. What is an arterial aneurysm?

An aneurysm is a focal dilatation of the artery, attaining a diameter of at least 150% of that expected for this segment. A true aneurysm comprises all layers of the vessel wall. It can be fusiform when affecting the arterial segment circumferen-

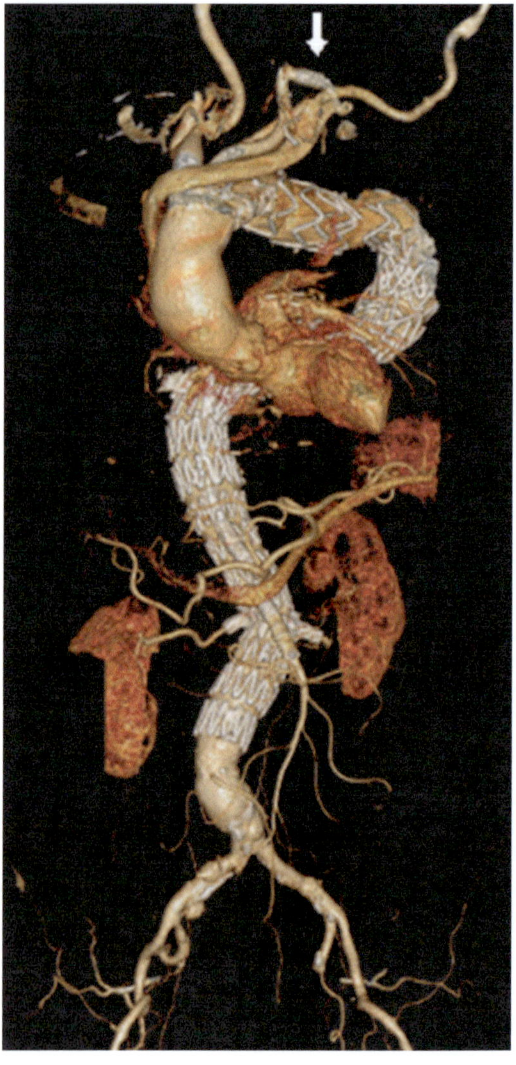

FIGURE 4 Postoperative CT angiography (3 months). Reconstruction showing patency of the subclavian-carotid bypass (*arrow*) and the visceral branches

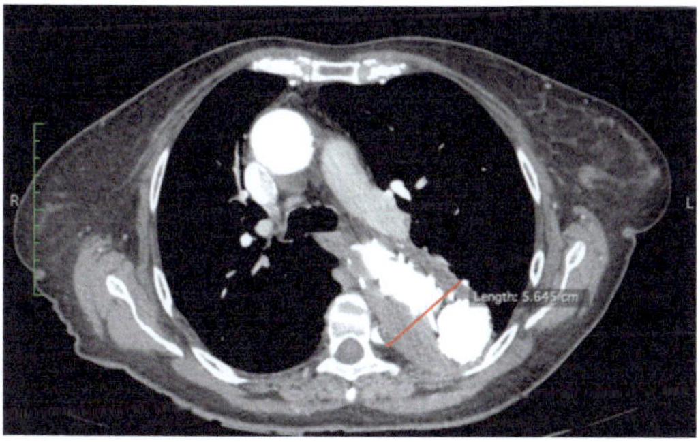

Figure 5 Postoperative CT angiography (3 months). Cross section showing the absence of endoleak and a slight decrease of the maximum transverse diameter of the thoracic aorta (5.6 cm) at the same point in Fig. 2

tially or vesicular when only a part of the circumference is involved.

The pseudoaneurysm occurs when there is an interruption of the arterial wall causing bleeding contained by the tissues surrounding the artery in question. Clinical examination shows a hyperpulsatile mass that resembles an aneurysm, but that body is not made up of all layers of the arterial wall, but the surrounding tissue, hence the name of a false aneurysm.

Complications associated with arterial aneurysm are rupture, distal embolization, and compression of neighboring structures. The frequency of each type of complication varies according to the location of the aneurysm. As an example, the aneurysm of the infrarenal aorta, the most common among aneurysms, has the main complication of rupture, with rare atheroembolism. In the popliteal artery, aneurysm is the reverse, getting atheroembolism as the most frequent complication and failure rare.

The main risk factor for rupture of an aortic aneurysm is its diameter: the greater the risk, the greater its maximum transverse diameter.

2. What is the cause of aneurysms?

The vast majority of aneurysms is the so-called degenerative aneurysms, which are related to risk factors for atherosclerosis, such as hypertension, diabetes, and smoking. About the risk of rupture, however, diabetes appears to be protective. Aortic aneurysms are more common in males, but the risk of rupture is higher among women.

Other diseases that are related to the emergence of arterial aneurysms and arterial dissection include Marfan syndrome, Ehlers-Danlos syndrome, infectious processes (infectious aneurysms, formerly called "mycotic"), fibromuscular dysplasia (especially aneurysms renal and carotid arteries), and trauma (pseudoaneurysm).

3. What are the most common signs and symptoms?

An aortic aneurysm is, in most cases, asymptomatic. Patients, especially those who are thinner, may notice a pulsating mass in the abdomen with a sense of having a "heart in the belly."

The pain symptom of aneurysm is extremely worrying, as it can reveal the verge of rupture or rupture already installed. The rupture of a thoracic or an abdominal aneurysm is a high mortality event in which more than half of patients do not arrive alive to the emergency room. When rupture occurs to the retroperitoneum, the bleeding can be stopped and the patient presents with low back pain and signs of hypovolemia, such as hypotension, tachycardia, and pallor.

Large aneurysms can cause the occurrence of symptoms by compressing the adjacent structures. Dysphagia, dyspnea, and cough may be associated with bulky thoracic aortic aneurysm. A major expansion of the abdominal aorta can lead to erosion of the lumbar vertebra and cause pain.

The atheroembolism and thrombosis of an aneurysm are rare in aortic aneurysm cases. The symptoms in these cases are ischemia of tissues due to arterial segment obstruction.

4. How is it diagnosed?

As the patient, in most cases, is asymptomatic, the diagnosis of an aneurysm arises when diagnosing other diseases.

The diagnosis of the thoracic aortic aneurysm can be hypothesized when there is mediastinal widening in simple chest X-ray. Abdominal ultrasound is an important method for the diagnosis and management of abdominal aortic aneurysms, having no value for the study of the thoracic segment.

As a rule, the main diagnostic methods are computed tomography angiography and magnetic resonance imaging. Angiography is not the most suitable method because besides being very invasive, it shows only the light of the vessels. As aneurysms have thrombus on its periphery, where the dilatation makes the blood flow turbulent, it leaves only the center of the vessel (which has laminar flow) patent. This exam very often generates images that do not show the actual dilatation of the vessel.

5. What are the indications for surgical treatment?

Small aortic aneurysms have a lower risk of rupture and should only be followed with serial imaging. The aneurysms with a big diameter or who have accelerated growth rate are indicated for surgical treatment.

As a rule, the operation is indicated for thoracic aortic aneurysms with a diameter greater than or equal to 6 cm. For the infrarenal aorta, surgical treatment is indicated for those aneurisms with a diameter of 5.5 cm or more, in women and in men. The growth of the aneurysm, that is, less than 0.5 cm in a 6-month interval, represents a marked expansion and indicates the need for surgical treatment. The clinical conditions, which have a direct impact on the surgical risk, of each patient influence the decision to operate or not the aneurysm.

Complications such as atheroembolism and/or compression of adjacent structures can also lead to the indication for invasive treatment.

A painful aneurysm means an imminent risk of rupture and is an indication for urgent treatment, as well as the ruptured ones. The ruptured aneurysms, of course, have an indication for immediate surgical treatment.

6. What are the surgical treatment options?

For surgical treatment, open surgery and endovascular approach are viable options.

The open operation consists of interrupting the bloodflow through the aneurysmal artery by clamping proximally and distally in order to prevent bleeding and reflow when performing surgery. Access depends on the position of the aneurysm being treated and may be a thoraco-phreno-laparotomy in thoracoabdominal aortic aneurysms, or a median, transverse, or even an extraperitoneal laparotomy access in the abdominals.

After clamping and opening the aneurysm, a synthetic vascular graft is sutured in a proximal segment and another distal free of aneurysmal disease. In thoracoabdominal aortic aneurysms, catheterization of the visceral arteries is often laborious and exposes the patient more to radiation, by using significant volumes of iodinated contrast, which has nephrotoxic properties. During the time of clamping, renal protection can be made with the intermittent infusion of cold crystalloid solution, for example, the solution comprising Ringer's lactate at 4 °C or 5 °C with 50 ml mannitol, 20% heparin 2500UI, and 200 mg methylprednisolone.

The synthetic vascular prosthesis is covered by the aneurysm, avoiding direct contact with other structures and preventing, for example, fistulation with the bowel.

The endovascular technique is based on the exclusion of the aneurysm by implanting a prosthesis comprising a metal frame similar to a stent but coated by synthetic tissue, the so-called endoprosthesis. This device is deployed from a distant artery aneurysm site (usually the femoral artery), which will navigate the intravascular space to the aneurysmal segment, where it is released. The endoprosthesis runs compressed within a catheter, expanding only after its release. Avoiding the open surgery approach of the chest and/or abdominal cavities by choosing the endovascular procedure is less aggressive for the patient. To be a viable option, the anatomy of the aneurysm should be favorable. The majority of aortic aneurysms can be treated by endovascular technique, due to the innovations on surgical and manufacturing terms.

7. What are the risks of the operation?

The main risks of a large operation are cardiovascular events and complications of respiratory and kidney failure.

Paraplegia is a concern primarily in the treatment of thoracoabdominal aortic aneurysms secondary to spinal cord ischemia. This is true for both the open operation, despite the revascularization of the intercostal arteries, and endovascular treatment. The greater the extent of the disease in the aorta, the greater the risk of paraplegia. Although the endovascular technique does not provide the revascularization of the intercostal arteries, the greater hemodynamic stability and less surgical aggression, avoiding the temporary interruption of blood flow, make the risk of paraplegia lower than the open operation.

The main measures to reduce the incidence of paraplegia in open operation are reimplantation of the intercostal arteries and aortic distal perfusion through total extracorporeal circulation, temporary axillary-visceral shunt, or atrial-femoral shunt. Monitoring the pressure and drainage of the cerebrospinal fluid is indicated, and should be extended for up to 36 h after the procedure. The goal is to keep the cerebrospinal fluid pressure around 10 mmHg, with careful surveillance.

8. What are the advantages and disadvantages of open and endovascular techniques in the treatment of aortic aneurysms?

The open operation involves an arguably greater tissue damage, starting with the surgical approach that in thoracoabdominal aortic aneurysms requires thoraco-phreno-laparotomy. Even in infrarenal aneurysms, transperitoneal access causes a slower recovery, which may present with paralytic ileus in the early days, delaying the reintroduction of oral diet, and respiratory disorders caused by postoperative pain. Another important aspect is that in the open technique is necessary to interrupt the blood flow through the aorta by positioning vascular clamps. This can causeischemia in the lower limbs and visceral hypoperfusion in proximal aneurysms cases. The broader dissection can cause inadvertent damage to other organs and structures.

The endovascular technique, in turn, requires continuous monitoring of the patient in the postoperative period, given the risk of stent graft migration and occurrence of leakage flow into the aneurysmal sac, called “endoleak,” which maintains the risk of rupture. The aneurysmal disease can progress to where the endoprosthesis is supported, being another cause of endoleak. In thoracoabdominal aortic aneurysms, catheterization of the visceral arteries is often laborious and exposes the patient more to radiation, by using significant volumes of iodinated contrast, which has nephrotoxic properties. Surgical aggression, however, is infinitely smaller, and you can treat large aneurysms through access to the femoral and eventually axillary arteries.

The higher cost of the stent relative to the vascular prosthesis used in the open operation is diluted by less need of blood transfusion, less time on intensive care unit, and lower total term of hospitalization provided by endovascular surgery.

Review About the Addressed Disease or Treatment

An aortic aneurysm is the 13th leading cause of death in the United States and the third cause of sudden death. The increase in life expectancy of men and women, as well as developments in diagnostic imaging methods, may explain the arising of the prevalence of this disease in the world population.

An aortic aneurysm is an insidious disease that develops and generates few or no symptoms but carries risks of life-threatening complications. The main one is the rupture of an aneursym, an event associated with a mortality of around 80%. The most commonly involved segment is the infrarenal aorta.

An aortic aneurysm is a multifactorial disease, whose pathogeneses include atherosclerosis, inflammation, extracellular matrix degradation, and genetic issues.

Over 90% of the aneurysms are classified as degenerative. Other less common causes are an infection, cystic necrosis of the medial layer, inflammatory diseases of the arteries, and connective tissue diseases.

Among the factors associated with increased risk of developing aortic aneurysm, the main ones are advancing age, smoking, hypertension, hypercholesterolemia, coronary heart disease, and family history of an aneurysmal disease. As for the rupture, which is the most feared complication of this disease, the factors related to a higher risk of this event are female, active smoking, hypertension, and especially the maximum transverse diameter of the aneurysm, which keeps a direct relation to the risk of rupture.

In most cases, the aortic aneurysm is asymptomatic, being diagnosed during palpation of the abdomen (especially in lean and tall patients) or by imaging studies performed for the investigation of other diseases. Too often, the aortic aneurysm is associated with the presence of aneurysms in other locations, especially the popliteal and iliac arteries. This association can be synchronous or metachronous.

The few times that an aortic aneurysm causes symptoms, these may be due to rapid expansion at break, atheroembolism, thrombosis, or compression of adjacent structures. The most frequent complication is a rupture.

Aneurysms, once diagnosed, can be stable for many years, with slow growth. An aortic aneurysm is, therefore, an important preventable cause of death. Once diagnosed, the patient should be monitored periodically. The recommended monitoring for abdominal aortic aneurysms is the ultrasound exam control every 6 months. For the thoracic aorta, computed tomography angiography or magnetic nuclear resonance angiography are the indicated methods, every 6 months.

The surgical correction can be done by open or endovascular means. The open track consists of a more definitive treatment but is a larger-sized procedure with increased perioperative morbidity and mortality as compared to endovascular technique. The lowest surgical aggression allows us to treat a greater number of patients, particularly those older and more comorbid conditions. If before the surgical risk of an open operation did not make them good candidates for open surgery, today due to lower morbidity and mortality of the endovascular technique, they are able to receive treatment.

This technical and technological progress advances in order to enable the treatment of longer aneurysms, including those that affect the origin of the visceral arteries. If once the endovascular technique was restricted to the infrarenal aneurysms or the thoracic aorta was isolated, today this possibility extends to thoracoabdominal aortic aneurysms and also involves the iliac arteries.

Bibliography

1. Crawford ES, Denatale RW. Thoracoabdominal aortic aneurysm: observations regarding the natural course of the disease. J Vasc Surg. 1986;3:578–82.
2. Reilly LM, Chuter TA. Endovascular repair of thoracoabdominal aneurysms: design options, device construct, patient selection and complications. J Cardiovasc Surg. 2009;50(4):447–60.
3. Safi HJ, Miller CC. Spinal cord protection in descending thoracic and thoracoabdominal aortic repair. Ann Thorac Surg. 1999;67:1937–9.
4. Verhoeven EL, Tielliu IF, Ferreira M, Zipfel B, Adam DJ. Thoracoabdominal aortic aneurysm branched repair.J. Cardiovasc Surg (Torino). 2010;51(2):149–55.

Hybrid Strategy on Aortic Arch Disease

Gabriel Lorente Mitsumoto, Henry Eiji Toma, Felipe Machado Silva, Luiz Antonio Rivetti, and Valquiria Pelisser Campagnucci

Clinical Presentation

A 77-year-old woman, born in São Paulo, was admitted in emergency department presenting intense chest pain for 15 days, radiating to the back associated with progressive shortness of breath, currently present even with minimum efforts.

Past medical history: systemic hypertension, chronic atrial fibrillation, class II obesity, and prior post-angiography pseudoaneurysm correction of the right femoral artery

The physical examination at admission was as follows. The patient was awake and alert, anxious, and afebrile, with no

G. L. Mitsumoto (✉) · H. E. Toma · F. M. Silva · V. P. Campagnucci
Santa Casa de Sao Paulo School of Medical Sciences (FCMSCSP)
São Paulo, SP, Brazil

L. A. Rivetti
Presidente do Instituto de Pesquisa e Inovação Tecnológica da
Santa Casa de São Paulo, São Paulo, SP, Brazil

R. M. S. Almeida, F. B. Jatene (eds.), *Cardiovascular Surgery*,
https://doi.org/10.1007/978-3-319-57084-6_7

Table 1 Pulse ratings

	Fe	**Po**	**aT**	**pT**
R	3+	3+	3+	2+
L	3+	3+	3+	2+
	Ax	**Br**	**Rd**	**Ul**
R	3+	3+	3+	3+
L	2+	2+	1+	1+

R right, *L* left, *Fe* femoral artery, *Po* popliteal artery, *aT* anterior tibial artery, *pT* posterior tibial artery, *Ax* axillary artery, *Br* brachial artery, *Rd* radial artery, *Ul* ulnar artery

signs of dehydration or cyanosis. The patient was in use of propranolol, substrate, furosemide, and alpha-methyldopa.

Vitals:

- Temperature: 36.6 °C (97.88 °F)
- Heart rate (HR): 92 bpm
- Respiratory rate: 16 bpm
- Blood pressure (BP): 110/80 symmetrical in upper and lower limbs both sides

Cardiovascular: Heart sounds with S1 and S2 with normal intensity, tachycardia, irregular rhythm, no murmurs. There was no hepatojugular reflux.

Pulse ratings at admittance (Table 1):

Respiratory: Breath sounds present and symmetrical, with no rales or wheezing and no signs of acute respiratory distress

Abdominal: Obese, normal bowel sounds, soft, no high-pitched or tinkling sounds, resonant to percussion, with pulsatile mass in mesogastric

Diagnosis, Assessment, and Treatment

Laboratory exams at admission are listed below (Table 2):

An ECG (Fig. 1a–d) was performed to assess heart's condition:

Table 2 Laboratory exams

Exams	Values
Hemoglobin	14 g/dL
Creatinine	0.8 mg/dL
Platelets	188,000 U/uL
Urea	28 mg/100 mL
Leukocyte	4700 U/uL
Neutrophils	67.4%
Segmented	67.4%
Lymphocytes	19.6%
Monocytes	7.7%
Eosinophils	4.7%
Basophils	0.6%
Total cholesterol	234 mg/dL
HDL	37 mg/dL
LDL	126 mg/dL
Triglyceride	354 mg/dL
Prothrombin activity (PA)	85%
INR	1.11
Activated partial thromboplastin time (APTT)	38.9 s
RT	1.34
High-sensitivity troponin	4.05 pg/mL

After the laboratory tests, ECG presenting atrial fibrillation and chest X-ray (Fig. 2) presenting an enlarged mediastinum suggesting an aorta enlargement, the main diagnostic hypothesis was acute aortic syndrome, and then it was decided to optimize antihypertensives especially beta blocker and analgesia. A computed tomography (CT) scan with reconstruction was also requested (Fig. 3a–c) to assess the aorta (Fig. 4a, b).

The 3D reconstruction of contrasted CT presented an aortic arch aneurysm and important tortuosity of descending aorta.

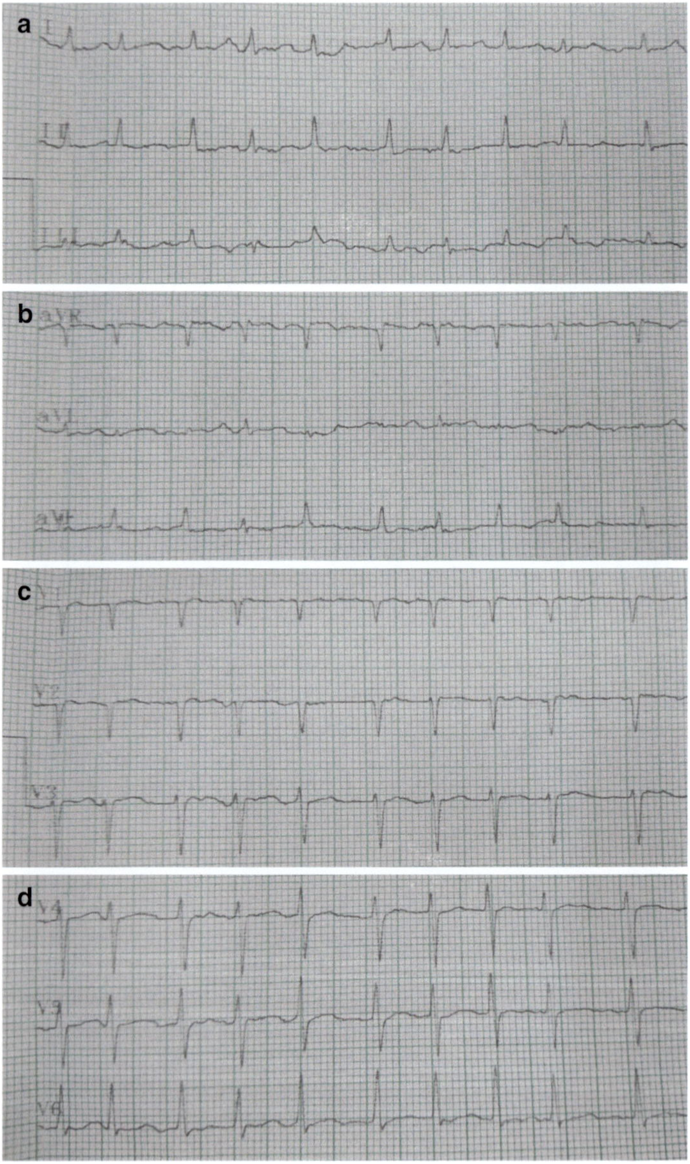

FIGURE 1 (**a–d**) ECG

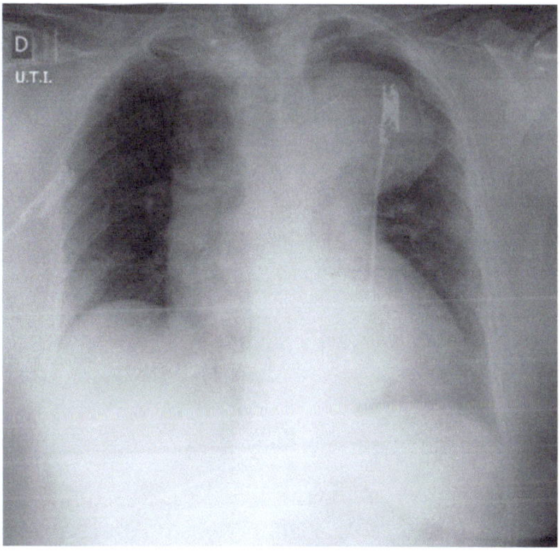

FIGURE 2 Chest X-ray

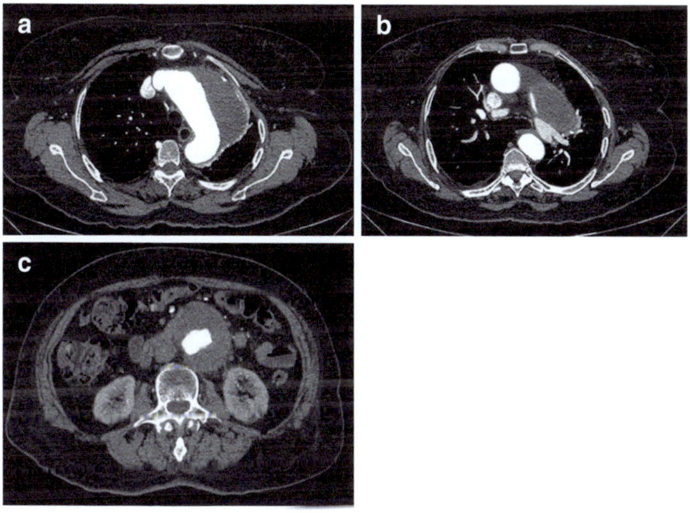

FIGURE 3 (**a**) Contrasted chest CT showing an enlarged aortic arch with mural thrombus. (**b**) Contrasted chest CT showing non-enlarged ascending aorta. (**c**) Abdominal contrasted CT showing an abdominal aortic aneurysm with mural thrombus

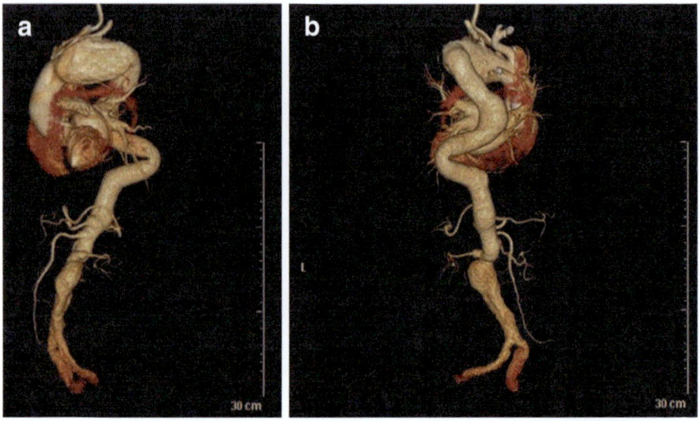

Figure 4 (**a**, **b**) 3D reconstruction of contrasted CT presenting an enlarged aortic arch and important tortuosity of descending aorta

Progression

The patient was stable and asymptomatic until surgery, being opted to pursue preoperative evaluation. She underwent an echocardiogram that showed anterior hypokinesia, 58% LVEF, and mild or moderate mitral regurgitation with no signs of pulmonary hypertension, not being possible to visualize the aortic arch.

The patient's EuroSCORE II was calculated: 6.49% (relative to the aortic arch surgery).

To evaluate the patient for coronary artery disease, a cardiac coronary arteriography was performed and showed diffuse parietal irregularities (Figs. 5 and 6).

The cardiac surgery determined the need for a surgical approach. Thus, a carotid Doppler ultrasound was performed revealing only small calcified plaque at the left carotid bulb without significant hemodynamic repercussions.

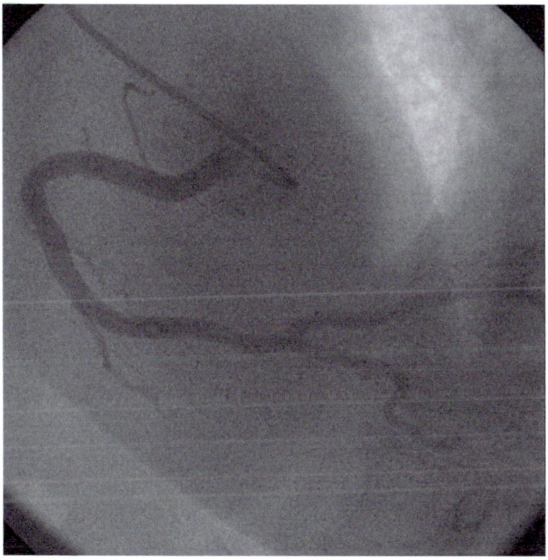

FIGURE 5 Right coronary artery showing the absence of stenotic lesions

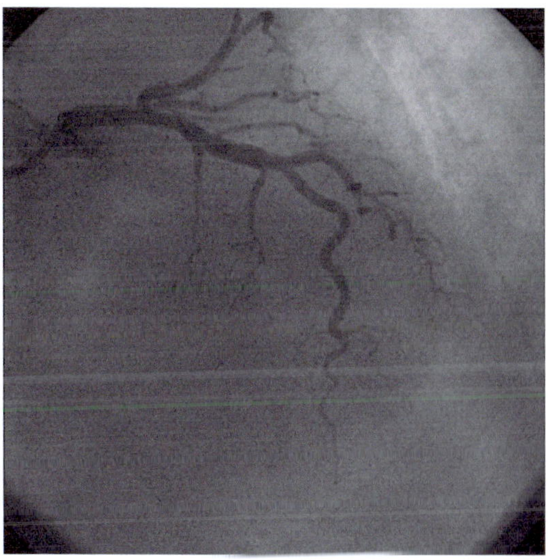

FIGURE 6 Main left coronary trunk and branches with no significant lesions

Surgery

Ascending aortic bypass was performed with a bifurcated tube for innominate artery and left carotid artery. The ascending aorta was partially clamped with an end-to-lateral anastomosis of the bifurcated prosthesis, followed by an end-to-lateral anastomosis of the bifurcated grafts to the innominate artery and the left main carotid artery, which were also partially clamped.

The patient had a good clinical-surgical evolution, was extubated in the immediate postoperative period and received norepinephrine for 24 h and dobutamine for 4 days as well as amiodarone EV and metoprolol for HR control. She was discharged from the ICU to the infirmary on the fifth postoperative day, where she waited for an endovascular procedure of the aortic arch aneurysm. Twenty days after the surgery, endovascular stent implantation beginning at the ascending, aorta until the descending thoracic aorta was performed.

The patient was then discharged from hospital 48 h after implantation of the endoprosthesis. The procedure is showed below (Fig. 7a–d).

Six months later, the patient performed a new aortic angiotomography (Fig. 8a, b), which can be seen below. Also, the patient had upper left arm compensated.

Questions

1. What are the life-threatening differential diagnoses of chest pain?

The life-threatening differential diagnoses of chest pain are an acute aortic syndrome, acute coronary syndrome, pneumonia, myocarditis, pulmonary thromboembolism, pericarditis, pneumothorax, and esophageal rupture.

2. What is the exam considered as the gold standard for diagnosis and to perform surgical strategic planning for cardiac surgeries?

The exam considered the gold standard is CT aortic angiotomography.

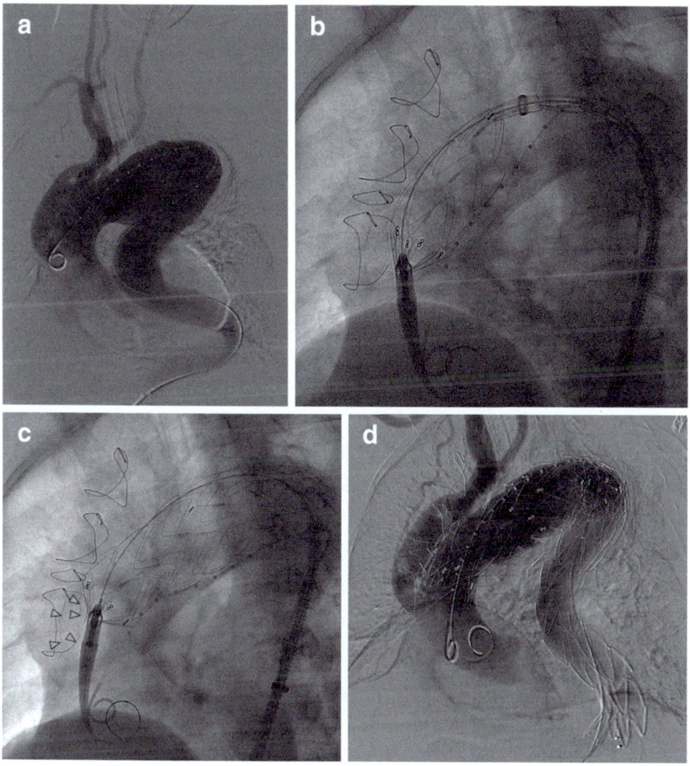

FIGURE 7 (**a**) Aortography showing aortic arch aneurism and supra-aortic branch bypass with good flow. (**b**) Chest X-ray of the endovascular procedure showing the deployment of the ascending aortic endoprosthesis with a closed free-flow tip (in order to avoid graft migration) just after the metallic clips (indicated by arrows' head in **c**) sutured around the ascending aortic graft. (**c**) Chest X-ray of the endovascular procedure showing the deployment of the ascending aortic endoprosthesis with a closed free-flow tip (in order to avoid graft migration) just after the metallic clips (indicated by arrows' head in the figure) sutured around the ascending aortic graft. (**d**) Final aspect of the endovascular procedure with contrast showing no endoleaks and good flow of the bifurcated graft

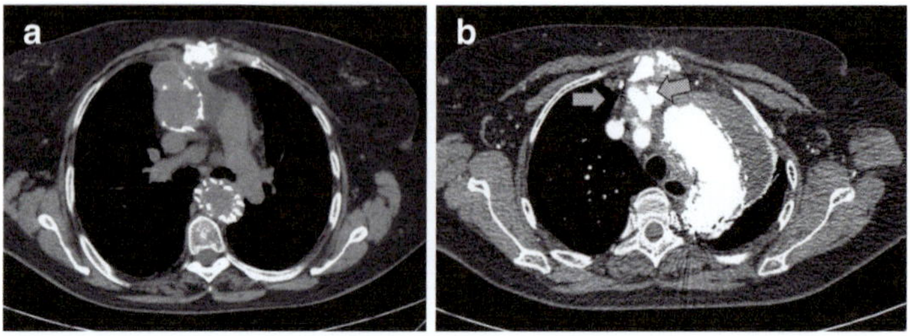

FIGURE 8 (**a**) Chest CT without contrast showing endoprosthesis in ascending and descending aorta as well as proximal origin of the bifurcated graft. (**b**) Contrasted chest CT showing both branches of the bifurcated graft anterior to the aorta (arrows)

3. What are the five groups of etiologies of aortic dissection and give some examples? Which of them is responsible for most cases?

The five groups and some examples are listed below:

- Arterial hypertension
- Inherited fibrillinopathies
  - Annuloaortic ectasia
  - Marfan syndrome (MFS)
  - Ehlers-Danlos syndrome (EDS)
- Hereditary vasculopathies
  - Aortic isthmus stenosis
  - Bicuspid aortic valve
- Inflammatory vascular diseases
  - Giant-cell arteritis
  - Takayasu arteritis
  - Rheumatic aortitis
  - Systemic lupus erythematosus
  - Behçet's disease
  - Syphilis
  - Mycotic aortitis
  - Ormond's disease (retroperitoneal fibrosis)
- Iatrogenic
  - Catheter procedures
  - Aortic/aortic valve surgery

- Vascular clamp
- Aortotomy
- Graft anastomosis

Among the acquired causes, arterial hypertension plays a leading role, accounting for 76.6% of the cases.

4. What is the typical clinical presentation for acute aortic dissection?

The typical clinical presentation is the presence of severe anterior chest pain in over 90% of patients, and most often there is a dorsal thoracic pain in approximately 70% of patients.

5. Describe the DeBakey classification of aortic dissection

There are three main types are as follows: types I and II which affect the ascending aorta and type III, distal dissection, which begins distal to the left subclavian artery, sparing the proximal arch and ascending aorta. DeBakey further distinguished type III dissection in types IIIa (down to or ending above the visceral segment) and IIIb (extending downward to involve the abdominal aorta and iliac arteries).

6. Describe the Stanford classification of aortic dissection and the purpose of the system

The Stanford classification divides dissections into two types: type A, which signifies involvement of the ascending aorta, and type B, in which the ascending aorta is not affected.

This system helps to delineate treatment. Usually, type A dissections require surgery, once the aortic valve is often involved, while type B dissections may be managed medically under most conditions and surgery reserved for any complications.

7. What diseases does acute aortic syndrome include?

Acute aortic syndrome is a condition that includes acute aortic dissection, intramural hematoma, aortic ulcer, and aortic trauma.

8. What is the hybrid strategy?

The hybrid strategy is a combination of tools available only in the catheterization laboratory (where the interventional cardiologist is the expert) with those available only in the operating room (where the cardiac surgeon is the expert) in order to gain maximum profit from both of them.

Review About the Addressed Disease or Treatment

This patient had a chest pain radiating to the back, and the diagnoses to be weighed are the differential diagnoses of chest pain: acute aortic syndrome, acute coronary syndrome, pneumonia, pulmonary thromboembolism, and esophageal rupture are some examples.

The acute aortic syndrome is a condition that includes acute aortic dissection, intramural hematoma, aortic ulcer, and aortic trauma.

Since there were no ECG signs of myocardial ischemia and cardiac enzymes also showed no signs of myocardial infarction, the most likely diagnosis is an acute aortic syndrome.

It is known that especially aortic dissection, for which there is a fairly consistent database called the International Registry of Acute Aortic Dissection, occurs more often in men and the average age is 61.5 (±14.6). The presence of severe anterior chest pain occurs in over 90% of patients with ascending aortic dissection (Stanford A) and in descending aortic dissection (Stanford B). Most often there is a dorsal thoracic pain in approximately 70% of patients. Hypertension is one of the associated or causal factors most often associated, being present in 76.6% of patients.

Regarding the complementary tests, chest X-ray is a quick examination, and mediastinal widening sign was present in 52% and 39% of X-rays in cases of aortic dissection in types A and B, respectively.

The ECG performed initially is a low sensitivity test for aortic dissection type A and B as it is normal in 30–47% of cases.

Besides ECG, an echocardiogram is often an examination of fast acquisition and easy availability especially in reference hospitals for the treatment of aortic dissections and is used as initial investigation exam of type B dissections in 11–16% and in type A in 23–49%. This happens because the exam considered the gold standard for diagnosis and to perform surgical strategic planning is CT aortic angiotomography.

CT has been indicated as the initial investigation in dissection of types A and B in 72.9% and 78.1%, respectively.

When the patient is stable, with improvement in symptoms, and dissection is not acute but, as in the case above, has passed more than 14 days, in other words chronic, further investigation should be conducted as completely as possible since performed with safety.

Still observing ECG, it was compatible with the patient's medical history; atrial fibrillation was observed where P waves were absent and RR intervals were irregular with the narrow QRS complex.

The images obtained by aortic angiotomography showed a significant aortic arch dilatation, in a way that is hard to define if there is dissection image with thrombus in the false lumen or just an aneurysm with mural thrombus. The aneurysm measured 7 centimeters in its largest diameter. A dissection of the abdominal aorta was also visualized which was considered an incidental finding since she was asymptomatic to this disease; hence this condition would be treated in the second moment.

Regarding the clinical treatment of acute aortic syndrome, some priority measures should be taken: pain control with powerful analgesics (parenteral opioids), heart rate and inotropic control with the use of beta-blockers, and strictly blood pressure control respecting a gradual decrease in patients with very high blood pressure. For the last one, parenteral vasodilators are usually used such as nitroprusside and nitroglycerin.

Other drugs are important in the clinical treatment of this patient, such as statins, once the patient had hypercholesterolemia and aortopathy; ASA may be indicated in this patient, but if you choose chronically by not doing anticoagulation for atrial fibrillation, such a definition should be taken based on the HAS-BLED indices and CHA_2DS_2-VASc scores, which will not be discussed in this chapter.

As mentioned above, the patient was stable and had passed the higher risk of death related to the first phase of the dissection of the ascending aorta (including arch), so it was opted to continue the diagnostic investigation. Whenever possible and if available, echocardiography should be performed for cardiac evaluation especially for the aortic valve and left ventricular contractility. The patient had segmental hypokinesia that is the reason why a coronary angiography was indicated despite the handling risks, which showed no significant coronary lesions.

After all diagnostic investigation, there was a high surgical risk patient with acute aortic syndrome progressing to chronic phase but with an "aneurysm/thrombosed dissection" arch, symptomatic of 7 cm in diameter; hence, the approach of the aorta was indicated.

It is known that clinical and surgical mortality of patients with aortic dissection gives special gravity to the disease, as can be seen below, according to the IRAD data related to hospital mortality.

This very IRAD registry brings positive results on the hybrid treatment and still poor results about the full endovascular treatment according to Table 3.

Thus, the patient having diseases that have worse prognosis and worse morbidity/mortality, it was chosen to undergo the hybrid treatment, being held through mini sternotomy to third intercostal space and inverted T and supra-aortic trunks debranching with bifurcated Dacron tube $16 \times 8 \times 8$ to the innominate artery and left carotid artery with ligature of these supra-aortic trunks in its origins. Due to technical difficulties, it was chosen not to realize bypass to the left subclavian artery during surgery.

Before hospital discharge, it was implanted a stent beginning at the ascending aorta, until the descending thoracic aorta, as seen in the images. The preparation by the previous debranching allowed the endoprosthesis landing zone to be the zero zone (Fig. 9).

Thoracic endovascular aortic repair (TEVAR) is a procedure that has currently been performed without previous aortic debranching with chimney technique.

So far there is no robust data in the literature to support the best treatment option for aortic arch disease whether

TABLE 3 Type A and type B management and mortality comparison

	Type A (n, 2952) management				Type B (n, 1476) management			
Category	Surgical	Medical	Endo	Hybrid	Surgical	Medical	Endo	Hybrid
n	2552 (86.4)	329 (11.1)	34 (1.2)	36 (1.2)	192 (13.0)	923 (62.5)	341 (23.1)	21 (1.4)
In hospital mortality*	502 (19.7)	188 (57.1)	24 (70.6)	5 (13.9)	33 (17.2)	80 (8.7)	42 (12.3)	3 (14.3)
Total mortality ($p < 0.001$)	721 (24.4)				158 (10.7)			

Values are n (%). *$p < 0.001$ for type A mortality between management types; p – 0.003 for type B mortality between management types

Endo endovascular

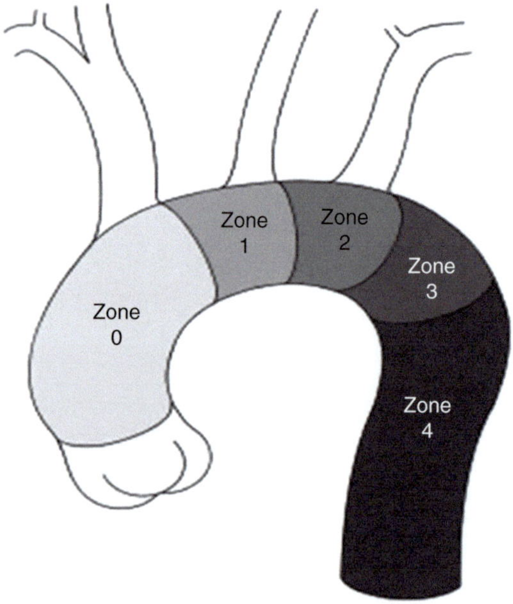

FIGURE 9 Zones of the aortic arch

totally endovascular, hybrid (debranching plus TEVAR), or open surgery. More long-term studies are needed for this to be set, but the reports so far suggest a tendency to percutaneous approach, whether hybrid or not.

Paola reported a study with 104 patients submitted to aortic arch debranching technique, obtaining satisfactory results. The 30-day death, stroke, and spinal ischemia rates were 5.7%, 3.8%, and 2.9%, respectively. There were, however, four retrograde dissections, two of which were fatal. At 1, 3, and 5 years, the survival rates were 89%, 83%, and 71%, and freedom from endoleak was 96%, 93%, and 88%.

The analysis of endovascular treatments should be evaluated not only by perioperative mortality and complications but also by long-term supra-aortic branch patency, endoleak rates, reinterventions, and changes in aneurysm diameter.

A review of the chimney procedure (or the snorkel technique) in supra-aortic branches identified 18 reports comprising 124 patients and 136 chimneys. The investigators reported a high primary success rate of more than 99%, with a mortality rate of 4.8% and a stroke rate of 4.5 %. A large number of different bare or covered stents were used. However, the overall endoleak rate was 18.5%.

The chimney technique in arch aneurysms remains untested and should not be used as an acceptable treatment other than for salvage.

There are branched prostheses for the aortic arch in the development and going through tests, and although the results are still not satisfactory, it is possible that this technique overcomes the chimney technique.

Bibliography

1. Criado F, Coselli J. Aortic dissection. Texas Heart Inst J. 2011;38(6):694–700.
2. De Rango P, Cao P, Ferrer C, Simonte G, Coscarella C, Cieri E, Pogany G, Verzini F. Aortic arch debranching and thoracic endovascular repair. J Vasc Surg. 2014;59(1):107–14.
3. Kirchhof P, Benussi S, Kotecha D, Ahlsson A, Atar D, Casadei B, Castella M, Diener H, Heidbuchel H, Hendriks J, Hindricks G, Manolis A, Oldgren J, Popescu B, Schotten U, Van Putte B, Vardas P. 2016 ESC guidelines for the management of atrial fibrillation developed in collaboration with EACTS. Eur J Cardiothorac Surg. 2016;50(5):e1–e88.
4. Kouchoukos N, Kirklin J. Kirklin/Barratt-Boyes cardiac surgery. Philadelphia: Elsevier/Saunders; 2013.
5. Moulakakis K, Mylonas S, Avgerinos E, Papapetrou A, Kakisis J, Brountzos E, Liapis C. The chimney graft technique for preserving visceral vessels during endovascular treatment of aortic pathologies. J Vasc Surg. 2012;55(5):1497–503.
6. Orr N, Minion D, Bobadilla J. Thoracoabdominal aortic aneurysm repair: current endovascular perspectives. Vasc Health Risk Manag. 2014;10:493–505.
7. Pape L, Awais M, Woznicki E. Presentation, diagnosis, and outcomes of acute aortic dissection: seventeen-year trends from the international registry of acute aortic dissection. J Vasc Surg. 2016;63(2):552–3.

Part II
Arrhythmias

Mitral Valve Disease and Atrial Fibrillation

Daniel Tomasi Keppen Sequeira de Almeida, Jéssica Nathiele Meotti, Mateus Fagundes, Evandro Luis Queiroz Flores, and Rui M. S. Almeida

Clinical Presentation

J.A.F.F.S, male, 28, brown, mason. History of dyspnea on efforts since 2003 that was never investigated during his teenage years. In 2014 he went to a local emergency care in his city, with complaints of pain in the epigastric region, dizziness, vomiting, and pain in the back of the neck. He was treated at the time with antibiotic therapy for *H. pylori*. In 2015, he went to a consultation at the health center and was evidenced systemic hypertension and systolic mitral murmur 4+/6+ and was referred to a cardiologist with prescription of Atenolol® and Furosemide®.

He was referred to a cardiologist, who diagnosed hypertension, and on a chest X-ray, a cardiomegaly has identified

D. T. K. S. Almeida (✉) · J. N. Meotti
M. Fagundes · E. L. Q. Flores
Assis Gurgacz Foundation University (FAG), Cascavel, PR, Brazil

R. M. S. Almeida
Department of Cardiology and Cardiovascular Surgery, University Center Assis Gurgacz Foundation, Cascavel, PR, Brazil

R. M. S. Almeida, F. B. Jatene (eds.), *Cardiovascular Surgery*,
https://doi.org/10.1007/978-3-319-57084-6_8

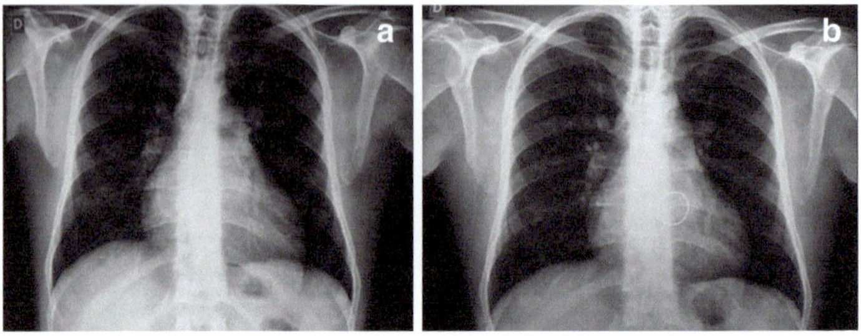

Figure 1 (**a**) Preoperatively chest X-ray exam evidencing cardiomegaly and pulmonary artery dilation. (**b**) Postoperative chest X-ray exam evidencing the presence of mechanic mitral valve prosthesis and reducing of pulmonary artery dilation

(Fig. 1). It was also performed an upper abdominal ultrasound that showed no abnormalities. An echocardiographic study was conducted, which concluded irregular heart rhythm, mitral valve insufficiency with signs of fibrosis and fusion of the commissures, and other atrioventricular and semilunar valves with no structural abnormalities. Normal wall thickness of the left ventricle. Marked severe dilation of the left atrium and moderate dilation on the left ventricle. Other cavity dimensions were normal as well as the ascending aorta. Segmental contractility with diffuse hypokinesia. Moderate systolic dysfunction of the left ventricle (Fig. 2). Doppler: signs of moderate to severe reflux for left atrium and discreet for right atrium. Concluding, a double mitral lesion, moderate pulmonary hypertension, moderate systolic dysfunction of the left ventricle (LV), and mild tricuspid insufficiency. In view of electrocardiogram study, an atrial fibrillation rhythm (AF) was confirmed.

Diagnosis, Assessment, and Treatment

The patient was then referred to the cardiac surgeon who, after analyzing the exams, carried out previously indicated surgical treatment. He was admitted to the hospital for surgery the next day. Atenolol® and Furosemide® medications

Measures	Pre-surgery	Post-surgery
Leftatrium (mm)	72	51
Aorticdiameter (mm)	29	24
Rightventricle (mm)	26	18
Leftventricle {diastole} (mm)	71	64
Leftventricle {systole} (mm)	47	42
Septum - thickness (mm)	10	10
P. Post left ventricle (mm)	10	10
Ejectionfraction (%)	61	62

FIGURE 2 Comparative table of echocardiographic measures between pre-surgery and post-surgery

that were already in use were maintained, except Warfarin® that was suspended. Laboratory tests didn't show any abnormalities, although the electrocardiogram identified an AF pattern.

A surgical procedure of mitral valve replacement was performed. This procedure was performed through median sternotomy with pericardial opening, standard heparin dose given, and cardiopulmonary bypass established with a 32 °C hypothermia. Cardioplegia cannula was introduced with subsequent infusion of blood St. Thomas cardioplegic solution, after aortic cross clamping. After that, there was the opening of the left atrium (LA) near the upper pulmonary vein and visualization of an insufficient, stenotic, and calcified mitral valve. It was decided to perform valve replacement with partial preservation of the sustaining apparatus; the prosthesis selected was a mechanical valve St. Jude® no. 31, fixed with separate points in the mitral annulus. In addition to performing mitral valve replacement, the left appendage was closed and a surgical ablation was performed with the Cardioblate® on the LA for correction of AF (Fig. 3). The LA was closed and the patient deaired and taken out of bypass. The heparin was reverted. A drain was placed in the anterior mediastinum. Then two pacemaker wires were positioned, one in the right ventricle and the other in the right atrial appendage. General

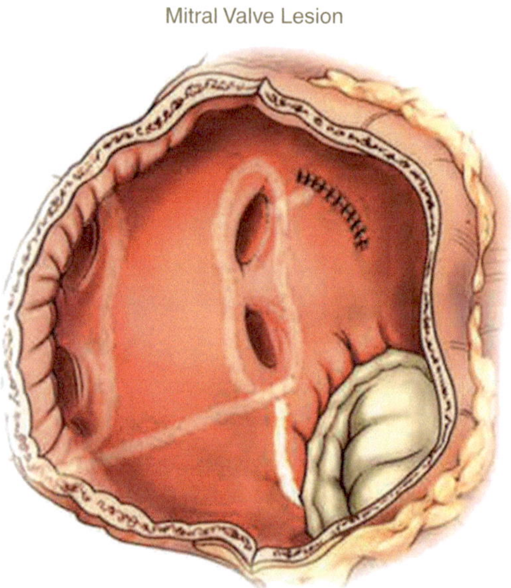

FIGURE 3 Ablation surgical technique to correct AF

review of hemostasis was performed and the pericardium was sutured. It was closed the sternum with steel wires and then the overlying plans. The heart rhythm was sinus.

Postoperatively the patient presented a good evolution, being the heart in sinus rhythm, confirmed by an electrocardiographic study. On the 30 day outpatient clinic consultation, the patient was in good general state, oriented in time and space. Cardiac auscultation: normophonetic rhythmic heart sounds in two times without murmurs. Pulmonary auscultation: vesicular murmurs present without adventitious sounds. In use of Warfarin®, Spironolactone®, and Atenolol®. It was carried out new control echocardiogram that showed mechanical prosthesis functioning normally, mild pulmonary hypertension, and increased left chambers (Fig. 1). Laboratory tests were normal with well-regulated anticoagulation. The X-ray showed decrease in pulmonary artery size (Fig. 2) and ECG showed sinus rhythm (Fig. 4).

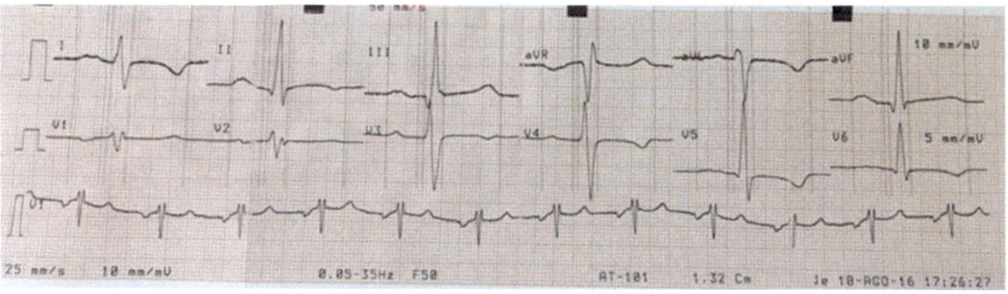

FIGURE 4 Post-surgery electrocardiogram evidencing the return of the sinus rhythm

Questions

1. What are the causes and conditions associated with atrial fibrillation (AF) in mitral valve disease?

AF associated with heart disease includes valvular heart disease (changes of the mitral valve is the most commonly found), coronary artery disease, and hypertension (particularly when associated with left ventricular hypertrophy). The AF may also be associated with hypertrophic cardiomyopathy, dilated cardiomyopathy, cardiomyopathy by deposition of glycogen, and congenital heart diseases. Potential etiologies include restrictive cardiomyopathies (amyloidosis, endomyocardial fibrosis, and hemochromatosis), cardiac tumors, and constrictive pericarditis as well. Other heart diseases such as mitral valve prolapse with or without associated regurgitation, mitral annular calcification, cor pulmonale, and idiopathic dilated right atrium have been associated with higher incidence of AF, as well as sleep apnea syndrome.

2. What are the objectives of catheter ablation in AF?

The surgical ablation, for the prevention of recurrence of AF, aims to eliminate triggers of the AF and modify the atrial substrate responsible for maintaining the arrhythmia, maintaining proper sinus rhythm, and controlling symptoms in these patients.

3. What are the recommendations for surgical treatment of AF?

Class I: patients with symptomatic AF that will be submitted for mitral valve surgery. Class IIB: surgery for exclusive treatment of AF in patients with symptomatic AF if the catheter ablation has failed or if it cannot be performed.

4. What is the main cause of mitral valve disease in Brazil?

Unlike most developed countries, the rheumatic fever is the main cause of valve disease in Brazil, responsible for 70% of cases. Studies conducted in the school population in some Brazilian cities have estimated the prevalence of rheumatic heart disease between 1 and 7 cases/1000, while in the USA, the prevalence is around 0.1 and 0.4 cases/1000 children. The most common rheumatic mitral valve disease is the double unbalanced dysfunction (insufficiency and stenosis at different stages of evolution) manifested between the second and fifth decades of life. Characteristically, mitral insufficiency (MI) is the acute injury, while the stenosis corresponds to the chronic injuries; however, it is possible that patients have varying degrees of stenosis and mitral insufficiency. In Brazil, mitral valve prolapse is the second cause of MI, the evolution of which is dependent on the intensity of the prolapse and has an average age of onset around 50 years.

5. What are the indications for surgical treatment in mitral stenosis?

As for the statement, this type of intervention is reserved for symptomatic patients (functional classes III–IV) with any of the following contraindications to balloon catheter mitral valvuloplasty (BCMV): unfavorable valve anatomy (Wilkins score greater than 8 associated with calcification and commitment of the subvalvular apparatus), presence of double mitral lesion with moderate to important insufficiency, concomitant tricuspid or aortic significant valve disease, and persistent left atrial thrombus (without resolution after adequate time for oral anticoagulation). Several world cardiological centers report good results with open commissurotomy. The average survival in 15 years is close to 96%, with free survival valvular complications around 92%. It is also possible the benefit of surgery in patients with moderate to important mitral stenosis in patients with embolic events despite adequate anticoagulation therapy and in those with functional class I to II, with severe pulmonary hypertension, without BCMV favorable anatomy. Patients with AF who will undergo valve surgery may benefit from concomitant surgical treatment of AF (as Maze surgery or radiofrequency ablation). The preservation of the mitral valve through surgical commissurotomy, although desirable, is not always feasible. The mortality related to valve replacement oscillates between 3% and 10%, being influenced by age, functional class, pulmonary hypertension, and the presence of concomitant coronary artery disease.

6. What are the levels of recommendation for echocardiography in mitral stenosis?

Regarding echocardiographic use recommendations: class I when used for diagnosis of MS with assessment of hemodynamic severity and evaluation of the size and function of the right ventricle; class I for the assessment of valve morphology to determine the suitability of percutaneous mitral valvotomy with balloon; class I when used for diagnosis and evaluation of concomitant lesions in the valves; class I when used for re-evaluation of patients with known MS and changed signs and symptoms; class IIa for the assessment of hemodynamic response of medium gradient and pulmonary arterial pressure, by Doppler echocardiography with stress, when there is discrepancy between hemodynamics at rest and clinical findings; class IIb when used in the re-evaluation of asymptomatic patients with moderate to severe MS to evaluate pulmonary arterial pressure; class III when used for routine revaluation of asymptomatic patients with mild MS and stable clinical findings.

7. What are the pharmacological treatment recommendations for mitral valve regurgitation (MR)?

Recommendation class I: intravenous vasodilator indication in acute MR, important and symptomatic, while awaiting surgical setting, having level B evidence.

Recommendation class I: Diuretics in severe chronic MR, symptomatic and with signs of congestion, while awaiting surgical setting. Having level C evidence

Recommendation class I: Oral vasodilators in severe chronic MR, symptomatic while awaiting surgical setting. Having level B evidence

Recommendation class IIa: Digitalis in control of ventricular rate in the high-response AF associated with severe chronic MR. Having level C evidence

Recommendation class IIb: Beta-blockers to control the ventricular rate in the high-response AF associated with severe chronic MR. Having level C evidence

Recommendation class IIb: Calcium channel blockers, nondihydropyridine for the control of ventricular rate in the high response AF associated with severe chronic MR. Having level C evidence

Recommendation class III: Vasodilators in chronic MR asymptomatic with normal ventricular function and in the absence of hypertension. Having level C evidence

8. How should anticoagulation be performed in patients with mechanical prosthesis?

It is generally agreed that the mechanical prostheses expose the patient to high risks of thromboembolism, regardless of heart rate. There is an estimated risk for thromboembolism of 12% per year for prosthesis in the aortic position and 22% in the mitral position, in the absence of oral anticoagulants. The patients with mechanical prosthesis, regardless of mitral/aortic implantation and heart rate, need antithrombotic prevention. For patients with implanted mechanical prosthesis in the mitral position, regardless of heart rate, prophylactic care against thromboembolism should be larger, recommending medium RNI of 3.0 (2.5–3.5). For patients with mechanical prosthesis in the presence of some risk factor for TE, as hypercoagulability blood, prior thromboembolism in the presence of adequate anticoagulation, or impaired ventricular function, it is recommended to add aspirin at a dose of 50–100 mg/day. The exceptions are people over 80 or those with a tendency to gastrointestinal bleeding.

9. What is the influence of pulmonary hypertension in patients with mitral valve injury?

Pulmonary hypertension is a common problem in heart valve diseases and worsens the prognosis of patients. In MS patients, severe pulmonary hypertension, defined as PASP ≥50 mmHg, is very common and can reach a prevalence of 40% and is the worst prognostic factor in these patients, leading to a median survival of 2.9 years in those who are not submitted to the surgical treatment. Early surgical mortality of MS patients without pulmonary hypertension ranges from 2.4% to 3.6%, while in patients with severe pulmonary hypertension may reach 10.5%. When pulmonary hypertension is suprasystemic, the surgical mortality approximates 30%. The survival in 5 and 10 years after surgical correction is approximately 80% and 65%, respectively. Right ventricular (RV) clinical dysfunction, RV hypertrophy and RV systolic pressure are considered independent predictors of operative mortality. The BCMV may be a safer alternative for the treatment of patients with MS and severe pulmonary hypertension. After the correction of MS (surgical or BCMV), immediate reduction in pulmonary hypertension levels occurs because of the decrease in LA pressure and reversal of pulmonary vasoconstriction in some patients. However, in patients with intrinsic changes of pulmonary arterioles (reactive pulmonary hypertension), the reduction of the pulmonary vascular resistance may occur over months, and, in most cases, it returns to normal blood pressure levels. In turn, in the patients with suprasystemic levels of pulmonary pressure, the residual pulmonary hypertension occurrence can reach 25%. Another cause of residual pulmonary hypertension is the presence of prosthesis-patient mismatch. In patients with mitral insufficiency (MI), the prevalence of severe pulmonary hypertension is approximately 25%. The pulmonary hypertension predictors are age, LA diameter, presence of AF, and CF III or IV. The presence of significant pulmonary hypertension increases the risk of overall mortality at six times and the risk of cardiovascular death, eightfold in patients kept under clinical treatment. The patients undergoing surgery who have pulmonary hypertension have twice the mortality at the end of 5 years compared to those with normal lung pressure.

Review About the Addressed Disease or Treatment

The mechanical valve prostheses have a low rate of structural failure, and with an appropriate anticoagulation, thromboembolic risk is similar to that observed with bioprosthesis without anticoagulation.

In this way, the mechanical prosthesis double brochure is a good option for a selected group of patients who are able to maintain appropriate control of anticoagulation, being indicated mainly in young adult patients, except for young women of childbearing age.

According to a study done by MARATIA et al. (1997, sp.), most of the patients operated for mitral lesion with chronic AF remain in AF, despite conventional therapy. Patients with mitral regurgitation and chronic AF associated with a LA diameter of less than 52 mm, had a better return rate to sinus rhythm after mitral valve surgery and concomitant surgical ablation.

We conclude that the present clinical case shows that even with a size greater than 52 mm, initially as the patient of this study, there is a possibility of returning to sinus rhythm when properly treated. The left atrium size of this patient was reduced from 72 mm to 51 mm, with a postoperative presenting good performance and sinus rhythm proven electrocardiographically.

Bibliography

1. Brandão CMA. Substituição valvar com próteses mecânicas de duplo folheto. 2000. Available at: http://www.scielo.br/pdf/%0D/rbccv/v15n3/3945.pdf (Accessed 28 Aug 2016).
2. Lorga FAM. Diretrizes Brasileiras de Antiagregantes Plaquetários e Anticoagulantes e Cardiologia. 2013. Available at: http://publicacoes.cardiol.br/consenso/2013/Diretriz_Antiagregantes_Anticoagulantes.pdf (Accessed 24 Aug 2016).
3. Maratia C.. Fatores preditivos de reversão a ritmo sinusal após intervenção na valva mitral em pacientes com fibrilação atrial crônica. 2016. Available at: http://www.scielo.br/scielo.php?script=sci_arttext&pid=S0102-76381997000100003 (accessed 28 Aug 2016).
4. Moreira HG. Complicações de ablação por cateter da fibrilação atrial: preditores e tendência temporal. 2009. Available at: http://cientifico.cardiol.br/cardiosource2/arritmias/int_artigo27.asp?cod=427 (Accessed 11 Aug 2016).

5. Pomerantzeff PM. "Diretrizes de Cirurgia nas Valvopatias. Arq Bras Cardiol. 82(suplemento V. 2004., Available at: http://www.scielo.br/pdf/%0D/abc/v82s5/19536.pdf (Accessed 17 Aug 2016).
6. Rodrigues AJ.. Substituição valvar isolada com próteses metálicas St. Jude Medical em posição aórtica ou mitral. Seguimento de médio prazo. 2009. Available at: http://www.scielo.br/scielo.php?script=sci_arttext&pid=S0066-782X2009000900014 (Accessed 28 Aug 2016).
7. Tarasoutchi F, Montera MW, Grinberg M, Barbosa MR, Piñeiro DJ, Sánchez CRM, Barbosa MM, Barbosa GV et al. Diretriz Brasileira de Valvopatias - SBC 2011 / I Diretriz Interamericana de Valvopatias - SIAC 2011. Arq Bras Cardiol. 2011; 97(5 Suppl 1): 1–67, available at: http://publicacoes.cardiol.br/consenso/2011/Diretriz%20Valvopatias%20-%202011.pdf (Accessed 11 Aug 2016).
8. Tarasoutchi F. Diretriz Brasileira de Valvopatias – SBC 2011/ I Diretriz Interamericana de Valvopatias - SIAC 2011. 2011. Available at: http://www.scielo.br/scielo.php?script=sci_arttext&pid=S0066-782X2011002000001 (Accessed 17 Aug 2016).
9. Zimerman LI, Fenelon G, Martinelli Filho M, Grupi C, Atié J, Lorga Filho A, e cols. Sociedade Brasileira de Cardiologia. Diretrizes Brasileiras de Fibrilação Atrial. Arq Bras Cardiol. 2009;92(6 Suppl 1):1–39, available at: http://publicacoes.cardiol.br/consenso/2009/diretriz_fa_92supl01.pdf. (Accessed 11 Aug 2016).

Late Arrhythmia After Fontan Repair

Anderson Berni Cristofari, Débora Cristina Haack Bassani, Letícia Lanzarin Gehm, and Basem Juma Abdalla Abdel Hamid

Clinical Presentation

The patient is an 18-year-old male patient, born in and a resident of Cachoeira do Sul, Rio Grande do Sul (RS), Brazil. The patient was born with the most prevalent cyanotic congenital heart defect and was submitted to surgical correction in a two-stage procedure. First, at 2 months old, the patient was submitted to pulmonary artery banding, and at 3 years old, the Fontan surgery was performed. Before the correction, echocardiography and computed tomography angiography (CT angiography) showed that superior and inferior vena cava anastomosed with pulmonary arteries and did not communicate with the atriums. Besides that, the pulmonary trunk was blind-ended, and there was a large interventricular and interatrial communication.

A. B. Cristofari (✉) · D. C. H. Bassani · L. L. Gehm
B. J. A. A. Hamid
Santa Cruz do Sul University (UNISC),
Santa Cruz do Sul, RS, Brazil

R. M. S. Almeida, F. B. Jatene (eds.), *Cardiovascular Surgery*,
https://doi.org/10.1007/978-3-319-57084-6_9

After the surgical procedures, the patient remained asymptomatic until 2014 when he sought medical care complaining of palpitations, malaise, and dyspnea, however without chest pain. During the physical exam, the patient presented diaphoresis and a rapid heart rate, approximately 160 beats per minute, and there was no cardiac souffle. An electrocardiogram was performed immediately, and continuous monitoring showed sustained tachycardia episodes in a row which required drug reversal in the emergency room several times.

Diagnosis, Assessment, and Treatment

After the results of echocardiography, CT angiography, and Holter monitoring, we chose to perform a therapeutic electrophysiological study with electroanatomic mapping system (Carto system), as shown in Fig. 1. Through the puncture of femoral vessels, catheters were positioned into the cardiac camaras, with a tridimensional reconstruction of the left atrium, right reminiscent atrium and pulmonary veins geometry. After the mapping, the arrhythmia was identified as shown in Fig. 2. The ablation of the arrhythmia was performed through sequential radio frequency, which succeeded to revert it (Fig. 3). After the procedure, the patient did not present anymore arrhythmic episodes, spending 20 months post-procedure without any symptoms.

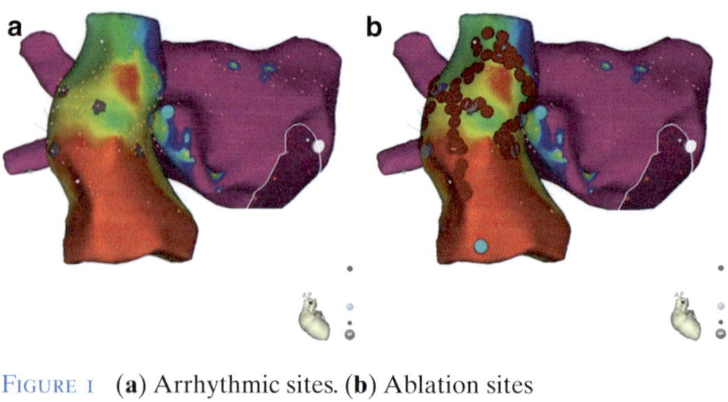

FIGURE 1 (**a**) Arrhythmic sites. (**b**) Ablation sites

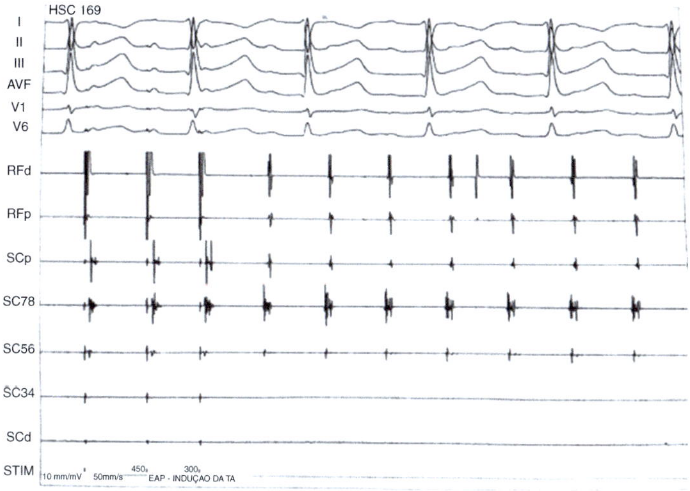

FIGURE 2 Tachycardia induction during electrophysiological study

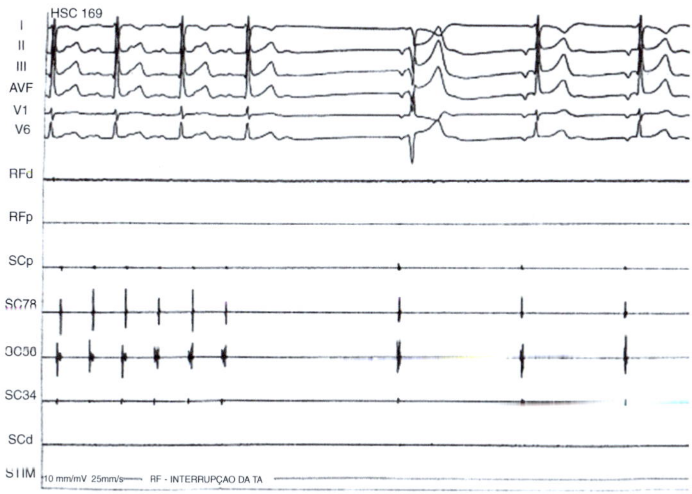

FIGURE 3 Arrhythmic event ablation

Questions

1. Which congenital heart disease did the patient have and what is its natural history?

Transposition of great vessels (TGV) is a congenital heart defect in which part of or the entire aorta arises from the right ventricle and part of or the entire pulmonary trunk arises from the left ventricle. This anomaly is known as ventriculoarterial discordance [6].

It is the most common cyanotic congenital heart disease, though with low prevalence (about 1%) among all the other congenital heart diseases [8].

TGV is widely known by its unfavorable natural history. If there is no blood mix between the two circulations, the condition becomes incompatible with life. Certain conditions allow a longer survival such as atrial communication and ventricular communication or great vessels (persistence of the ductus arteriosus) [4].

Among the patients who are not operated, 32% evolve to congestive heart failure and have 25% probability of death when they are close to the fourth decade of life. The specific surgical technique to correct it depends on an extensive variety of anatomical characteristics and the surgical team's experience [5].

2. Would the surgical procedure would be traditionally indicated for this heart defect?

Jatene's arterial repair is traditionally performed for TGV correction. In this procedure, the arterial switch and the coronary artery translocation to the neoaorta are performed. With the vessel's inversion, the coronary arteries anastomose to the vessel that arises from the left ventricle, receiving arterial blood. The surgery seeks to restore the normal heart anatomy and physiology and to establish ventriculoarterial concordance [4].

3. Why the traditional surgical procedure for this heart disease was not performed?

Fontan surgery was the preferred operation because the patient had only one ventricle (pulmonary trunk was blind-ended).

Fontan procedure, described first in 1971, is performed nowadays to approach univentricular hearts by making an atriopulmonary connection. It diverts the blood flow directly to the lungs, without passing through the right ventricle [7]. The two most frequently used ways to do this is through an extracardiac conduit or through hemi-Fontan procedure [6].

Hemi-Fontan surgery is similar to a cavopulmonary shunt, creating a superior vena cava and pulmonary artery connection. The difference is that it is used hypothermia and extracorporeal circulation during the procedure. Both can be used in TGV treatment, with considerable variations and adaptations depending on the service. Moreover, there are no clear indications regarding which is the best procedure to perform [6].

4. Which surgical procedure could be performed at 2 months old and what are its benefit?

Patients with univentricular hearts who are candidates to be submitted to Fontan surgery usually have to go through palliative procedures to avoid pulmonary hyperflux previous to the operation.

Pulmonary artery banding allows better and early pulmonary vascular disease control; thereby, Fontan surgery can be performed later [1].

5. Which are the main postoperative complications regarding the surgical procedures used to correct this heart disease?

In the last decades, sophisticated corrective procedures improved the quality of life and life expectancy of patients with congenital heart defects. Nevertheless, due to surgical procedure healing, the use of patches and suture lines, and consequent fibrosis, the development of arrhythmias is increasingly common in this population. Atrioventricular heart block is the main postoperative arrhythmia after cardiac surgeries, and insertion of a pacemaker is mandatory in 80% of cases [2].

Loss of sinus rhythm may be associated with complex etiologies. The development of arrhythmias does not depend on the type of Fontan procedure [6].

Arrhythmias are poorly tolerated after Fontan procedure due to limited cardiac reserve and low cardiac output [7]. Moreover, atrial muscle presents macroscopic and microscopic changes. Atrial wall thickening – and not fibrosis – would be responsible for the development of arrhythmias after the surgery [10]. Other known causes are suture lines, patches, and anatomic barriers.

Furthermore, patients who went through Fontan procedure have dilated right atriums, extensive low-voltage areas, and high prevalence of fractionated potentials compared to other groups who corrected TGV by other techniques. Those are the main characteristics associated with the recurrence of arrhythmias after the ablation [10].

6. Which arrhythmia (Fig. 2) did the patient present years after the procedure?

The patient presented sustained intra-atrial tachycardia episodes. Studies show that the frequency of arrhythmias in patients who are submitted to heart surgery can vary between 7% and 60%. In Fontan surgery the prevalence described is 42% of arrhythmic events, reaching a prevalence of 100% after 26 years.

A study that analyzed patients who were previously submitted to correction of congenital heart defects found 62 different types of atrial arrhythmia. The most common types of atrial arrhythmia are the typical atrial flutter; reentrant intra-atrial tachycardia involving sutures, scar tissue, and prosthetic materials; and focal atrial tachycardia [3].

Other references consider the terms "intra-atrial reentrant tachycardia" and "incisional tachycardia" as synonyms, to distinguish them from typical atrial flutter that occurs in structurally normal hearts. Generally, intra-atrial reentrant tachycardia tends to be slower than the typical flutter, with atrial rates in the range of 150–250 per minute [9].

Between these, the most prevalent is intra-atrial reentrant tachycardia (about 66%) [7]. Reentrant arrhythmia is the most prevalent, 34% being due to typical atrial flutter and 44% due to reentrant intra-atrial tachycardia [3].

7. What are the treatment options for postoperative arrhythmias developed after TGV correction?

Several therapies are suggested to treat arrhythmias in these cases such as reoperations, antiarrhythmic medications, and ablation of the electric circuit that provokes the arrhythmia.

Although it can still be prescribed in selected cases, pharmacological therapy has been discouraged, once the results are disappointing even when potent agents such as amiodarone are used [9].

Ablation has been considered the treatment of choice for arrhythmias [10] in patients with congenital heart defects and corrective surgeries. In patients with reentrant atrial tachycardia, ablation is successful in 70% of cases [3, 9].

If pharmacological measures and ablation fail to prevent new episodes, or if the patient is returning to the emergency room unstable, consideration should be given to morphologic heart surgery, known as atrial maze operation. Patients with the most refractory variety of intra-atrial reentrant tachycardia are usually the ones who need this procedure, which is often combined with a revision of the Fontan connection [9].

8. What is the importance of continued clinical follow-up of these patients?

The long-term following of the patients with TGV is extremely important due to substantially increased mortality in this group after developing an arrhythmia, about 50% compared to patients without arrhythmia [9].

The risk of postoperative arrhythmia is particularly high (nearly 40%) among Fontan patients, who tend to have the largest number of intra-atrial reentrant circuits and thicker and larger atriums.

Besides that, due to increased longevity and better quality of therapeutic procedures, it is possible that the number of patients with postoperative arrhythmias increases with time.

Review About the Addressed Disease or Treatment

Patients submitted to Fontan surgery can present significant late complications, for that reason, they must keep clinical following through life. Among the main complications, there are atrial arrhythmias (atrial flutter and paroxysmal atrial tachycardia), as cited before, with variable incidences depending on the study, from 0.4% to 13.9% per year. Thromboembolic events can also occur, such as vena cava or pulmonary artery thromboembolism [1, 6].

Other examples are systemic venous collateralization and protein-losing enteropathy. The first one is common in bidirectional Glenn, and the collaterals usually originate from the vena cava and hepatic veins. The second one occurs due to the increase in systemic venous pressure which causes lymphangiectasis, with the passage of albumin and protein into the gastrointestinal tract as a result. The diagnosis is made when there is ascites, edema of lower extremities, diarrhea, low serum albumin, and an increase in fecal alpha-1-antitrypsin. Some patients may need cardiac transplantation due to late complications related to left ventricular dysfunction after Fontan surgery [1, 6].

Bibliography

1. Croti UA, Mattos SS, Pinto VC Jr, Aiello VD. Cardiologia e Cirurgia Cardiovascular Pediátrica. 2nd ed. São Paulo: Ed Roca; 2008.
2. Daudt SN. Acompanhamento tardio das cardiopatias congênitas. Rev Soc Cardiol do RS. 2004;13(1):1–4.
3. De Groot NM, Zeppenfeld K, Wijffels MC, Chan WK, Blom NA, Van der Wall EE, Schalij MJ. Ablation of focal atrial arrhythmia in patients with congenital heart defects after surgery: role of circumscribed areas with heterogeneous conduction. Heart Rhythm. 2006;3(5):526–35.
4. Jatene MB, Jatene FB, Monteiro AC. Correção cirúrgica da transposição das grandes artérias: 30 anos de operação de Jatene. Rev Med (São Paulo). 2005;84(3–4):113–7.
5. Karl TR. The role of the Fontan operation in the treatment of congenitally corrected transposition of the great arteries. Ann Pediatr Cardio. 2011;4(2):103–10.
6. Kouchoukos TN, Blackstone EH, Hanley FL, Kirklin JK. Kirklin/Barratt-Boyes cardiac surgery, expert consult-online and print. 4th ed: Elsevier Health Sciences; 2012.
7. Quinton E, Nightingale P, Hudsmith L, Thorne S, Marshall H, Clift P, de Bono J. Prevalence of atrial tachyarrhythmia in adults after Fontan operation. Heart. 2015;101(20):1672–7.

8. Song MK, Bae EJ, Kwon BS, Kim GB, Noh C, Choi JY, Kim WH, Lee JR, Kim YJ. Intra-atrial reentrant tachycardia in adult patients after Fontan operation. Int J Cardiol. 2015;187:157–63.
9. Walsh EP, Cecchin F. Arrhythmias in adult patients with congenital heart disease. Circulation. 2007;115:534–45.
10. Yap SC, Harris L, Downar E, Nanthakumar K, Silversides CK, Chauhan VS. Evolving electroanatomic substrate and intra atrial reentrant tachycardia late after Fontan surgery. J Cardiovasc Electrophysiol. 2012;23(4):339–45.

Paroxysmal Atrial Fibrillation Due to Repeated Episodes of Severe Hypoglycemia in Patient with Type I Diabetes Mellitus

Letícia Oliveira and Edmo Atique Gabriel

Clinical Presentation

C.D.R.O, 55 years and 6 months, female, Brazilian, married, Catholic, born in Poloni-SP, covenant-health: Own. She was admitted to the emergency department with tachycardia and discomfort of sudden onset (3 h of symptoms), without hemodynamic instability, unrelieved factors, or injury. The patient reports that she was at home and chatting with her family when she noticed palpitations and trembling hands and was feeling unwell abruptly, referring to sense that the heart was "out of her mouth." The accompanying concerns have offered (30 min after the onset of symptoms) a glass of soda for the mother to drink, thinking it is another episode of hypoglycemia. Two months ago, due to NPH insulin resistance, her endocrinologist promoted a therapeutic adjustment, replacing NPH by glargine, a rapid-acting insulin. As a result of

L. Oliveira (✉) · E. A. Gabriel
Grandes Lagos Faculty (UNILAGO),
São José do Rio Preto, SP, Brazil

R. M. S. Almeida, F. B. Jatene (eds.), *Cardiovascular Surgery*,
https://doi.org/10.1007/978-3-319-57084-6_10

insulin adjustment, the patient in question has to present repeated episodes of severe hypoglycemia (including night, reaching 30 mg/dL detected in blood glucose test) sometimes with the presence of warning signs. The patient has type I diabetes mellitus for 50 years and high blood pressure for 20 years with severe distal sensory-motor peripheral neuropathy in upper and lower limbs (newly diagnosed) resulting from diabetes mellitus which is difficult to control and denies smoking, drinking, illicit drug use, acute myocardial infarction and previous stroke, and drug allergy regarding day vaccination. The patient has negative serology tests for HIV and hepatitis and no recent trips and denies previous similar frames, denies thyroid changes, and denies known cardiac pathologies.

In regular use: losartan, 50 mg/day (early); furosemide, 40 mg/day; metformin, 850 mg (2×/day – lunch/dinner); regular insulin, 30–30-30UI lunch/breakfast and dinner. Insulin prolonged action (glargine), 90UI by morning; amitriptyline, 75 mg/day; quetiapine, 50 mg/day; gabapentin, 300 mg (3×/day); thioctacid; diazepam, 10 mg (night); simvastatin, 40 mg

Vital signs at admission:

Blood pressure, 120 × 80 mmHg; heart rate, 160 beats for minute; respiratory rate, 22 breaths per minute; axillary temperature, 36.0 °C; Sat O_2 = 93%

Capillary blood glucose: 57 mg/dL

In the emergency room, an emergency electrocardiogram was performed (shown in Fig. 1).

Diagnosis, Assessment, and Treatment

Conduct: was established with attack dose amiodarone (300 mg) (in peripheral access). There was no reverse clinical condition. Correction of glucose was made with an infusion of dextrose and heparin was held for antithrombotic prophylaxis. The patient was referred to the hospital for amiodarone impregnation. Arrhythmia was reversed in 24 h.

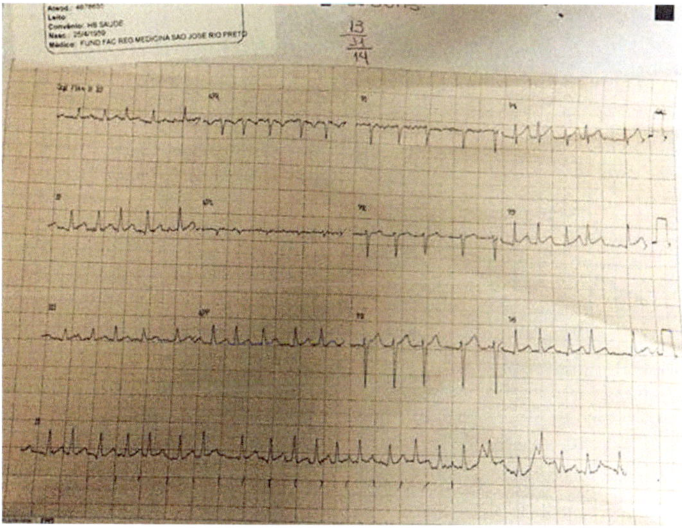

FIGURE 1 ECG performed on arrival compatible with atrial fibrillation with high ventricular response. Absence of electrocardiographic changes suggesting myocardial ischemia

The patient in good general condition was discharged and guided in searching for cardiologist for a clinical follow-up.

An echocardiography was performed with post-reversion of atrial fibrillation for investigation of cardiac structural alterations:

A patient with sinus rhythm presents the following results:

Diameter of aorta artery: 32 mm
Diameter left atrium: 41 mm
Diastolic diameter of the right ventricle: 18 mm
The thickness of the septum: 10 mm
Wall thickness: 10 mm
Diastolic diameter of the left ventricle: 48 mm
Systolic diameter of left ventricle: 28 mm
%D: 41.7
Left ventricular ejection fraction (LVEF) (Teich): 72.5%
Rel AO/LA: 0.78

Rel septum/wall: 1.00
Weight LV: 196.9 g
Rel. volume/weight: 0.52

Septum of the left ventricle (LV)	Wall of LV
Movement: normal	Movement: normal
Thickness: normal	Thickness: normal

Cavity of left ventricle	Segmental contraction
Size: normal	Movement: normal
Function: preserved	

Valves	
Mitral: normal aortic, normal tricuspid, normal	Pulmonary: normal

LA: mild elevation	RV: normal
RA: normal	Aorta: normal
Pericárdio: normal	

LV = left ventricle; LA = left atrium; RV = right ventricle; LV = left ventricle; AO = aorta;

Doppler

Mitral regurgitation flow, minimum ("valvar escape physiological")

Reviews

- Parietal thickness of the left ventricle of the ceilings of normal
- Contractile function of the normal
- LV of the global point of view left atrium volume = 61 mL
- Volume of the left atrium corrected by body surface area = 30 ml/m^2

Conclusion

Echocardiography is normal under the anatomical aspect.

The patient was discharged with guidelines to follow in outpatient follow-up and performed exams of Holter monitoring and echocardiography, without amendments. After 2 years of follow-up, the patient presented no new episodes of tachyarrhythmia.

Diagnostic hypothesis

Paroxysmal atrial fibrillation due to repeated episodes of severe hypoglycemia in patients with type I diabetes mellitus reverted after antiarrhythmic therapy and stabilization of blood glucose.

Questions

1. What are the risk factors for atrial fibrillation?

Atrial fibrillation (AF) occurs when electrophysiological abnormalities alter the atrial tissue and promote training/spread of abnormal electrical impulse. Many clinical risk factors are associated with increased risk of AF, and in addition to the classic factors like hypertension, diabetes, valvular heart disease, myocardial infarction, and heart failure, potential new factors may be mentioned.

Among them are obstructive sleep apnea, obesity, alcohol use, physical exercise, strenuous work, family history, and genetic factors. In this case, we report a patient who presented with paroxysmal atrial fibrillation caused by recurrent episodes of hypoglycemia in deriving an antidiabetic treatment rigorously.

2. What are the electrocardiographic criteria that define AF?

The electrocardiogram, the absence of atrial depolarization crime is reflected with the replacement of the P-waves, characteristics of the sinusal rhythm, by an earthquake of high frequency from the baseline of the electrocardiogram that varies in shape and size. This change is associated with a fast and erratic ventricular rate that occurs only in the presence of atrioventricular node integrity and without the action of drugs that impair their ability to drive.

3. What is the association between hypoglycemia and cardiac arrhythmias?

Hypoglycemia is a common event that typically occurs in diabetic patients. In this context, hypoglycemia usually results from an imbalance among diabetic therapy, level of activity, and dietary intake. Therefore, management of hypoglycemia has become "scripted": glucose administration, followed by adjustments in insulin or oral medications or diet. The mechanisms by which hypoglycemia induces such arrhythmias are unknown but may include the direct effect of hypoglycemia, hypokalemia, and increased secretion of noradrenaline on a possible background of specific myocardial disease and cardiac autonomic neuropathy. Hypoglycemia may be proarrhythmic via a number of mechanisms (see Figs. 2 and 3). The direct effect of low glucose on the human ether-a-go-go-related gene ion channel, hypokalemia, and catecholamine release prolongs cardiac repolarization, increasing the risk of early after depolarizations and ventricular arrhythmias. Since arrhythmias can be triggered by a transient change in sympa-

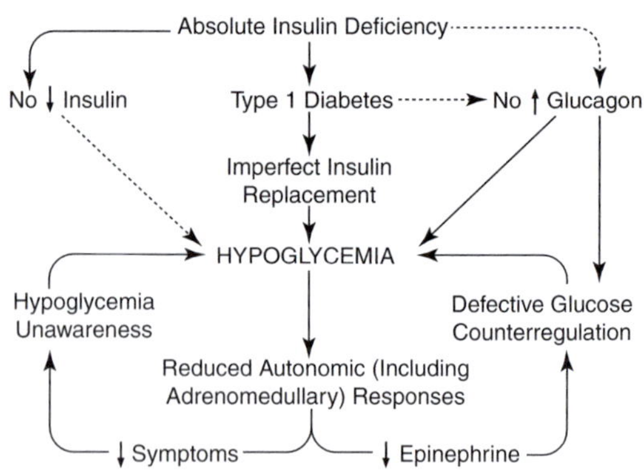

FIGURE 2 Diagrammatic representation of the concept of hypoglycemia-associated autonomic failure in diabetes

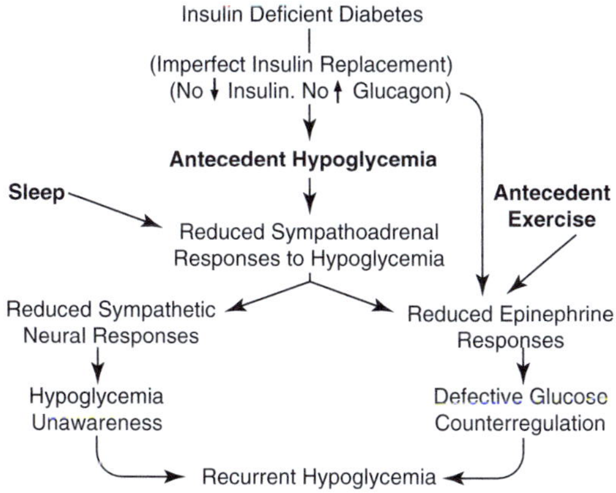

FIGURE 3 Hypoglycemia-associated autonomic failure in type I diabetes

thovagal balance, it also seems worthwhile exploring the effect of hypoglycemia on autonomic tone.

4. What other effects are printed by the hypoglycemia on the cardiovascular system?

Increased myocardial oxygen demand is causing a sympathetic surge, releasing counterregulatory hormones, such as epinephrine, norepinephrine, cortisol, glucagon, and growth hormone, which have immediate adverse cardiovascular effect by increasing afterload, inotropic, and chronotropic status of the myocardium. These adrenergic hormones also cause coronary vasoconstriction, impairing coronary blood flow and myocardial oxygen supply. In addition, hypoglycemia and coronary vasoconstriction limit the delivery of substrate (glucose and free fatty acids) to the myocardium, which further deteriorates the imbalance of myocardial energy supply and demand. Previous case reports regarding hypoglycemia-induced myocardial infarction mostly focused on ST-segment elevation myocardial infarction.

5. What the current recommendations for adequate glycemic control in patients with diabetes mellitus?

Intensive glycemic control during 3 and 5 years did not reduce cardiovascular mortality in recent trials, and the

Action to Control Cardiovascular Risk in Diabetes (ACCORD) trial was terminated early owing to increased mortality in patients with type II diabetes at high cardiovascular risk. It is well-known that intensive glycemic control increases the risk of hypoglycemia. This was strongly associated with an increased downstream risk of vascular events and death, but evidence of a direct causal link is lacking.

There have been sporadic case reports of supraventricular and ventricular arrhythmias associated with hypoglycemia. Among supraventricular arrhythmias, transient atrial fibrillation is most frequently reported.

6. On the hypoglycemia without alarm signals

The high prevalence of asymptomatic hypoglycemia is striking and probably reflects diminished counterregulatory responses associated with long disease duration and with nocturnal episodes where hypoglycemia occurred during sleep in a supine posture. Asymptomatic hypoglycemia can contribute to an excess of arrhythmic risk, and these episodes may be frequent and go unnoticed.

The hypoglycemia is a proarrhythmic condition with a risk higher than during euglycemia or hyperglycemia. The electrophysiological conditions during hypoglycemia could contribute to the initiation of ventricular tachyarrhythmias in a number of ways.

7. What prognosis of patients with atrial fibrillation (AF)?

In individuals over 65 years, mortality associated with AF is of 10.8% at 30 days after the diagnosis of arrhythmia, reaching 42% in 3 years of follow-up. Patients aged 65 years presented a relative risk of death of 4.88 for women and 3.07 for men in 1 year. The AF is a significant predictor of all-cause mortality in the presence of renal failure, cancer, and chronic obstructive pulmonary disease. Epidemiological studies show a clear association between AF and risk of stroke, ischemic or hemorrhagic stroke, and mortality. Cognitive changes, heart failure (HF), and socioeconomic implications are also important consequences of AF. In clinical studies involving patients with HF, the AF was considered an independent risk factor for mortality. Heart failure and atrial fibrillation coexist in a high percentage of patients (22–42%).

8. What would be the most appropriate management to reverse the AF in the patient described?

Previous cases reported of AF for hypoglycemia were promptly reverted with the intravenous infusion of glucose (dextrose), without which the administrations of antiarrhythmic drugs have been required. However, we observed failures with the management of sudden onset of atrial fibrillation, when sometimes hypoglycemia is ignored, even in patients without previous history of arrhythmias or heart diseases. The objective of the presented case is to guide professionals in an emergency, to trace hypoglycemia, and to promote immediate correction in order to avoid complications, reducing morbidity and mortality of these patients.

Bibliography

1. Celebi S, Celebi OO, Aydogdu S, Diker E. A peculiar medical cardioversion of atrial fibrillation with glucose infusion--a rare cause of atrial fibrillation: hypoglycemia. Am J Emerg Med. 2011;29:134.e1–3.
2. Khunti K, Davies M, Majeed A, Thorsted BL, Wolden ML, Paul SK. Hypoglycemia and risk of cardiovascular disease and all-cause mortality in insulin-treated people with type 1 and type 2 diabetes: a cohort study. Diabetes Care. 2015;38:316–22.
3. Hsueh YC, Lee WH, Huang YY, et al. Hypoglycemia-induced non-ST segment-elevation myocardial infarction: an unusual complication of diabetes mellitus. Acta Cardiol Sin. 2012;28:148–51.
4. Nordin C. The proarrhythmic effect of hypoglycemia: evidence for increased risk from ischemia and bradycardia. Acta Diabetol. 2014;51:5–14.
5. Mellbin LG, Rydén L, Riddle MC, et al.; ORIGIN Trial Investigators Does hypoglycaemia increase the risk of cardiovascular events? A report from the ORIGIN trial. Eur Heart J. 2013;34:3137–3144.

Part III
Cardiac Tumors

Cardiac Leiomyosarcoma

Matheus Duarte Pimentel, Caroline Cleophas Lobo Leite, Joely Nataly Silva, José Glauco Lobo Filho, and Heraldo Guedis Lobo Filho

Clinical Presentation

A 65-year-old man was admitted with mild weakness and dyspnea on exertion. The patient had no history of hypertension, type II diabetes mellitus, dyslipidemia, or any other medical or familial conditions. Physical examination revealed the presence of a diastolic murmur 2+/6+, most evident in the mitral area, radiating to the axillary region. No other abnormal signs were identified.

Diagnosis, Assessment, and Treatment

A transthoracic echocardiography (TTE) was requested to evaluate the diastolic murmur, and it revealed an increase of the left atrium diameter, with a tumor (3.7 × 3.4 cm) attached

M. D. Pimentel (✉) · C. C. L. Leite · J. N. Silva
J. G. Lobo Filho · H. G. Lobo Filho
Federal University of Ceará (UFC), Fortaleza, CE, Brazil

R. M. S. Almeida, F. B. Jatene (eds.), *Cardiovascular Surgery*,
https://doi.org/10.1007/978-3-319-57084-6_11

to the anterior leaflet of the mitral valve, with thickening of this structure, moderate mitral valve stenosis with an average diastolic gradient of 15 mmHg, and moderate valvular regurgitation. Left ventricular function was normal. A transesophageal echocardiography (TEE) was also requested, showing more details of the tumor connection to the mitral valve and to the lower portion of the interatrial septum, with an initial suspicion that it would be a cardiac myxoma (Fig. 1). Due to the size of the tumor and its adherence to important structures, cardiac magnetic resonance imaging (MRI) was requested to decide the best approach for treatment.

The findings previously described were confirmed in the cardiac MRI, and the tumor showed iso-signal intensity compared to the myocardium on the T1-weighted image, high signal intensity compared to the myocardium on the T2-weighted image, heterogeneous washout with late enhancement, and the presence of first-pass myocardial perfusion (Fig. 2).

2D Doppler echocardiogram revealed significant dilatation of the left atrium and presence of a rounded, large, and echogenic mass, with heterogeneous texture, measuring 4.0 × 3.6 cm in the left atrium. It was mobile and was oscillating into the mitral valve ostium during diastole, resulting in a moderate mitral stenosis.

Cardiac MRI also showed significant dilation of the left atrium, and presence of a mass located in the left atrium,

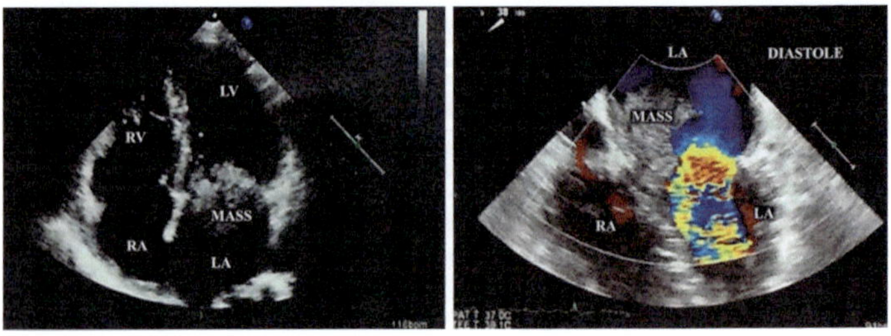

Figure 1 Transesophageal echocardiographic examination

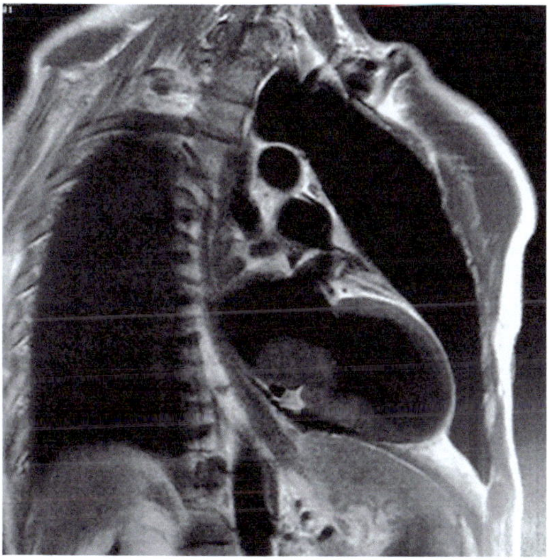

FIGURE 2 Aspect of the mass in the left atrium as seen in cardiac MRI

appended to the interatrial septum and adhered to the mitral valve, with restriction of the valve opening.

Considering the potential complications related to the presence of the left atrial tumor, although the patient was asymptomatic at diagnosis, surgery appeared to be the best therapeutic approach to managing the case.

The surgical procedure was performed through a median sternotomy, followed by installation and start of the cardiopulmonary bypass (CPB) circuit, and then proceeded to the aortic cross-clamp and infusion of blood cardioplegic solution. Left atriotomy was made, and the exposure of the interior of the atrial cavity revealed the presence of a large, smooth, broad-based mass, firmly attached to the anterior leaflet of the mitral valve and to the lower portion of the atrial septum, thereby restricting valve opening and causing septal strain.

In order to obtain complete resection of the mass, the mitral valve and the lower portion of the interatrial septum were resected with surgical margins (Fig. 3). It was proceeded then to

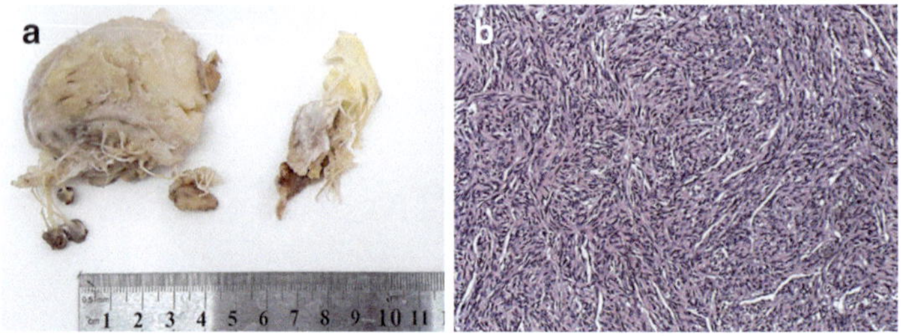

FIGURE 3 Macroscopic (**a**) and histological (**b**) aspects of surgically excised leiomyosarcoma

implantation of a biological mitral valve prosthesis and reconstruction of the interatrial septum with bovine pericardium. After closure of the atrial incision, release of the aortic clamping, removal of the CPB, and synthesis of the initial surgical incision, the patient was transferred to an intensive care unit (ICU).

The excised atrial tumor tissue was sent for histopathological analysis, which showed the presence of a pattern of fusiform cells, with moderate mitotic activity, hyperchromasia, polymorphism, moderate anaplasia, and mild necrosis, concluding the diagnosis of high-grade sarcoma. Immunohistochemical analysis showed high positivity for antibodies to smooth muscle actin, desmin, and calponin, specifying the diagnosis of a leiomyosarcoma (Fig. 3).

(a) Macroscopic appearance of a malignant tumor shows tawny nodular mass adhered to the mitral valve leaflets with apparent macroscopic invasion. (b) Histological appearance of the leiomyosarcoma shows neoplastic proliferation of spindle cells with moderate mitotic activity, arrangement in bundles interspersed with lush vascularization, and moderate rate of mitosis and focal areas of necrosis.

Postoperative echocardiogram showed no signs of the tumor in the left atrial cavity, and revealed presence of a normal functioning bioprosthetic mitral valve (Fig. 4). The patient had an uneventful recovery and was discharged on the 8th day of hospitalization, being actually in follow-up 1 month after surgery.

Bidimensional postoperative *echocardiogram illustrates the presence of biological prosthesis in mitral position. There are no signs of masses on the left atrium cavity.*

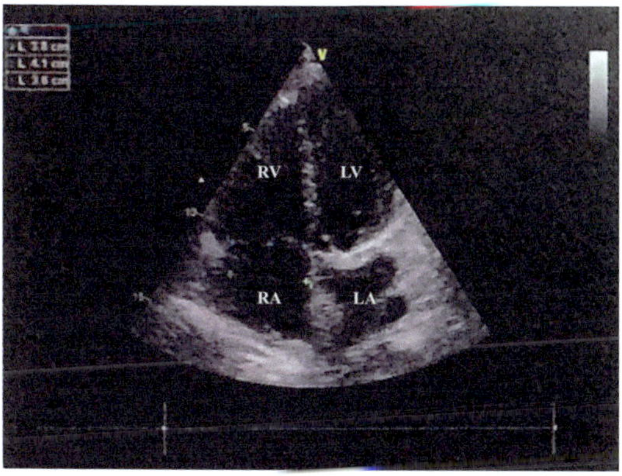

FIGURE 4 Postoperative *echocardiogram*

Questions

1. What is the incidence of cardiac tumors?

In general, primary cardiac tumors are a rare group of disorders, with data obtained from autopsy series showing its prevalence between 0.0017% and 0.03% of the subjects [1–3]. Reynen in 1996, reviewing 22 autopsy series, found the presence of 157 cardiac tumors, including benign and malignant, in 731,309 cases of autopsies illustrating an estimated prevalence of 200 tumors for every million of autopsies [1–7].

2. What is the classification of the cardiac tumors?

Cardiac tumors can initially be classified as primary or secondary. The primary group is constituted of those originating from the heart and the pericardium cells, while the secondary are those derived from other tissues that later migrate and proliferate in cardiac tissues. The primary cardiac tumors can also be classified as benign or malignant and according to their histological characteristics [3, 8, 9]

Benign primary cardiac tumors are a benign group of tumors that are confined exclusively to the heart at the time of their diagnosis. The primary malignant cardiac tumors are a group of tumors with insidious development until the appearance of signs of severity and may cause congestive heart failure in weeks [8, 9].

3. What are the most common types of primary benign cardiac tumors and of primary malignant cardiac tumors?

Among the different varieties of primary benign tumors, the main ones are myxoma, rhabdomyoma, papillary fibroelastoma, fibroma, lipoma, and hemangioma, among other variables of rare tumors. Cardiac myxoma deserves special mention for being the most prevalent among all cardiac tumors, accounting for almost 80% of all tumors surgically excised [3, 9].

The most common type of primary malignant cardiac tumor is the angiosarcoma, and other types include undifferentiated pleomorphic sarcoma, rhabdomyosarcoma, osteosarcoma, leiomyosarcoma, fibrosarcoma, and cardiac lymphomas [4, 8].

4. How tumors from other tissues spread to the heart?

Regarding secondary cardiac tumors, it is noteworthy that they are about 30 times more frequent than primary malignancies and spread to the heart via three routes, by lymphatic tissue, by direct extension, or through the blood, on this last situation, usually from the inferior vena cava or the pulmonary veins [3, 9].

Lung carcinomas and its metastasis are the main types of tumors that spread to the heart, followed by lymphomas, breast carcinomas, stomach carcinomas, and leukemias. Theoretically, sarcomas from any part of the body can spread through the blood to the heart [4].

5. How is the clinical presentation of cardiac tumors?

Cardiac tumors are neoplasms that, although uncommon, have considerable complexities in its diagnosis and management, clinical and surgical, because of the possibility to resemble other cardiac pathologies, presenting in very variable ways [2, 3, 5, 9].

In up to 12% of the cases, cardiac tumors do not show clinical symptoms, being diagnosed during a routine evaluation or during the diagnostic investigation of another condition. In general, the presentation of these tumors depends on factors such as location, size, involvement, or extension to adjacent structures, in addition to detecting the presence of metastases. In this context, chest pain, thromboembolic events, arrhythmias, syncope, hemoptysis, and congestive heart failure are possible to be diagnosed in patients with cardiac tumors. In rare cases, these neoplasms may also be associated with the presence of constitutional symptoms such as fever, weight loss, asthenia, leukocytosis or leukopenia, and hypergammaglobulinemia [2, 3, 5, 8, 9].

The pericardium is commonly affected by these tumors, which even can be primarily originated in this structure. Thus, the presence of pericardial effusion, cardiac tamponade, and pericarditis should always be investigated in clinical evaluation [2, 5].

6. How is the diagnostic approach in patients with cardiac tumors?

Since cardiac tumors are infrequent and may be present asymptomatically until they grow and/or sufficiently infiltrate the myocardial tissue to cause symptoms, a high degree of clinical suspicion for the diagnosis at an early stage is necessary. Given the low specificity of the clinical signs, complementary tests have a prominent role in the evaluation of patients presenting cardiac tumors [2, 3, 5, 8, 9].

The ECG may show heart rhythm disorders, with atrial fibrillation, present in 16% of patients with malignant cardiac tumors, and ventricular tachycardia, present in 7% of patients, emerging as the most common findings. Laboratory tests do not have great specificity but may show the presence of high levels of inflammatory markers [2, 3].

To increase the accuracy of diagnosis, imaging studies have an important role. Echocardiography, computed tomography, and cardiac MRI are those with greater sensitivity and specificity in the detection and differentiation of these lesions in early stages, allowing adequate surgical and therapeutic planning. Coronary angiography is usually required in patients over 40 years, especially in the presence of associated coronary artery disease [1, 2, 5].

Histopathological and immunohistochemical evaluation after tumor resection eventually confirm the classification of the tumor and help to assess the need for neoadjuvant therapies [2, 3].

7. What are the characteristics of the tumors with the classification of the one reported in this case?

Leiomyosarcomas are tumors that have a mesenchymal origin, presenting smooth muscle differentiation. These neoplasms have no gender preference, affecting individuals with a mean age of 40 years. They are a group of rare and aggressive tumors that account for about 10% of all cardiac sarcomas [2–4].

These sarcomas are located predominantly in the left atrium, often invading the mitral valve and the pulmonary veins, and in some cases, even the lung infundibulum can be stricken [2, 5, 8, 9]

Macroscopically the tumors usually have grayish, firm, and sessile aspect. Histologically, the presence of fusiform bundles with cores and blunt ends and areas of tumor necrosis and high mitotic activity are common findings [4, 6, 10].

In immunohistochemical analysis, leiomyosarcomas have strong positivity for the presence of smooth muscle actin, desmin, and vimentin [4, 6, 10].

8. What is the best therapeutic approach in cases like the one described above?

The treatment is not standardized, especially due to the rarity of these tumors and to the lack of specific guidelines; however, an approach which usually consists of surgical resection of the tumor is preferable for the possibility of improved prognosis and relief of the patient's symptoms. Complete resection of the tumor with adequate surgical margins, both laterally and in depth, is recommended, but in cases of very large tumors or with a high degree of infiltration, this approach is challenging [3, 4, 9].

The use of chemotherapy or adjuvant radiotherapy is shown as recommended and systemic therapy indicated in patients with advanced disease or evidence of tumor recurrence. Heart transplantation is not discarded in cases in which there is no evidence of distant metastases [2, 5, 8, 9].

Review About the Addressed Disease or Treatment

Columbus, in the sixteenth century, made the first description of a cardiac tumor. Centuries have passed, and, until Barnes diagnosed, for the first time, a primary cardiac sarcoma in 1934 and Crawford in 1954 performed surgical resection of a myxoma, almost all cardiac tumors were diagnosed only after the death of patients at autopsy. This was a reality that has changed only during the second half of the twentieth century due to the comprehensive development of echocardiography and important advances in cardiovascular surgery [3, 8, 9].

As previously reported, in this case, the clinical presentation of this neoplasm depended on factors such as location, size, extension, and involvement of adjacent structures. Because of the left atrial and mitral valve involvement, dyspnea and fatigue were presented as the main symptoms resulting from the presence of the leiomyosarcoma. If the diagnosis was not established early, increased systolic pulmonary artery pressure, atrial arrhythmias, and worsening of mitral stenosis as a result of growth and tumor infiltration could occur, leading to deterioration of cardiac function and worsening of patient's prognosis [1, 4, 6, 10].

Echocardiography is shown as the method of choice in the evaluation start, allowing evaluation of the size, shape, and location of the tumor consistency [1, 10]. In CT scans, it can be noted that leiomyosarcomas usually arise in the posterior wall of the left atrium, presenting as hypoattenuating irregular masses [1]. MRI can also be used for detection and tumor staging evaluation, usually depicting a mass isointense in T1 mode, and hyperintense on T2, especially after contrast application, findings consistent with the illustrated in the case [1].

Due to the aggressive nature of the tumor, with rapid invasion of adjacent structures, surgical resection is basically palliative, in order to alleviate the symptoms resulting from the clogging of valves or blood vessels of great importance, and most patients have died less than 1 year after the onset of symptoms [3, 8, 9].

Chemotherapy and radiation therapy in adjuvant character associated with extensive surgical resection and subsequent neoadjuvant chemotherapy could promote improvement of long-term prognosis of this patient that actually is in oncological monitoring [4, 6, 10].

Bibliography

1. Araoz PA, Eklund HE, Welch TJ, Breen JF. CT and MR imaging of primary cardiac malignancies 1. Radiographics. 1999;19(6):1421–34.
2. Burazor I, Aviel-Ronen S, Imazio M, Markel G, Grossman Y, Yosepovich A, Adler Y. Primary malignancies of the heart and pericardium. Clin Cardiol. 2014;37(9):582–8.
3. Butany J, Nair V, Naseemuddin A, Nair GM, Catton C, Yau T. Cardiac tumours: diagnosis and management. Lancet Oncol. 2005;6(4):219–28.
4. Maraj S, Pressman GS, Figueredo VM. Primary cardiac tumors. Int J Cardiol. 2009;133(2):152–6.
5. Orlandi A, et al. Cardiac sarcomas: an update. J Thorac Oncol. 2010;5(9):1483–9.
6. Pessotto R, Silvestre G, Luciani GB, Anselmi M, Pasini F, Santini F, Mazzucco A. Primary cardiac leiomyosarcoma: seven-year survival with combined surgical and adjuvant therapy. Int J Cardiol. 1997;60(1):91–4.
7. Reynen K. Frequency of primary tumors of the heart. Am J Cardiol. 1996;77(1):107.
8. Shanmugam G. Primary cardiac sarcoma. Eur J Cardiothorac Surg. 2006;29(6):925–32.
9. Shapiro LM. Cardiac tumours: diagnosis and management. Heart. 2001;85(2):218–22.
10. Wang JG, Cui L, Jiang T, Li YJ, Wei ZM. Primary cardiac leiomyosarcoma: an analysis of clinical characteristics and outcome patterns. Asian Cardiovasc Thorac Ann. 2015;23(5):623–30.

Part IV
Coronary Insufficiency

Intra-aortic Balloon Pump in Acute Myocardial Infarction and Ischemic Mitral Insufficiency

Luciana Baltazar da Silveira de Araujo, Maria Tereza de Magalhães Andrade, Thainá de Lima Quinteiro, Roque Aras Júnior, and André Maurício Souza Fernandes

Clinical Presentation

A 71-year-old woman was referred for a cardiologic evaluation, with a report of chest pain in the last 24 h. The chest pain started at dawn and was characterized as burning, radiating to the jaw and back, associated with diaphoresis and nausea. The patient sought the emergency unit at 10 am of the same day, and she was hemodynamically stable, breathing spontaneously in a comfortable pattern, referring nausea. She vomited while in the emergency room. Her medical history was positive for arterial hypertension, type 2 diabetes mellitus, and dyslipidemia. She was a smoker for 30 years, and she had also obesity class II (BMI 37.4). She was also sedentary. Her family history was not reported. She didn't have any abnormalities at physical exam.

L. B. da Silveira de Araujo (✉) · M. T. de Magalhães Andrade
T. de Lima Quinteiro · R. A. Júnior · A. M. S. Fernandes
Federal University of Bahia (UFBA), Salvador, BA, Brazil

R. M. S. Almeida, F. B. Jatene (eds.), *Cardiovascular Surgery*,
https://doi.org/10.1007/978-3-319-57084-6_12

Diagnosis, Assessment, and Treatment

At the emergency unit, electrocardiography (ECG) showed ST elevation in inferior and anterior walls (Fig. 1). Therefore, acute coronary syndrome (ACS) protocol was initiated and transfer requested, with no report of thrombolysis. In addition, the patient had attended an emergency unit with similar painful episode 5 days prior, when ECG was performed, but the patient was discharged. An ECG analysis showed an ST elevation in D2, D3 (D3 > D2), aVF, V5, V6, V7, V8, V3R, and V4R, compatible with right coronary injury with impairment of the right and left ventricles' posterior wall. Then she was referred to the emergency hemodynamics service.

A coronarography was performed at about 11:30 AM, which showed an occlusion of the middle segment of right coronary artery (RCA) with thrombus image, an occluded circumflex artery, and anterior descending artery (ADA) with middle segment lesion 50–75% and 90% average distal lesion. It was prescribed anticoagulation for 7 days, after which another coronarography would be performed, in order to evaluate the possibility of percutaneous transluminal angioplasty of the RCA. At about 9:30 PM, patient started fast clinical deterioration, with hemodynamic instability, tending to hypotension and

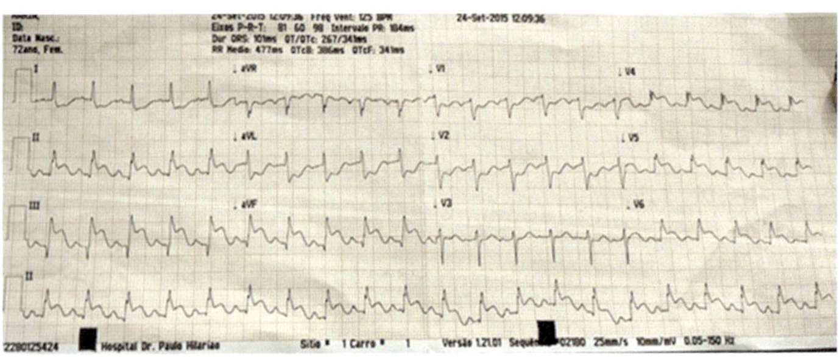

Figure 1 ECG accomplished at 12h09, on September 24. It shows a ST elevation in D2, D3 (D3 > D2), aVF, V5, V6, V3R, and V4R, which means that a right coronary injury with impairment of right ventricular and left ventricular posterior wall occurred

uncomfortable ventilation pattern, using an O_2 catheter to keep $SatO_2$ within limits. After starting noninvasive ventilation, the patient presented with worsening of hypotension and need for vasoactive drugs (norepinephrine and dobutamine).

At 00:00 AM of the following day, she was submitted to the second coronarography, which showed a severe three-vessel obstructive pattern, with diffuse involvement of coronaries: RCA with an apparently recent occlusion and severe mitral insufficiency with significant opacification of the left atrium and pulmonary veins (mechanical complication of acute myocardial infarction). An intra-aortic balloon pump was introduced, and the surgical team was contacted. She maintained unstable hemodynamics in use of noradrenaline 35 ml/h and dobutamine 10 mcg/kg/h and maintained a comfortable ventilation pattern on mechanical ventilation and good gas exchange analysis. An echocardiogram was performed on the morning of the same day, which showed mild aortic and tricuspid insufficiency, moderate mitral regurgitation with moderate regurgitation fraction, lower akinesia of the left ventricle, mild/moderate pulmonary hypertension, and left ventricular ejection fraction (LVEF) (Simpson) of 55%.

After discussion with the surgical team, conservative treatment was chosen. The patient remained in hemodynamic instability, even in use of intra-aortic balloon pump, requiring high doses of vasoactive drugs. Nonresponsive to treatment, she evolved with presented with anuria, pulmonary congestion and a drop in blood pressure, refractory to vasoactive amines with subsequent cardiac arrest. The patient died at 7:23 PM of the following day.

Questions

1. How can one classify chest pain according to the Coronary Artery Surgery Study (CASS)? What are the possible differential diagnoses for each of the ratings?

Once the history of the pain is obtained, the physician makes a global assessment of the symptom. This classification scheme for chest pain classifies it into three groups: typical angina, atypical angina, or noncardiac chest pain. According to this, typical angina presents when someone has the following: (1) substernal chest discomfort with a characteristic quality and duration; (2) pain that is triggered by exertion or emotional stress; (3) pain that is relieved by resting or using nitroglycerin (NTG). Atypical angina occurs when only two of these are present, and the chest pain is considered noncardiac when only one or none of the above is present [3].

2. What is the pathophysiology of STEMI? Which typical symptoms of STEMI this patient presented? What are the most prevalent findings on physical examination of a patient with STEMI?

Myocardial infarction is the death of cardiomyocytes caused by prolonged ischemia, which spreads from the sub-endocardium to sub-epicardium [5]. The ischemia is usually caused by a sudden rupture, thrombosis, and/or vasospasm of an inflamed atherosclerotic plaque. A smaller portion is associated with atherosclerotic plate erosion [8]. A persistent and intense left chest pain, radiating to the left arm, which does not improve or only has partial relief with rest or sublingual nitrates, characterizes the typical presentation of a STEMI. Irradiation to jaw, right upper limb, back, shoulders, and epigastrium is also possible. In patients with diabetes, in elderly or those in postoperative period, the STEMI may occur in the absence of pain, but with nausea, dyspnea, tachycardia, or confusion. This patient reported chest pain lasting for about 24 h, characterized as burning, with radiation to the jaw and back, associated with diaphoresis and nausea [5]. Although there was no alteration found at physical examination of this patient, frequently cardiac auscultation may reveal tachycardia (associated with a worse prognosis), valvular murmurs (due to ischemic valvular dysfunction), and a third heart sound (associated with acute ventricular failure). Hypotension may be an early symptom of cardiogenic shock [5].

3. Which is the importance of STEMI risk factors?

Risk factors for STEMI include previous cardiovascular diseases (coronary artery disease, brain vascular disease, and occlusive peripheral artery disease), subclinical atherosclerosis, previous artery revascularization procedures, diabetes mellitus, arterial hypertension, dyslipidemia, chronic kidney disease, age, and smoking [10]. Some of these factors are included in STEMI classification parameters through TIMI risk score, which considers age (≥75 years old), history of arterial hypertension, diabetes mellitus, and angina. This classification allows determining patient management, estimating the degree of ventricular dysfunction, and evaluating the prognosis of STEMI [4].

4. Why is it important to analyze the biochemical markers of myocardial injury in the diagnosis of ACS? Which biochemical markers should be analyzed?

Biochemical markers of myocardial injury are essential to assist in the diagnosis and prognosis of patients with acute coronary syndrome (ACS). In patients with suggestive symptoms of ACS, biochemical markers are useful to confirm the diagnosis of myocardial infarction. They also provide important prognostic information, since there is a direct association between elevated serum markers and the risk of cardiac events in short and medium term [2].

Myoglobin is a very early marker of myocardial necrosis, preceding the release of CK-MB in 2–5 h, but it is not a cardiac-specific marker, so its main advantage is the early detection of ACS in patients at a high level of suspicion [2]. CK-MB is still widely used in clinical practice, although it's major limitation is the rise after damage in no cardiac tissues (false positives), with 97% sensitivity and 90% specificity for the diagnosis of AMI. The subforms of CK-MB were employed as early markers of myocardial injury [2]. The troponins are proteins of the complex of myofibrillar regulation, which are not present in smooth muscle. There are three subunits: troponin T (TnTc), troponin I (TnIc), and troponin C. Troponin C is co-expressed in skeletal muscle fibers of slow contraction and is not considered as a cardiac-specific marker. Troponins' main advantages compared to CK-MB are (1) increased specificity for myocardial injury and (2) ability to detect small amounts of myocardial damage not detectable by CK-MB tests. TnTc and TnIc are currently the biochemical markers of choice for detection of myocardial necrosis in patients with suspected ACS. Cardiac troponins remain high after 24 h of onset of symptoms [2]. Although the troponins are also important prognostic risk factors, they should not be used alone to set the risk of patients with ACS. The majority of patients who develop complications starts with normal troponins. No biochemical marker is perfectly accurate to determine myocardial damage [2].

5. Which are the indications for coronarography? In this case, why coronarography was indicated for the patient?

Coronary angiography is defined as the radiographic visualization of the coronary vessels after the injection of radiopaque contrast media. It is performed to evaluate or confirm the presence of luminal obstruction of the coronary arteries and to determine the necessity of surgical treatment (coronary angioplasty or cardiac surgery) [7].

This test is indicated for those patients classified as high and intermediate risk. According to ACC/AHA guidelines for coronary angiography, a patient is considered at high risk when at least one of the following features is present: (1) prolonged ongoing (>20 min) chest pain; (2) pulmonary edema, most likely related to ischemia; (3) angina at rest with dynamic ST changes ≥1 mm; (4) angina with new or worsening MR murmur; (5) angina with S3 or new/worsening rales; and (6) angina with hypotension. Intermediate risk is defined by no high-risk features but has one of the following features: (1) prolonged (>20 min) angina at rest, resolved, with moderate or high likelihood of CAD; (2) angina at rest (>20 min or relieved with rest or sublingual nitroglycerin); (3) nocturnal angina; (4) angina with dynamic T-wave changes; (5) new-onset CCSC III or IV angina in the past 2 weeks with moderate or high likelihood of CAD; (6) pathological Q waves or resting ST depression ≤1 mm in multiple lead groups (anterior, inferior, lateral); and (7) age > 65 years [7].

Patients classified as low risk are characterized by no high- or intermediate-risk features. For those patients, coronary angiography is not indicated, and these patients are stratified by noninvasive methods [7]. The patient of the case presents some features that include her as high risk: prolonged ongoing chest pain (about 24 h) and the angina at rest with dynamic ST changes ≥1 mm. Therefore, coronary angiography is indicated for this patient.

6. Why was an intra-aortic balloon pump introduced on this patient?

The intra-aortic balloon pump (IABP) improves diastolic coronary blood flow and reduces myocardial work. These physiological effects of the IABP are especially helpful in patients with STEMI with ongoing or recurrent ischemic discomfort, hypotension from ischemia-mediated LV dysfunction who do not respond to other interventions, and cardiogenic shock that is not quickly reversed with pharmacological therapy [1]. Therefore, it is a useful stabilizing measure for patients in whom cardiac catheterization and revascularization are considered. It should be used in addition to medical therapy for these patients [1]. As the patient of the case presented hemodynamic instability, even with vasoactive drugs, tending to hypotension and with uncomfortable ventilation pattern, it is possible to include her on the indications for introduction of IABP.

7. How should be the electrocardiographic evaluation of a patient admitted with complaints of chest pain?

The assessment of electrocardiographic examination should be performed ideally in less than 10 min of presentation to the emergency, and it is the center of the initial decision-making in patients with suspected AMI. It is important to evaluate serial tracings in a short period of time (5–10 min), if the patient remains symptomatic, due to the possibility of nonspecific ECG changes, and this reevaluation strongly increases the sensitivity of the method. After therapy has been instituted, the ECG should be repeated 3, 6, 9, and 12 h after admission and daily until discharge from the coronary care unit [4].

8. What is the pathophysiology of ischemic mitral regurgitation?

Ischemic mitral regurgitation is a frequent complication of left ventricular global or regional pathological remodeling due to chronic coronary artery disease. It isn't a valve disease but represents the valvular consequences of increased tethering forces (papillary muscles displacement leading to a more apical position of the leaflets and their coaptation point) and reduced closing forces (reduced contractility, dyssynchrony of the papillary muscles, intra-left ventricular dyssynchrony). Although mitral regurgitation has an unloading effect and reduces impedance, the volume overload causes further left ventricular dilatation and increases ventricular wall stress, leading to worsened performance. The volume overload due to MR contributes to a vicious circle: the more remodeled the LV, the more severe the MR which triggers further LV dilatation and, thus, further MR. This cycle has important effects on LV geometry, leading to a rather spherical LV [6].

9. What impact in mortality does the surgical treatment have? What are the main indications?

Current studies have documented that there are better clinical outcomes with lower mortality after the surgical treatment of MR with revascularization. Current research demonstrates that combined mitral valve repair and revascularization resulted in less postoperative mitral regurgitation and a similar 5-year survival when compared with revascularization alone [9].

Bibliography

1. Antman EM, et al. ACC/AHA guidelines for the management of patients with ST-elevation myocardial infarction. Circulation. 2004; 110(5):588–636. Available at: http://www.ncbi.nlm.nih.gov/pubmed/15289388.
2. Avezum Junior Á, et al. V Diretriz da Sociedade Brasileira de Cardiologia sobre Tratamento do Infarto Agudo do Miocárdio com Supradesnível do Segmento ST. Arq Bras Cardiol. 2015;105(2 Suppl 1):1–121. Available at: www.arquivosonline.com.br
3. Committee on Management of Patients With Chronic Stable Angina. ACC/AHA/ACP-ASIM practice guidelines ACC/AHA/ACP-ASIM guidelines for the management of patients with

chronic stable angina committee members task force members. J Am Coll Cardiol. 1999;33(7):2092–197.
4. O'Gara PT, et al. 2013 ACCF/AHA guideline for the management of st-elevation myocardial infarction: a report of the American college of cardiology foundation/American heart association task force on practice guidelines. J Am Coll Cardiol. 2013;61:e78.
5. Pesaro AEP, Serrano CV Jr, Nicolau JC. Infarto agudo do miocárdio: síndrome coronariana aguda com supradesnível do segmento ST. Rev Assoc Med Bras. 2004;50(2):214–20.
6. Piérard LA, Carabello BA. Ischaemic mitral regurgitation: pathophysiology, outcomes and the conundrum of treatment. Eur Heart J. 2010;31:2996.
7. Scanlon PJ, et al. ACC/AHA guidelines for coronary angiography: executive summary and recommendations. J Am Coll Cardiol. 1999;33(6):1756–824.
8. Stefanini E, Ramos RF. Infarto Agudo do Miocárdio com Supradesnivelamento do Segmento ST: Avaliação Clínica e Laboratorial. Tratado de Cardiologia SOCESP. 2009:893–908.
9. Tarasoutchi F, et al. Diretriz Brasileira de Valvopatias – SBC 2011/ I Diretriz Interamericana de Valvopatias – SIAC 2011. Arq Bras Cardiol. 2011;97(5):01–67.
10. Xavier HT, et al. V Diretriz Brasileira de Dislipidemias e Prevenção da Aterosclerose. Arq Bras Cardiol. 2013;101(4):01–22. Available at: www.arquivosonline.com.br.

Diagnosis and Management of Takotsubo Syndrome (Broken Heart Syndrome)

Mariana Vano Galvão Almeida França, Nilton Freire de Assis Neto, Isadora Simão Almeida Liberato, and Fernando Augusto Alves da Costa

Clinical Presentation

Female patient, 70 years old, admitted to the emergency of Beneficencia Portuguesa Hospital, in April 2016, with a typical chest pain for 2 h associated with pain in the left shoulder and dyspnea on moderate exercises, with progressive worsening on the last 30 min.

On physical examination, the patient was in regular general condition, oriented, with intense sweating, also being observed jugular stasis. Cardiac auscultation showed regular rhythm, in two stages, with normal sounds and without heart murmur, and lung auscultation revealed bilateral vesicular murmur with rales/crackles in bases, without lower limb edema. Her heart rate was 86 beats per minute, blood pressure of 160/90 mmHg, respiratory rate of 17 cycles per minute, and axillary temperature of 36 °C.

M. V. G. A. França (✉) · N. F. de Assis Neto
I. S. A. Liberato · F. A. A. da Costa
Anhembi Morumbi University (UAM), São Paulo, SP, Brazil

R. M. S. Almeida, F. B. Jatene (eds.), *Cardiovascular Surgery*,
https://doi.org/10.1007/978-3-319-57084-6_13

Diagnosis, Assessment, and Treatment

The initial management requested an electrocardiogram (Fig. 1), which indicated a left branch block and atrioventricular block of first degree. Laboratory tests showed elevated cardiac enzymes (Table 1), and a chest X-ray showed a pulmonary congestion. The patient developed acute pulmonary edema, requiring diuretic administration and nitroprusside.

The patient was managed initially as presenting an acute coronary syndrome and admitted for more exams. The transthoracic echocardiography showed an ejection fraction of 0.35, akinesia of the septal wall, anterior mid-apical hypokinesia, and lower middle-basal hypokinesia. After 5 days of hospitalization, an angiography was performed that showed a slight obstruction of 40% in the proximal third of the right coronary artery (Fig. 2).

After 11 days of hospitalization, it was requested a new transthoracic echocardiography that showed a systolic dysfunction on the left ventricle with a diffuse hypokinesia and

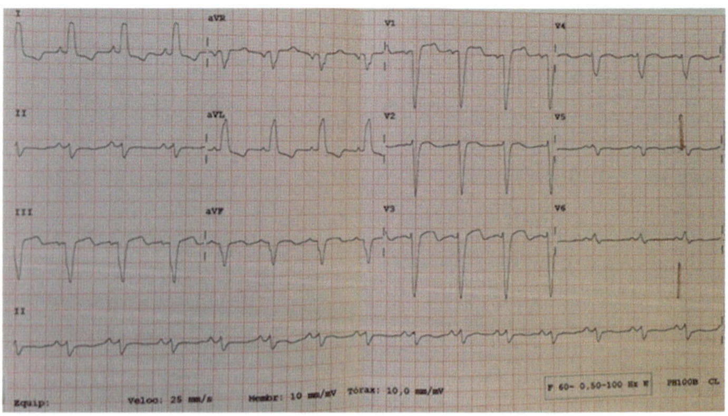

Figure 1 Electrocardiogram. (Source: prepared by the authors (2016))

TABLE 1 Cardiac enzymes

	April 21, 2016 21h23min	**April 22, 2016 2h10min**	**April 22, 2016 5h53min**
CK (U/l)	34	30	298
Troponin (ng/ml)	<0.100	0.295	0.098
BNP	–	4658	5623
CK-MB (ng/ml)	9.1	8.2	30

Source: prepared by the authors

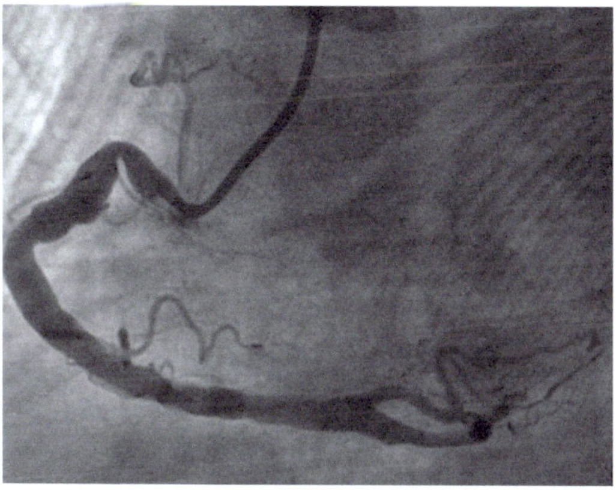

FIGURE 2 Coronary angiography. (Source: prepared by the authors (2016))

asynchrony of the septal wall, and an ejection fraction of 0.60, indicating a rapid ventricular recovery.

The patient obtained good clinical outcome with supportive treatment, and after 13 days in the hospital, she was asymptomatic and discharged home with the following medications: acetylsalicylic acid, isosorbide mononitrate, statin, and spironolactone.

Questions

1. What is the main differential diagnosis of Takotsubo syndrome?

Acute coronary syndrome. The clinic points to an acute coronary syndrome. The patient has chest pain associated with shortness of breath and adrenergic symptoms with elevated cardiac markers [1, 2].

2. What is the clinical difference between acute coronary syndrome and sindrome Takotsubo?

Takotsubo courses with a rapid evolution of the ventricular function. The reasoner this event, is the release of catecholamines with sympathetic stimulation, leading to spasms of the epicardial coronary arteries and vascular spasms. Because of these spasms, the ventricular function can be recovered quickly.

3. In the acute phase, which is done to ensure the diagnosis?

Coronary angiography is the major exam used in the acute phase. We are talking about a disease in which there are vascular spasms, so angiography is the great test to assess if there is obstruction, the level of obstruction, and what can be done to reverse the condition.

4. What is the principle pathophysiological mechanism related to microvascular spasm and myocardial injury?

The release of catecholamines leads to an exacerbated sympathetic activation. Faced with this adrenergic discharge, the ventricle beats disorderly, for not keeping up with the pace that has now been demanded. With all this disorganization, there are vascular spasms in the epicardial arteries and microvascular spasms.

5. Who are the suspected patients?

Postmenopausal women with acute coronary syndrome that do not correspond to electrocardiographic changes and biomarkers.

6. What sex is more affected?

Although it is still little elucidated, the disease happens to be detected in the patient after the menopause, which causes us to associate the hormonal load related to the female. By virtue of this, the female sex is the most affected.

7. What is the need for the echocardiogram in the investigation of the disease?

The great benefit of the echocardiogram is related to the measurement of the ejection fraction. After following the values, you can follow an evolution of the ventricular function. As we know that the disease is present with a rapid improvement of the ventricular function, in the quality of the control, we can guarantee the safety of the diagnosis.

8. What is the pharmacological therapy for a disease?

Antiplatelet to prevent the formation of thrombi and vasodilator to avoid spasms. If the patient has developed pulmonary edema, a diuretic is necessary.

Thematic Thread Discussion

The Takotsubo syndrome was described initially in Japan, known as a transitional left ventricular dysfunction in the absence of obstructive coronary artery disease, and is associated in most cases with psychological stressors [3, 4]. The similarity of the clinical manifestation from the Takotsubo disease with myocardial infarction causes the underdiagnosis of this disease.

The patient had a chest pain associated with dyspnea and sweating imitating coronary syndrome, with elevation of cardiac enzymes. The echocardiogram performed 1 day after the symptoms, showed a previous medium-apical hypokinesia and mid-basal hypokinesia on bottom of the left ventricle, and an ejection fraction of 0.35. The second echocardiogram performed 11 days after the first one, indicated an ejection fraction of 0.60, showing a significant improvement and rapid recovery of the ventricle. In addition, coronary angiography showed no significant obstructions to justify the clinical conditional.

The pathophysiological mechanisms are not well elucidated, but it is known that there is a significant increase in catecholamines, and this sympathetic stimulation can lead to ventricular hypokinesia contributing to spasms of the epicardial coronary arteries, microvascular spasm, or injury to myocardial cell.

The diagnosis of Takotsubo cardiomyopathy should be suspected in women after menopause who have an acute coronary syndrome in the clinical manifestations, and ECG abnormalities are disproportionate to the degree of elevation of cardiac biomarkers. Apical ballooning or mid-ventricular hypokinesia is usually seen on the left ventriculography or echocardiography.

As a transitional disease, the patient evolves with rapid recovery of left ventricular function in a few weeks [5, 6].

References

1. Magalhães CC, Serrano, Júnior VC, Consolim-Colombo NF, Fonseca F, Helfenstein AF, Ferreira MFJ. Treaty of cardiology SOCESP. 3rd ed. São Paulo: Manole; 2015.
2. Braunwald E. Treaty of cardiovascular diseases. 9nd ed. Rio de Janeiro: Elsevier; 2013.
3. Lemos TEA, Araújo JLA, Lemos MT, Belém SL,Filho VCJF, Barros BR. Síndrome do Coração Partido (Síndrome de Takotsubo). Available at: <http://www.arquivosonline.com.br/2008/9001/pdf/9001012.pdf>.
4. Hoekstra EB, Reis SSE, Ribeiro B, Costa CAM. Takotsubo Disease (Broken Heart Syndrome): an Underdiagnosed Disease? Available at: <http://www.rbconline.org.br/artigo/doenca-de-takotsubo-sindrome-do-coracao-partido-uma-doenca-subdiagnosticada/>.
5. Silva GLLV, Hisano KD, Aquino RTR, Magliari REM, Almeida FAJ, Almeida DJ, Almeida LA, Kadri T, Franken AR. Broken heart syndrome (Takotsubo Syndrome, Stress-Induced Cardiomyopathy): case report. Available at: <http://www.fcmsantacasasp.edu.br/images/Arquivos_medicos/2008/53_3/vlm53n3_7.pdf>.
6. Rihl FM, Haas P, Holthausen SR. Takotsubo cardiomyopathy: case report. Available at: <http://www.amrigs.org.br/revista/59-01/07_1384_Revista%20AMRIGS.pdf>.

Kawasaki Disease with Coronary Artery Bypass Grafting

Maikon Augusto Vogado Aranda Florenciano, João Vitor Ferreira Carvalho, Jéssica Krieger de Souza, and Marcos Antonio Cantero

Clinical Presentation

NSG patient, female, 5-year-old, black, native of Rio Brilhante, was admitted to the Hospital Benevolent Association of Rio Brilhante, in 2002, referring abrupt onset of fever, polymorphous rash, arthralgia, and rash desquamation on hands and feet. Initially, it was suspected of being the case of meningitis and rheumatoid arthritis as diagnostic hypotheses. Without further clarification, the patient was referred to the University Hospital of Campo Grande – MS, being hospitalized for 11 days. In this period, additional tests were done such as transthoracic echocardiography and electrocardiography (ECG), suggesting the clinical finding of Kawasaki disease. The patient was discharged by treatment with acetylsalicylic acid 100 mg daily for 4 months.

M. A. V. A. Florenciano (✉) · J. V. F. Carvalho · J. K. de Souza
M. A. Cantero
Federal University of Grande Dourados (UFGD),
Dourados, MS, Brazil
e-mail: maikonflorenciano@outlook.com

R. M. S. Almeida, F. B. Jatene (eds.), *Cardiovascular Surgery*,
https://doi.org/10.1007/978-3-319-57084-6_14

At age 17, the patient had chest pain in distress, severe dyspnea, sweating, nausea, and vomiting, being transmitted to Evangelical Hospital in Dourados – MS, on December 2014. At the time, denied dyslipidemia, hypertension, smoking, and diabetes mellitus. On admission, the patient had Hb = 12.8 g/dL, Ht = 37.2%, SO_2 = 99.3%, BP = 120/80 mmHg, and HR = 102 bpm. In the anteroposterior (AP) chest radiograph, an increased and irregular hilar and pulmonary vasculature was revealed and the heart area was on the upper limit of normality. In the hemodynamic study, the patient presented left ventricle with normal contraction; coronary calcification; coronary aneurysms in the left main coronary artery (greater inner diameter 8.03 mm) and proximal left anterior descending (larger inner diameter 9.28 mm), circumflex (higher internal diameter 5.32 mm), and right coronary artery (greater inner diameter of 11 mm and outer diameter 14.5 mm); and right coronary dominance, setting coronary insufficiency. The ECG was normal (Fig. 1).

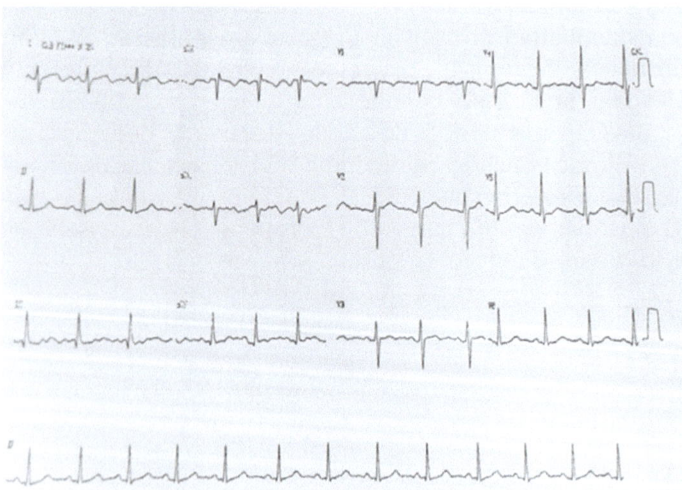

FIGURE 1 Electrocardiogram unchanged. (Source: prepared by the authors)

Diagnosis, Assessment, and Treatment

In the AP chest radiograph, an increased and irregular hilar and pulmonary vasculature was revealed and the heart area was on the upper limit of normality. In the hemodynamic study, the patient presented left ventricle with normal contraction; coronary calcification; coronary aneurysms in the left main coronary artery (greater inner diameter 8.03 mm) and proximal left anterior descending (larger inner diameter 9.28 mm), circumflex (higher internal diameter 5.32 mm), and right coronary artery (greater inner diameter of 11 mm and outer diameter 14.5 mm); and right coronary dominance, setting coronary insufficiency. The ECG was normal.

After a hemodynamic study, there were absences of structural pathologies of the arteries of the proximal superior and mammary limbs, being necessary to opt for the surgical conduction, with revascularization of the myocardium. Laboratory evaluation showed changes in LDL (166.20 mg/dL), total cholesterol (242 mg/dL), AST (41.1 U/L), ALT (49.2 U/L), and glucose (106.3 mg/dL). Lactate, urea, creatinine, C-reactive protein, and coagulation tests were normal.

After 5 days of hospitalization, the patient underwent complete revascularization of the myocardium. Held dissection of the left internal thoracic artery and right and left saphenous vein. Continuing, the anastomosis of the right internal thoracic artery was performed to the left anterior descending artery with 7-0 prolene, anastomosis of the left internal thoracic artery to the marginal coronary artery with 7-0 prolene, anastomosis of saphenous vein segments with posterior descending artery with continuous polypropylene 7-0, and anastomosis between the saphenous vein and the ascending aorta. Postoperatively started dobutamine and sodium nitroprusside. The patient progressed in good general condition (GGC) with MAP = 95 mmHg, HR = 70 bpm, and $SO_2 = 100\%$. On the first postoperative day progressed hemodynamically stable GGC, afebrile, good ventilation, and good SpO_2 standard. Still, the patient showed good diuresis, uneventfully. Physical examination showed the lungs had vesicular murmurs present with adventitious sounds and normal cardiac rhythmic with two sounds, without murmurs. On the second postoperative day, the use of sodium nitroprusside was interrupted, remaining the use of dobutamine. In the third postoperative day, medications in use were removed and was prescribed hospital discharge.

Questions

1. What is the incidence of chest pain in children?

According to some studies, the pediatric population with chest pain complaint is from 0.3% to 0.6% of the consultations, both in clinics and in emergency services.

2. What are the most common causes of chest pain in children?

Although it is quite a frequent complaint, chest pain in this age group rarely has a cardiovascular origin, which, according to some studies, ranges from 1% to 7%. The most frequent causes are musculoskeletal disorders, arising from trauma, costochondritis, muscle strain, and other causes, followed by idiopathic, respiratory (pneumonia, asthma, pneumothorax), psychogenic (anxiety, depression), and gastrointestinal (reflux, peptic ulcer) diseases. Cardiovascular causes, although quite unusual, are considered the most serious, standing out myocardial ischemia due to angina, coronary anomaly, family atherosclerosis, and Kawasaki disease, among others. There are still other cardiac chest pain causes, such as myocarditis, cardiomyopathy, and aortic dissection.

3. What is the incidence of Kawasaki disease?

Kawasaki disease has universal occurrence and affects all pediatric groups, and 85% of cases are in patients up to 5 years old. It has a higher incidence in boys, around 1.5:1 in relation to girls. Regarding ethnicity, the prevalence is higher in Asian individuals. The occurrence is rare in patients over 8 years old.

4. What are the most common clinical manifestations?

Kawasaki disease consists on a generalized systemic vasculitis predominantly affecting the medium-caliber vessels, particularly coronary arteries. It is characterized by a fever, rash and conjunctival and oral erosion, hands and feet edema, erythema of the palms and soles, scaly rash, cervical lymphadenopathy, and polymorphous rash. The untreated can lead to the development of cardiovascular sequelae such as aneurysms and stenosis and development of acute myocardial infarction frame by rupture or thrombosis evolving to sudden death.

5. How to evaluate? Which tests should be asked?

After the suggestive clinic, the first test to be considered is the coronary echocardiography, which has high specificity and sensitivity to show changes in the proximal segments of the coronary arteries, which can show a coronary arteritis before aneurysm formation. Another complementary examination option is the magnetic resonance imaging that has the advantage when compared with echocardiography in detecting changes in the distal segments of the coronary arteries. Angioresonance and computed tomography may also be required. Angiography is the gold standard to assess cardiac impairment.

6. How is the treatment?

The treatment of acute phase seeks to reduce inflammation and prevent complications of vasculitis, aneurysms, and stenosis. Myocardial ischemia and infarction are complications that treatment also seeks to prevent. Intravenous immunoglobulin (IVIG) is used to decrease the duration of symptoms as well as the frequency of abnormalities of the coronary arteries. It is relevant to be administered at the very beginning of the acute phase, since late IVIG therapy (after 10 days of onset of disease) does not prevent vessel changes. Acetylsalicylic acid (ASA) is used in high doses, with an anti-inflammatory effect, which also enhances the effect of IVIG. Corticosteroids are used in refractory cases.

7. In what conditions should the operation occur?

Surgical treatment of revascularization is indicated when there is the presence of severe occlusion of the common trunk or proximal segment of the left coronary artery. It is also shown when more than one main coronary artery and/or when collaterals are shown to be at risk.

8. Which technique is ideal?

In coronary artery bypass grafting (CABG), the most indicated grafts are the internal mammary arteries, since they reveal growth capacity in agreement with the somatic growth of the patient. It is suggested that this type of artery is spared from atherosclerosis, thereby contributing to endothelial function. Saphenous vein grafts showed good results in the right coronary circulation.

Review About the Addressed Disease or Treatment

Kawasaki disease is characterized by a generalized vasculitis framework, which mainly affects the vessels of medium caliber. It has universal occurrence with predominance in Asian boys. In all cases, 85% are aged up to 5 years old, being rare before 6 months and after 8 years. Its etiology is still unclear but suggests a delayed hypersensitivity reaction against a previously characterized antigen, which leads to the production of autoantibodies against the endothelial and smooth muscle cells, resulting in acute vasculitis. Generally, it is a self-limiting condition characterized by presentation of acute fever, erythema and conjunctival and oral lesions, swelling in hands and feet, the palms and soles erythema, desquamation rash, and cervical lymphadenopathy. The main complication is cardiac lesions by the involvement of the coronary arteries, corresponding to 20% of cases. This portion, which ultimately leads to the formation of aneurysms, acute myocardial infarction, and heart failure, corresponds to cases that do not receive effective and early treatment, mainly consisting of intravenous immunoglobulin administration (IVIG) at high dose (2 g/kg as an infusion only for 10 h) and acetylsalicylic acid (100 mg/kg/day for 14 days followed by 3–5 mg/kg/day for several weeks) in the acute phase of the disease to reduce the prevalence of abnormalities of the coronary arteries. Currently, the correct and early management brought down the rate of cardiac complications to 4%. The cases that progress to coronary artery disease undergo majority to CABG.

Bibliography

1. Castro PA, Urbano LMF, Costa IMC. Kawasaki disease. Brazilian Ann Dermatol. 2009;84(4):317–31.
2. Metze K. Blood and lymphatic vessels. In: Filho GB, editor. Bogliolo: pathology. Rio de Janeiro: Guanabara Koogan; 2011. p. 507.
3. Mitchel RN, Schoen FJ. Blood vessels. In: Kumar V, Abbas AK, Fausto N, Aster JC, editors. Robbins & Cotran: Patologia – pathological basis of disease. Rio de Janeiro: Elsevier; 2010. p. 523.
4. Pfeiffer MET. Chest pain in children and adolescents: why, when and how to evaluate the heart? Revista do DERC. 2012;18(3):86–90.
5. Santos V, Simões AS, Teixeira A, Abecasis M, Loureiro M, Anjos R. Coronary artery bypass surgery after Kawasaki disease. Portuguese Journal of Cardiology. 2011;31(6):433–7.

Stable Angina and Revascularization in Type 1 Diabetic Patient

Carolina Kuchenbecker Soares, André Gorle de Miranda Chaves, Gabriel Prado Saad, Graziela Chequer, and Jéssica Silva de Paula

Clinical Presentation

D.G.L, female, 38 years old, from Belo Horizonte, Minas Gerais, Brazil, presented to her cardiologist with stabbing precordial chest pain complaint, that started almost 1 year ago. Pain lasts 10–15 min, does not radiate, is associated with dyspnea, occurs in times of stress or exercise and is relieved with rest.

Past medical history (PMH): type 1 diabetes mellitus since 7 years old with diabetic nephropathy diagnosed 8 years ago (stage IV, pre-dialysis) and retinopathy nonproliferative in monitoring. Hypertension for 16 years and hypothyroidism for 13 years.

In use of the following:

- Levothyroxine 100 mcg once a day
- Furosemide 40 mg twice a day

C. K. Soares (✉) · A. G. de Miranda Chaves · G. P. Saad
G. Chequer · J. S. de Paula
Minas Gerais Federal University (UFMG),
Belo Horizonte, MG, Brazil

R. M. S. Almeida, F. B. Jatene (eds.), *Cardiovascular Surgery*,
https://doi.org/10.1007/978-3-319-57084-6_15

- Amlodipine 5 mg twice a day
- Enalapril 5 mg twice a day
- AAS 100 mg once a day
- Allopurinol 150 mg once a day
- Atorvastatin 20 mg once a day
- 20 IU NPH insulin in the morning, 12 UI at lunch, and 4UI at night

Family history (FH): Father with high blood pressure and cardiac arrhythmia (with implantation of pacemaker 2 years ago). Mother who is morbidly obese, with type 2 diabetes mellitus type 2 and high blood pressure.

On examination:

Blood pressure (BP): Sitting 134 × 92 mmHg, lying 132 × 84 mmHg, and after 3 min standing 132 × 88 mmHg. Heart rate: 88 bpm. Respiratory rate: 16 bpm. Normal remaining exam.

Diagnosis, Assessment, and Treatment

Previous exams:

- Echocardiography with Doppler: left ventricle and right ventricle with normal conformation and preserved function. Mitral and tricuspid discrete regurgitation. Ejection fraction of 68%.
- Stress test: Stopped at 04 min and 27 s of the Bruce protocol due to exhaustion. The absence of chest pain or other clinical abnormalities on stress. Depressed chronotropic response and pressor response within physiological limits. Reaches 73% of maximum heart rate expected for age. The absence of arrhythmias. ST segment depression 1.5 mm in DII, DIII, V5, and V6 C5M until hit effort. Functional capacity is considered very poor according to criteria of the American Heart Association (AHA). Reached 4.5 metabolic equivalents (METs) of test.
- Myocardial scintigraphy stress (Fig. 1): transient myocardial ischemia in the anterior wall of the left ventricle with moderate length and marked degree, left ventricular ejection

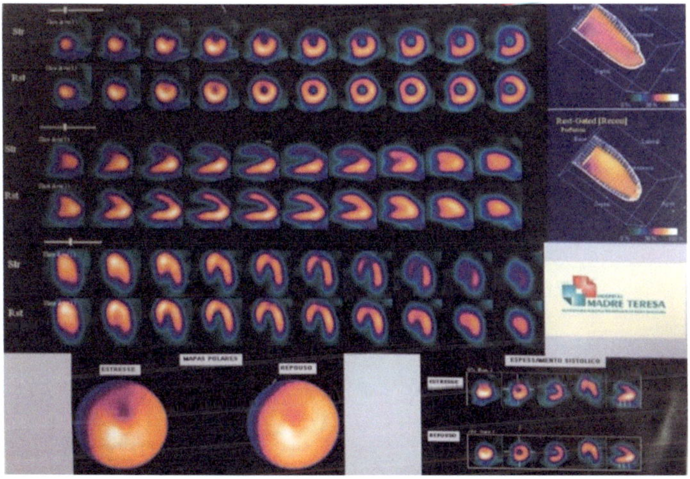

Figure 1 Myocardial scintigraphy stress test showing transient myocardial ischemia in the anterior wall of the left ventricle with moderate length and marked degree

fraction (LVEF) of 72% at rest, and transient ischemic dilation index (TID) 0.81 (reference value <1.20). Pharmacological stress test: 4 min after drug injection reached heart rate (HF) 125 bpm (an increase of 42% compared to baseline) and started limiting dizziness coincident with electrocardiographic changes suggestive of ischemia (ST segment depression in CM5, aVL, V3, V4, and V5).

Diagnosis: Stable angina CCS 2

Conduct: Prescribed atenolol 25 mg twice a day and prompted cardiac catheterization. In the following appointment, the patient reported improvement of the episodes of chest pain after initiation of beta-blocker and brought the result of catheterization that revealed severe coronary atherosclerosis: left coronary artery free of obstructions. Severe segmental injury (70%) in the proximal third of left anterior descending artery (LAD) and in the ostium of first diagonal (70%). Circumflex artery (CX) with severe obstruction (80%) in thin gauge segment. Right coronary artery free of obstructions (Figs. 2 and 3). In spite of angina remission with beta-blocker therapy, exertion

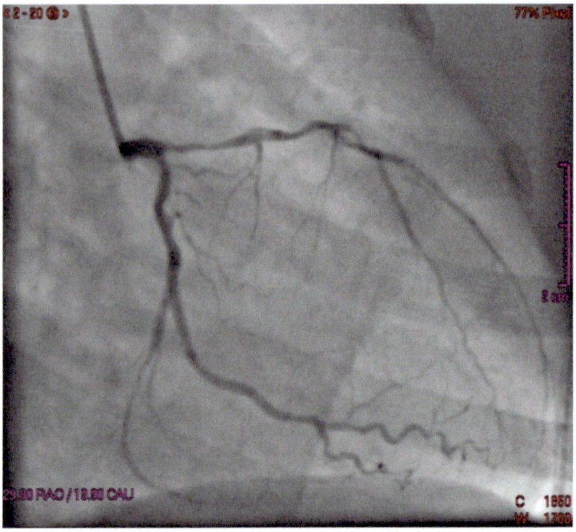

Figure 2 Coronary angiography showing severe segmental injury (70%) in the proximal third of the left anterior descending artery and severe obstruction (80%) in thin gauge segment of the circumflex artery

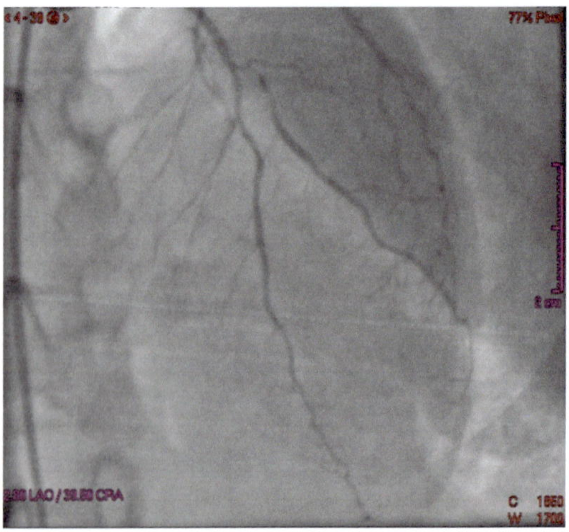

Figure 3 Coronary angiography showing severe obstruction in the ostium of first diagonal branch (70%)

ECG and myocardial scintigraphy show severity parameters. Pharmacological stenting was performed in the left descending artery, and the diagonalis branch was left untreated.

Questions

1. What type is the patient's angina and what is her pretest probability of coronary artery disease (CAD)?

The pain is classified as atypical angina [3]. Stable angina is defined when symptoms haven't changed lately and are precipitated by a reasonably predictable exertion level and relieved with rest and nitrates. On the other hand, a low pain threshold associated with frequency, intensity, or symptom duration progression predicts the unstable angina diagnostic [4]. Typical angina is defined by a positive answer to three simple questions: (1) Is substernal discomfort present? (2) Is it precipitated with exertion? (3) Is it relieved by nitrates? Two positive answers indicate atypical angina, and one or none indicates noncardiac pain. Atypical angina is more common in women, who frequently have a variable pain threshold and present atypical pain in unconventional locations. The patient's pretest probability would be 2–39% as can be seen on the Diamond/Forrester and CASS Data.

2. What are the indications to carry out the exercise test in this case?

Stronger recommendation for exertion diagnostic test is for patients with an intermediate pretest probability (10–90%) of CAD. It is less useful for diagnostic in patients with high or low pretest probability. It is contraindicated in patients with an abnormal ECG at rest (e.g., left bundle branch block, ST segment elevation or depression, digitalis use, Wolff-Parkinson-White syndrome, electrolytic abnormalities) that does not allow appropriate evaluation of ST segment alterations.

3. What are the findings in the exercise test that support the indication for scintigraphy?

Myocardial scintigraphy is indicated for patients who present with atypical thoracic pain and a normal ECG at rest or nondiagnostic exertion ECG, as happened in the case [4]. Commonly the exertion ECG may be complemented with perfusion imaging for a more precise diagnostic or replaced by an alternative diagnostic approach.

4. What are the findings on scintigraphy that support the indication for catheterization?

Coronary angiography is the standard to evaluate presence and severity of CAD, being necessary to choose and guide revascularization procedures [1]. Coronary anatomy must be identified to make a proper choice of treatment. Cardiac catheterization can also be used to perform ventriculography, helpful in defining CAD prognostic and extension, as well as left ventricle dysfunction, as these are the main long-term determinants for patients with angina, clinical evidence of heart failure and severe ventricular arrhythmia, and who were resuscitated after cardiac arrest.

5. What are the findings in the catheterization that support the indication for revascularization?

Coronary artery bypass graft (CABG) has a grade IA recommendation in ≥50% obstruction in proximal AD [1]. The presented patient has a severe segmental injury (70%) in the proximal third of AD and in the ostium of first diagonal (70%) and CX with severe obstruction (80%) in thin gauge segment, fulfilling the formal indications for intervention (Table 1).

6. Why we opted for percutaneous revascularization instead of surgery?

Anatomically, the presence of CAD in the left coronary trunk or proximally in the left descending artery is important in the revascularization strategy definition [1]. In this setting (left descending artery disease), CABG has been shown to provide better long-term survival rates when compared to medical therapy alone and to have similar results to those of percutaneous coronary intervention (PCI). CABG has been shown to be superior to PCI when considering diabetic patients with multivascular disease. Therefore, in the presented cases, the choice between the two procedures comes down to the reference service expertise and evaluation of comorbidities.

Table 1 Revascularization to improve symptoms with significant anatomic (≥50% Left main or ≥70% non-Left Main CAD) or physiological (FFR ≤0.80) coronary artery stenoses

Clinical setting	COR	LOE
≥1 significant stenosis amenable to revascularization and unacceptable angina despite GDMT	1 – CABG 1 – PCI	A
≥1 significant stenosis and unacceptable angina in whom GDMT cannot be implemented because of medication contraindications, adverse effects, or patient preferences	IIa – CABG IIa – PCI	C C
Previous CABG with ≥1 significant stenosis associated with ischemia and unacceptable angina despite GDMT	IIa – PCI IIb – CABG	C C
Complex 3-vessel CAD (e.g., SYNTAX score >22) with or without involvement of the proximal LAD artery and a good candidate for CABG	IIa – CABG preferred over PCI	B
Viable ischemic myocardium that is perfused by coronary arteries that are not amenable to grafting	IIb – TMR as an adjunct to CABG	B
No anatomic or physiological criteria for revascularization	III: Harm – CABG III: Harm – PCI	C C

Adapted from "ACCF/AHA/ACP/AATS/PCNA/SCAI/STS guideline for the diagnosis and management of patients with stable ischemic heart disease" (Fihn et al. 2012, p. 415)

CABG coronary artery bypass graft, *CAD* coronary artery disease, *COR* class of recommendation, *GDMT* guideline-directed medical therapy, *LOE* level of evidence, *PCI* percutaneous coronary intervention, *TMR* transmyocardial revascularization

7. To what extent does the diabetes mellitus influence the indication of revascularization type in CAD?

Diabetic patients, especially those with advanced disease and insulin-dependency, customarily present intense and diffuse atherosclerotic process [4], with involvement of various segments of the coronary bed and multivascular disease. The CABG surgery is able to effectively treat this form of multivascular disease, which is why it is the preferred treatment modality for such patients. The CABG revascularization allows a larger area than coronary angioplasty and is not subject to complications such as the formation of intra-stent or peri-stent thrombus. Furthermore, in cases where there is multicoronary involvement, a common complication in diabetic patients, studies have indicated reduced mortality, less occurrence of myocardial infarction, and a reduced need for re-operating when CABG is performed, comparing with PCI. The SYNTAX score, calculated on anatomical basis and vascular involvement and assessed by coronary angiography, is used as a basis to define the best procedure. In patients with a score >32, the surgical option presents results clearly favor CABG, while lower scores show uncertain benefit. The issue is still hotly debated, but what is clear is that, based on the evidence currently available, the most effective approach option for multivascular diabetic patients is CABG. In case of a single-artery approach, the two options can be considered. It is always important to individualize the choice according to the preference of the patient and the experience of the multidisciplinary team to define the best approach according to particular variations.

8. What is the pharmacological optimization indicated for patients as exemplified?

The key treatment goals of CAD include the following: (1) prevent myocardial infarction and reduce mortality and (2) reduce the symptoms and the occurrence of myocardial ischemia, providing a better quality of life [2]. As for drug therapy, antiplatelet agents; lipid-lowering drugs, particularly statins; beta-blockers after myocardial infarction; and inhibitors of angiotensin-converting enzyme I (ACEI) reduce the incidence of heart attack and increase survival.

(a) Aspirin: remains the antiplatelet of excellence and should always be prescribed – except in rare cases of contraindications (allergy or intolerance, active bleeding, hemophilia, active peptic ulcer disease) or high likelihood of gastrointestinal or genitourinary bleeding. Aspirin is indicated for all patients. Class I, Level of Evidence A.
(b) Thienopyridine derivatives: studies comparing the antiplatelet effects of this drug to aspirin only included patients with AMI, stroke, and/or peripheral arterial disease, but not specifically evaluated the patients with chronic coronary disease. Thus, the use of clopidogrel is indicated in absolute contraindication to the use of aspirin and associated with aspirin after intervention with stents, for at least 30 days. Class I, Level of Evidence B. Similarly, the use of ticlopidine is indicated in absolute contraindication to the use of aspirin and associated with aspirin after intervention with stents, for 30 days. Class IIa, Level of Evidence B.
(c) Dipyridamole: dipyridamole, in the treatment of CAD, is not indicated. Class III, Level of Evidence B.
(d) Anticoagulants: in high-risk patients, aspirin association with warfarin, in the prevention of myocardial infarction and cardiovascular death, was more effective than monotherapy of these drugs. The warfarin use can be considered as a substitute for aspirin in the total intolerance to the latter, as are the other antiplatelets. In patients with CAD, INR values should be kept around 2.0 in isolated or combined use with aspirin in high-risk patients. Its use is so indicated in the presence of high-thrombotic risk associated with aspirin, especially after myocardial infarction. Class I, Level of Evidence A. And also as an alternative to complete intolerance to aspirin. Class IIa, Level of Evidence A.
(e) Statins: are the best therapeutic option for the control of serum levels of LDL-c, and the drug of choice to reduce it in adults, and also assist in the stabilization of atherosclerotic plaques. In patients with CAD, they should be used at full doses.

(f) Fibrates: are indicated in the treatment of endogenous hypertriglyceridemia, when there is a failure of lifestyle changes or when hypertriglyceridemia is very high (>500 mg/dL).
(g) ACE inhibitors: the benefits of ACE inhibitors in the treatment of CAD have been proven from clinical trials that included asymptomatic patients with reduced EF and patients with ventricular dysfunction after myocardial infarction. In individuals with increased risk, especially in the presence of diabetes mellitus, it decreased rates of death and adverse events. Thus, the benefit of ACEI is confirmed even in a population with CAD considered lower risk. The benefits are significant for ACEI as a class and so considered. Its use is recommended routine when there is ventricular dysfunction and/or heart failure (pode apagar esse failure na minha opinião - Gabriel). Degree of recommendation I, Level of Evidence A. And routine in all patients with CAD. Class IIa, Level of Evidence B.
(h) Angiotensin receptor blockers: are alternative for patients who cannot tolerate ACE inhibitors, since no studies have been conducted with this group of drugs in stable coronary disease. In other situations, no benefit accruing is compared to ACE inhibitors, which reduce infarction.

Review About the Addressed Disease or Treatment

Angina pectoris is an episodic clinical syndrome due to transient myocardial ischemia and a symptomatic manifestation of CAD [1]. When we said that angina is stable, it considers that the symptoms are not changed recently, and these are precipitated by a degree of predictable effort, relieved with rest and faster with nitroglycerin. The typical presentation is characterized by:

1. Sternal discomfort
2. Provoked by exertion or emotional stress (or after large meals)
3. Relief use at home or nitrate (in 1–3 min)

The angina is considered as atypical when the patient reports only two of the above criteria – common in women, the elderly and diabetics – and noncardiac chest pain when the patient reports only one criterion.

Angina is caused by variations combined with increase in demand infarction, decreased perfusion, and coronary artery disease [3]. The determinants of O_2 supply are coronary flow, diastolic blood pressure, and the diastolic time. On the other hand, determinants of O_2 demand are myocardial contractility, heart rate, and tension in the ventricular wall [influenced by preload (diastolic volume final) and afterload (systemic blood pressure)].

In clinical presentation, the typical patient with angina describes a sense of weight/pressure/constriction/suffocation in the chest (visceral). As Cecil et al. [3] added, a patient finds the discomfort on the sternum, usually hand in hand (Levine sign). In general, increasing the pain-decreasing pattern features, lasting 2–5 min, it may be referred to on shoulders and arms (also interscapular region, neck, jaw, and dental arch epigastrium). One must always remember that in women and diabetic patients, angina may have atypical location [2]. Ischemic pain does not radiate to the trapezius muscle, and in the setting of chest pain radiating to the trapezius, acute pericarditis should be suspected. It should be investigated also in careful history for anginal equivalent: dyspnea, nausea, fatigue, and fainting (more common in the elderly and diabetics):

- Dyspnea – drop in LV ejection fraction, leading to pulmonary congestion
- Fatigue, dizziness, and feeling faint – low cardiac output
- Transient mitral regurgitation – ischemia of the papillary muscles

- Palpitations – tachyarrhythmias induced by ischemia
- Nausea, vomiting, sweating, and pallor – neurovegetative symptoms

Bibliography

1. Fihn SD, et al. ACCF/AHA/ACP/AATS/PCNA/SCAI/STS Guideline for the Diagnosis and Management of Patients With Stable Ischemic Heart Disease: A Report of the American College of Cardiology Foundation/American Heart Association Task Force on Practice Guidelines, and the American College of Physicians, American Association for Thoracic Surgery, Preventive Cardiovascular Nurses Association, Society for Cardiovascular Angiography and Interventions, and Society of Thoracic Surgeons. Circulation. 2012;126(25):354–471.
2. Armaganijan D, Bodanese LC, Cesar LA, Ferreira JF, Gowdak LH, Mansur AP, et al. Diretriz de Doença Coronária Estável. Arq Bras Cardiol. 2014;103:1–59.
3. Cecil RL, Goldman L, Schafer AI. Cecil medicine. 24th ed. Rio de Janeiro: Elsevier; 2014.
4. Windecker S, et al. ESC/EACTS Guidelines on myocardial revascularization. European Heart Journal. 2014;35(37):2541–619.

Unusual Mechanism of Myocardial Infarction in Prosthetic Valve Endocarditis

Armindo Jreige Júnior, Felipe Bezerra Martins de Oliveira, Larissa Lucas Schloicka, Fernando Antibas Atik, and Claudio Ribeiro da Cunha

Clinical Presentation

A 46-year-old man presented with a history of dyspnea and fatigue exacerbated by a recent hospitalization related to pulmonary edema. The diagnosis was confirmed by echocardiography, which revealed the presence of a bicuspid aortic valve with a mixed lesion, predominantly stenotic. The left ventricle had moderate systolic dysfunction and severe concentric hypertrophy. Past medical history was consistent with hypertension. Surgery was indicated for symptomatic severe aortic stenosis. A preoperative coronary angiogram did not reveal any abnormalities. The patient was submitted to aortic valve replacement with a stented bioprosthesis. The operation and his postoperative recovery were uneventful. He was

The original version of this chapter was revised. A Correction to this chapter can be found at https://doi.org/10.1007/978-3-319-57084-6_41

A. Jreige Júnior (✉) · F. B. M. de Oliveira · L. L. Schloicka
F. A. Atik · C. R. da Cunha
Cardiology Institute of Federal District (ICDF), Brasília, DF, Brazil

R. M. S. Almeida, F. B. Jatene (eds.), *Cardiovascular Surgery*,
https://doi.org/10.1007/978-3-319-57084-6_16

prescribed the following medications to take at home: enalapril 5 mg twice daily, carvedilol 6.25 mg twice daily, furosemide 20 mg daily, and ferrous sulfate 300 mg daily (orally).

Approximately 1 month later, the patient returned, complaining of a high-grade fever and chills for a few days. He was admitted to the emergency department with acute-onset chest pain, dyspnea, and vomiting. On physical exam, he was lethargic, febrile, pale, and hemodynamically unstable, with cold extremities and faint pulses.

Diagnosis, Assessment, and Treatment

The admission electrocardiogram (ECG) is shown in Fig. 1. Laboratory values on admission demonstrated remarkable elevation of cardiac enzymes. The cardiologist on call interpreted the patient as having non-ST elevation acute coronary syndrome and treated him with aspirin, clopidogrel, morphine, and heparin. An emergent coronary angiogram (Fig. 2) revealed a long, complex lesion on the left main coronary artery (80% lumen obstruction) with tapering contour, suggesting extrinsic compression. Due to ongoing myocardial

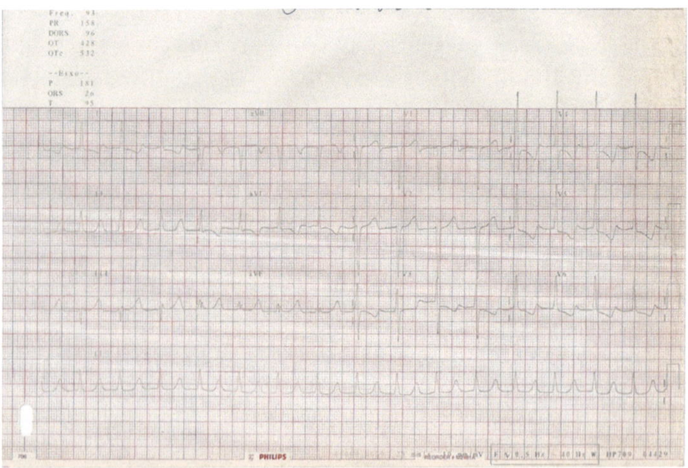

FIGURE 1 Admitting electrocardiogram

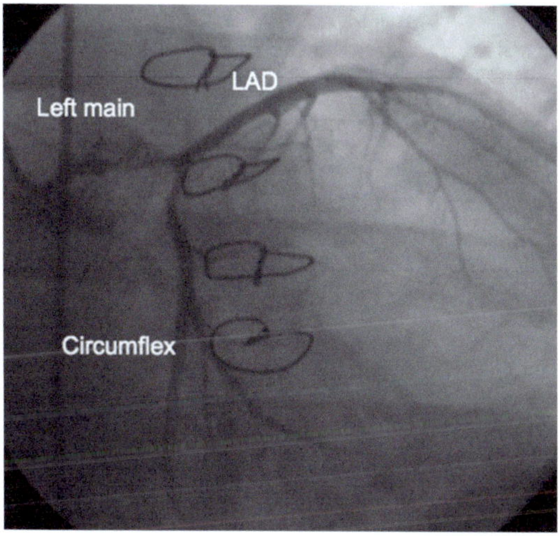

FIGURE 2 Coronary angiogram in the right anterior oblique showing a complex obstruction of the left main coronary artery (Abbreviation: LAD, left anterior descending)

ischemia and hemodynamic compromise, an intra-aortic balloon pump was inserted. The patient was further managed with intravenous fluids, inotropes, and mechanical ventilation. Blood cultures were drawn and identified as oxacillin-resistant *Staphylococcus epidermidis*. Before the blood cultures' results were available, broad-spectrum antibiotics (vancomycin, rifampicin, and imipenem) and also an antifungal drug (amphotericin B) were initiated empirically. Renal function was impaired. Transesophageal echocardiography showed vegetations attached to the prosthesis, aortic root abscess, and an aortic-to-right-atrium fistula. Left ventricle ejection fraction was 36%, and there were wall motion abnormalities on lateral and anterior walls. Chest computed tomography (Fig. 3) suggested that left main compression was due to aortic root abscess or hematoma.

Urgent reoperative aortic valve replacement was indicated. Postoperatively, the patient had acute renal failure requiring hemodialysis, sepsis, transient liver failure, prolonged mechanical ventilation and complete atrioventricular

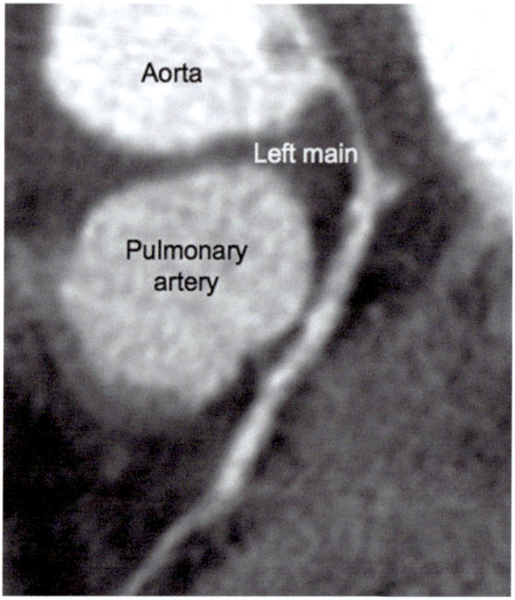

FIGURE 3 Chest computed tomography showing a long obstruction of the left main coronary artery due to extrinsic compression

block requiring permanent pacemaker. Antibiotic therapy, as previously mentioned, was initiated empirically with vancomycin, rifampicin, imipenem, and amphotericin B. Rifampicin was discontinued on the second day of use due to mild liver failure. Imipenem was used until the 14th postoperative day. Vancomycin was replaced by teicoplanin shortly after the operation due to acute renal failure, and it was used until the 30th postoperative day. Amphotericin B was used until the 34th postoperative day. Then, it was replaced by fluconazole, which was continued for a year thereafter.

A month after the operation, the left ventricular function had improved (ejection fraction of 58%) with a mildly dilated ventricle and a normal aortic valve function. The patient was discharged home 6 weeks after surgery in good condition, with no signs of active infection. At 36-month follow-up, the patient is currently in New York Heart Association functional class I

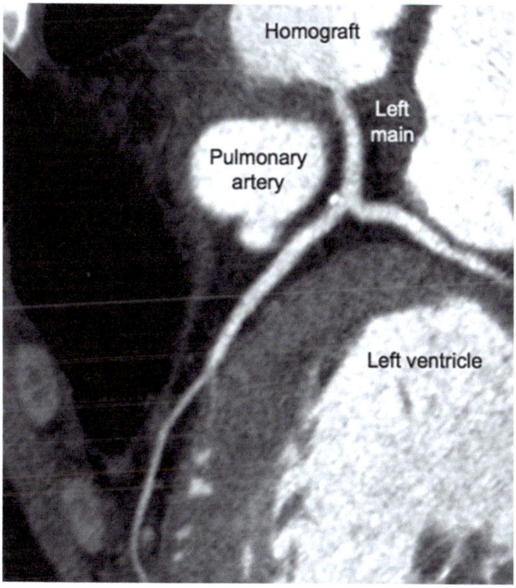

FIGURE 4 Late postoperative chest computed tomography revealed a patent left coronary artery after homograft root replacement

with no recurrent infection, and the ventricular function is normal. The left main is widely patent and the saphenous vein graft is occluded on control chest computed tomography (Fig. 4).

Questions

1. Report the ECG in Fig. 1

Admitting electrocardiogram revealed normal sinus rhythm, signs of left ventricle hypertrophy, and ST depression on posterior and lateral leads.

2. What are the complications of prosthetic valve endocarditis?

Although infrequent (1–4% in the first year), infective endocarditis may occur after aortic valve replacement [8]. Prosthetic valve endocarditis is associated with elevated hospital mortality (approximately 40%) [4] and morbidity dependent on the infecting pathogen, duration of illness prior to therapy, and underlying comorbidities.

The main complications of endocarditis, by prevalence, are occurrences of cardiac complications (severe heart failure, valve injury, pericarditis, acute myocardial infarction, conduction abnormalities, fistulous communication, perivalvular abscess, and others), neurologic complications (cerebral embolism, mycotic aneurysms, meningitis, stroke, intracranial hemorrhage, cerebral abscess, and others), septic complications (infection unresponsive to treatment, persistent fever, disseminated intravascular coagulation, and others), renal complications (renal failure, nephrotic syndrome), extracranial systemic arterial complications, septic pulmonary embolisms, three splenic infarctions or abscesses, and some other complications associated with infective endocarditis [6].

3. What is the clinical presentation of acute coronary syndromes in patients with endocarditis?

Clinical presentation of acute coronary syndromes in patients with endocarditis is similar to those with coronary artery disease. As systems attempt to meet stringent door-to-balloon initiatives, it becomes imperative that a detailed history and physical exam be performed in this narrow time window in order to avoid unnecessary tests and/or therapeutic regimens.

4. What investigation is most likely to be diagnostic in this case?

The diagnostic workup of a patient with a clinical history of high-grade fever and chills within a month after a straightforward aortic valve replacement with known absence of coronary artery disease includes, firstly, a transesophageal echocardiography [5]. It has a sensitivity and a specificity for abscess detection of 87% and 95%, respectively [2]. Coronary angiogram in this particular patient was indicated based on a misdiagnosis of coronary artery disease. Although the angiographic appearance is typical (complex and long lesion that often disappears on diastole), a coronary angiogram should be avoided because it may cause dislodgement of septic fragments, which fortunately did not occur in this particular case.

5. What are the most likely mechanisms responsible for myocardial infarction during infective endocarditis?

The present case describes a rare complication of prosthetic valve endocarditis, an aortic root abscess causing external coronary artery compression and acute myocardial infarction. Acute coronary syndromes are uncommon in prosthetic valve endocarditis, with a prevalence of between 1% and 3% [1]. The most likely mechanisms responsible for myocardial ischemia during infective endocarditis are the presence of preexisting coronary artery disease and coronary emboli from aortic vegetations. Other less frequent mechanisms have been described, such as obstruction of the coronary ostium due to large vegetation and severe aortic insufficiency [1, 3]. External coronary artery compression due to infective endocarditis is also a described mechanism but is a rare occurrence with only a few cases reported in medical literature [3, 9].

6. Why did this patient receive empiric antibiotic therapy?

The isolation of the causative organism of prosthetic valve endocarditis is essential, and antibiotic therapy should be delayed pending the blood culture results in cases of patients who are hemodynamically stable with an indolent clinical course. However, patients presenting hemodynamic instability or acute disease should receive empiric broad-spectrum antibiotic therapy promptly [7]. Therapy should be subsequently adjusted according to the culture results. The American Heart Association (AHA) and the European Society of Cardiology (ESC) guidelines recommend that prosthetic valve endocarditis should be treated for at least 6 weeks with an adequate bactericidal agent.

7. How do you justify the urgent operation despite the patient's condition?

Although the patient was a very high-risk surgical candidate, the urgent operation was justified due to patient's age and treatable heart problems, despite the presence of active infection, aortic root invasion, and abscess.

8. How should the patient be managed in the urgent operation?

The operation was performed with the aid of hypothermic cardiopulmonary bypass with aortic and bicaval cannulation. Myocardial protection was achieved with cold blood cardioplegia delivered through the coronary ostium and coronary sinus. An oblique aortic arteriotomy revealed a large anterior aortic root abscess, which had invaded the left and right coronary cuspids. The bioprosthesis was removed, and the abscess was evacuated; complete debridement of all infected material was also performed. Both coronary buttons were carefully mobilized and cleaned of all infected tissue. The aortic annulus was severely destroyed by the infection. Aortic root replacement with cryopreserved homograft was performed using interrupted monofilament sutures. The coronary buttons were directly reimplanted on the homograft with continuous sutures. The aortic-to-right-atrium fistula was closed with an autologous pericardium patch. Additionally, a coronary artery bypass grafting with a reversed saphenous vein graft to left anterior descending artery was performed. Prolonged cardiopulmonary bypass and mediastinal bleeding were problems in the operating room, requiring vigorous transfusion and delayed chest closure on the next day. Cultures drawn in the operating room were negative.

Bibliography

1. Attias D, Messika-Zeitoun D, Wolf M, Lepage L, Vahanian A. Acute coronary syndrome in aortic infective endocarditis. Eur J Echocardiogr. 2008;9:727–8.
2. Daniel WG, Mugge A, Martin RP, Lindert O, Hausmann D, Nonnast-Daniel B, Laas J, Lichtlen PR. Improvement in the diagnosis of abscesses associated with endocarditis by transesophageal echocardiography. N Engl J Med. 1991;324:795–800.
3. Harinstein ME, Marroquin OC. External coronary artery compression due to prosthetic valve bacterial endocarditis. Catheter Cardiovasc Interv. 2014;83:E168–70.
4. Hoen B, Duval X. Infective endocarditis. N Engl J Med. 2013;369:785.
5. Horton CJ Jr, Nanda NC, Nekkanti R, Mukhtar O, Mcgiffin D. Prosthetic aortic valve abscess producing total right coronary

artery occlusion: diagnosis by transesophageal three-dimensional echocardiography. Echocardiography. 2002;19:395–8.
6. Mansur AJ, Grinberg M, Da Luz PL, Bellotti G. The complications of infective endocarditis. A reappraisal in the 1980s. Arch Intern Med. 1992;152:2428–32.
7. Manzano MC, Vilacosta I, San Roman JA, Aragoncillo P, Sarria C, Lopez D, Lopez J, Revilla A, Manchado R, Hernandez R, Rodriguez E. Acute coronary syndrome in infective endocarditis. Rev Esp Cardiol. 2007;60:24–31.
8. Millaire A, Van Belle E, De Groote P, Leroy O, Ducloux G. Obstruction of the left main coronary ostium due to an aortic vegetation: survival after early surgery. Clin Infect Dis. 1996;22:192–3.
9. Zoffoli G, Gherli T. Images in cardiovascular medicine. Periaortic valve abscess presenting as unstable angina. Circulation. 2005;112:e240–1.

Part V
Congenital Heart Disease

Atrioventricular Septal Defect with Pulmonary Hypertension After the First Year of Life

Raphaella von Sohsten Calabria Lima, Laryssa Alves de Farias, Assiane Gabriela Anceles da Rocha, and Pedro Rafael Salerno

Clinical Presentation

A female infant, 1 year and 10 months old with Down syndrome, arrived at the emergency room. The mother reported that her child was presenting fatigue on efforts and cyanosis since birth and suffering from repeated respiratory infections but never was seen by a cardiologist. She also reported cough, runny nose, and nasal obstruction for the last 5 days.

Upon admission, physical examination revealed regular general condition. She was ruddy, hydrated, and dyspneic and had perioral and peripheral cyanosis. Respiratory rate was 66 ipm, with a bilateral vesicular murmur, normal capillary filling, and oxygen saturation (SaO_2) of 87% on ambient air. Heart rate was 160 bpm and cardiac auscultation revealed regular heart rhythm with a systolic murmur +6/+6 on the left sternal border, while second heart sound was hyperphonetic.

R. von Sohsten Calabria Lima (✉) · L. A. de Farias
A. G. A. da Rocha · P. R. Salerno
Catholic University of Pernambuco (UNICAP), Recife, PE, Brazil

R. M. S. Almeida, F. B. Jatene (eds.), *Cardiovascular Surgery*,
https://doi.org/10.1007/978-3-319-57084-6_17

The patient also presented flaccid abdomen, liver at 5 cm from the right costal margin, spleen not palpable, and the presence of bowel sounds.

Diagnosis, Assessment, and Treatment

The chest X-ray showed enlarged cardiac area with global cardiomegaly and signs of increased pulmonary flow. There were also signs of bronchopneumonia (Fig. 1). The electrocardiogram (ECG) showed sinus rhythm, delayed right ventricular conduction, left anterior fascicular block, left ventricular hypertrophy with repolarization abnormality, ST elevation, and prolonged QT (Fig. 2). The echocardiogram showed an atrioventricular septal defect (AVSD) type A of Rastelli, significant tricuspid valve insufficiency, persistent ductus arteriosus (PDA), severe pulmonary hypertension, and mild pericardial effusion. Systolic pulmonary artery pressure was estimated as 90 mmHg by the ECG.

At the intensive care unit (ICU), laboratory exams showed compatible signs of infection. She began treatment with ceftriaxone 100 mg/kg/day once a day and furosemide

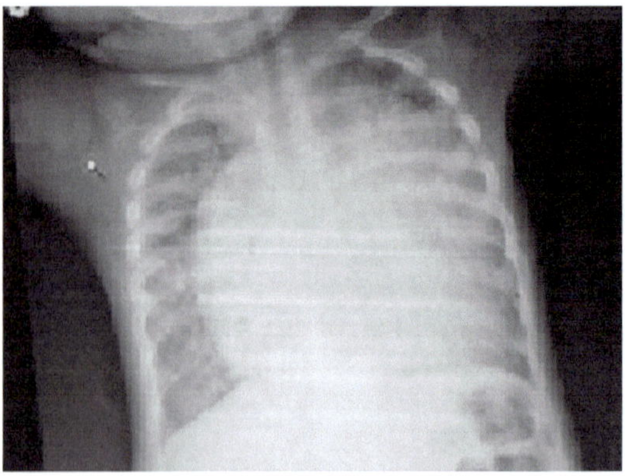

Figure 1 Chest X-ray showing increased cardiac area by right cameras and dilated pulmonary artery

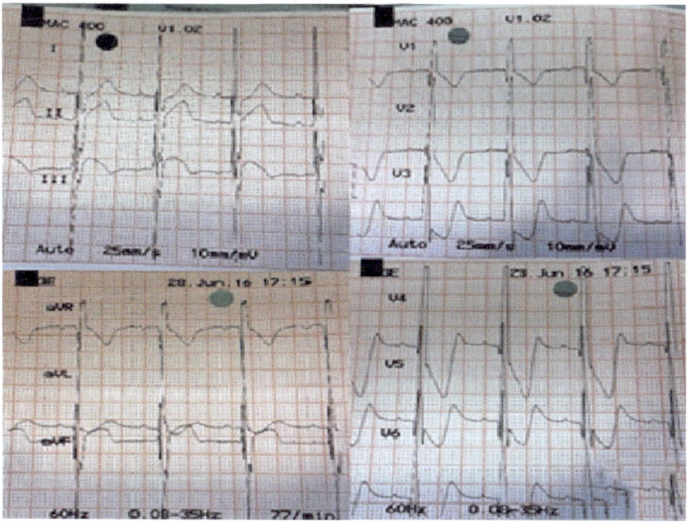

FIGURE 2 EKG shows sinus rhythm, delayed right ventricular conduction, left anterior fascicular block, left ventricular hypertrophy with repolarization abnormality, ST elevation, and prolonged QT

2 mg/kg/day four times a day. ICU stay was uneventful and the patient was discharged in good clinical condition. Cardiac catheterization was requested and presented as conclusions total atrium-ventricular septal defect, important failure of atrioventricular (AV) valve, small patent ductus arteriosus, pulmonary hypertension, high pulmonary vascular resistance (PVR), and vasoreactivity test response with a decrease of 92% in PVR and an increase of 4,3% of the pulmonary artery mean pressure. On ventilation with $FiO_2 = 100\%$, the PVR was 0,64 UW and Qp/Qs was 20,62:1. (Fig. 3).

Surgical treatment of AVSD was chosen. The total correction was performed with moderate hypothermic (28 °C) cardiopulmonary bypass (CPB). The monitoring was held by EKG, pulse oximetry, and mean arterial pressure through right radial catheter. Proper asepsis was performed.

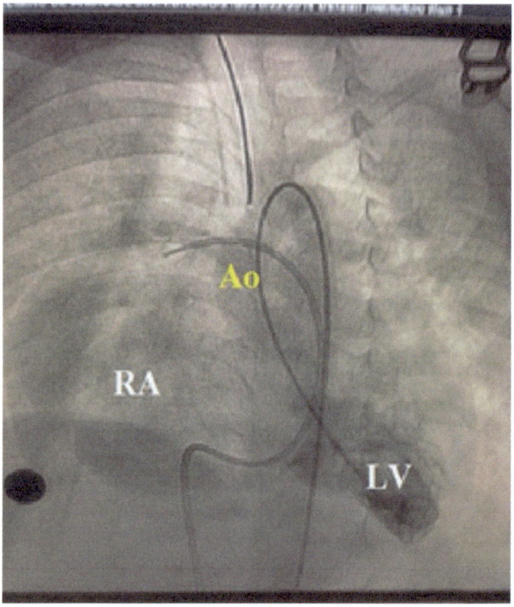

FIGURE 3 Cardiac catheterization shows dilated right atrium, left ventricle with final diastolic volume and contractile function preserved, goose neck signal, and ascendent aorta with reduced caliber

The surgical technique consisted in a transsternal median thoracotomy and pericardiotomy spotting an enlarged cardiac area 3+/4+ related to increased right cavities and dilated pulmonary trunk. Afterward, dissection of the ductus arteriosus was performed, followed by ligature with cotton thread. Preparation for CPB was done by lowering temperature to 28 °C and using blood cardioplegia at 8 °C, which was repeated every 30 min.

The aorta was clamped. A right atriotomy was performed, evidencing thickened walls and an AVSD with large atrial septal defect (ASD). All the strings of the posterior leaflet presented at the top of the septum and a wide slit and dilation of the left AV valve ring were found. On the anterior portion of the leaflet, the strings were repaired with continuous suture Prolene 6.0. A flap of bovine pericardium was sutured, dividing the leaflet into left and right valves. The closure of left valve cleft was performed with 5.0 Prolene. Testing the valves with saline solution, both proved competent. The ostium primum ASD atrioseptoplasty was performed with a bovine pericardium patch, and the ostium secundum ASD was partially closed, leaving a 4 mm aperture, finishing the procedure with right atrial suture. Removal of air cavities was done and the recovery rate was in sinus rhythm. The temperature was normalized and the patient was removed from CPB and cannulas. Protamine was done, hemostasis reviewed, and two pacemaker wires installed on the right ventricle (RV). Lastly, mediastinal drainage with 18 drain and curative were performed.

The patient was transferred to the ICU. Prophylactic and therapeutic vancomycin was initiated. Platelets, vasoactive drugs, and vitamin K were needed. The patient was submitted to a new chest X-ray that showed decreased cardiac area and less pulmonary congestion (Fig. 4). A new echocardiogram was performed showing no residual defects and decreased pulmonary artery hypertension.

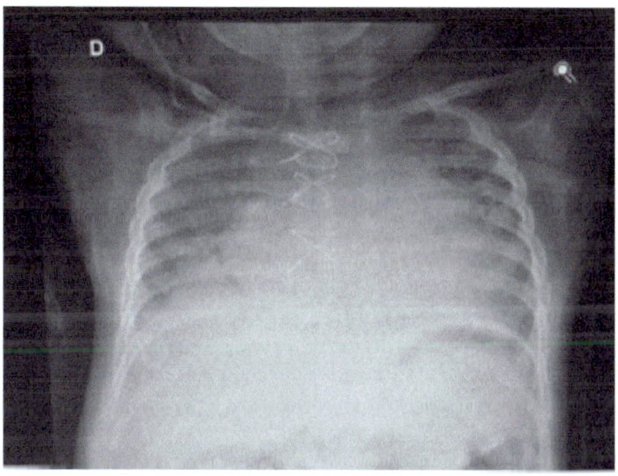

FIGURE 4 Chest X ray after surgical treatment. Considerable reduced size of right atrium and pulmonary congestion is observed

Questions

1. The case describes a congenital heart defect diagnosed at 1 year and 10 months. Why does the time of this diagnosis affect the actual severity of the disease?

The late diagnosis of this disease is directly related to the progress of anatomical and functional changes. The left-right shunt due to both the ASD and the VSD leads to pulmonary hyperflow and, over time, the presence of pulmonary hypertension, heart failure, pneumonia, and arrhythmias, including atrial premature contractions, supraventricular tachycardia, and atrial fibrillation. The magnitude of the shunt increases with age, and the continuous increase in vascular pressure leads to a remodeling of the pulmonary vessels and right ventricular failure. All this can lead to pulmonary complications high resistance type, such as pulmonary vascular occlusive disease.

2. Early diagnosis of congenital heart disease is essential to prevent or treat pulmonary hypertension in early stages. How could it be done?

Structural malformations usually occur in the first trimester of pregnancy and are not always detected by routine ultrasonography. Only fetal two-dimensional Doppler echocardiography can determine more accurately the presence of a heart problem. The AVSD with all its morphological variants are among the diseases most easily detected by fetal echocardiography. It is important to note that the identification of the common atrioventricular valve, usually with a septal defect of the ostium primum and often with an inflow tract ventricular septal defect (VSD), is the registered trademark of the defect. The presence of systolic regurgitation of one or both components of the atrioventricular valve is the rule, with a possible detection by both pulsed Doppler and the color flow mapping. Early diagnosis combined with effective surgical treatment is primarily responsible for the reduction of morbidity and mortality in this population. In this matter, it is important to consider the difficulty of access to health care because this patient lives in the countryside of Brazil, and despite the high incidence of cardiac malformations and progression to pulmonary hypertension in people with Down syndrome, she was never forwarded to the mandatory investigation of congenital heart disease, although it has shown symptoms of this condition from birth.

3. What anatomophysiological factor could justify a worse prognosis in patients with Down syndrome, when compared with another patient suffering from the same heart disease, however, with no syndrome?

The atrioventricular septal defect is basically characterized by pulmonary hyperflow in the first weeks of life, but symptoms and signs of this disease may be absent in the first days of life. However, several authors have suggested that children with Down syndrome develop earlier and more rapidly progressive pulmonary vascular changes than children who do not carry the syndrome. A possible explanation for this is that patients with Down syndrome often have enlarged tongue and nasal turbinate hypertrophy, which leads to a state of hypoventilation added to the hyperflow. Thus, chronic hypoxia is a potent promoter of pathological vascular remodeling. This patient also has an aggravating factor for pulmonary hypertension, patent ductus arteriosus, which also causes hyperflow. However, in some cases, children with Down syndrome may also have no earlier symptoms, as in this case. Therefore, it is worth noting that pulmonary hypertension in patients with Down syndrome may be influenced by many factors such as chronic airway obstruction, abnormal growth of the pulmonary vasculature, alveolar hypoventilation, decreased number of alveoli, and thinner pulmonary arterioles, among others.

4. Atrioventricular septal defect (AVSD) is currently classified in the group of acyanogenic congenital heart diseases. What would be the explanation for this patient to present peripheral and perioral cyanosis?

The presence of moderate cyanosis (oxygen saturation 80–85%) in patients with AVSD is suggestive of pulmonary vascular obstructive disease or Eisenmenger syndrome. Thus the defect of AVSD is considered an acyanogenic heart disease, but some complications of this disease can cause cyanosis. As the pulmonary vascular resistance increases, the flow resistance into the pulmonary circulation possibly exceeds the resistance to flow into the systemic circulation, leading to the right-left shunt, resulting in varying degrees of cyanosis. The Eisenmenger syndrome is particularly common in patients with AVSD and Down syndrome. In this case, probably the perioral and peripheral cyanosis was associated with respiratory infection, as well as pulmonary hyperflow.

Are there differences between AVSD with and without Down syndrome?

Most patients with Down syndrome have more of a heart structural defect concomitantly. The highest prevalence is AVSD associated with tetralogy of Fallot and patent ductus arteriosus. While in patients without Down syndrome, the AVSD appears more associated with the right ventricular double-outflow tract and the double aortic arch.

Surgical correction of AVSD should be performed preferably between 4 and 12 months old. What were the surgical criteria for this patient?

If the patient still has symptoms of heart failure (tachypnea, little weight gain, hepatomegaly) and cardiac catheterization shows typical angiogram, Qp/Qs = 1.67, and PVR = 6.5 U/m^2, surgical treatment should be done despite the cyanosis and high strength. Patients with complete atrioventricular septal defect associated with left-right shunt signals with lower pulmonary vascular resistance than 6 U/m^2 may be considered candidates for surgical treatment. The long-term monitoring of patients with ventricular septal defect and superior resistance to 6 U/m^2 has shown good results in 79% with a significant reduction in the pulmonary pressure. A comprehensive analysis of previous clinical and laboratory data surgery can guide the appropriate management.

What types of surgery are available to correct AVSD?

There are the corrective and palliative surgical treatments for AVSD. The corrective surgical treatment aims to close the atrial septal defect, close ventricular septal defect, avoid damage to the conduction tissue, and create two atrioventricular valves. This treatment should be carried out using two flaps of autologous or bovine pericardium, and the cusps sutured. If the valves are not viable, the patient may be required to return for an implantation of a cardiac prothesis. The palliative procedure consists in pulmonary artery banding, reducing blood flow to the lungs. However, a drop in blood oxygenation arises, especially after a few months when the child grows, increasing demand for oxygen. At this time, there will be the need for reoperation to remove the pulmonary banding and perform corrective surgery.

What is the relation between the types of surgical techniques and mortality?

The first surgical experiences for correction of this defect were associated with high mortality rates often due to conduction tissue injuries, severe regurgitation of the atrioventricular valve, and subaortic stenosis. Although surgical mortality in the correction of AVSD has declined significantly in the last decade, surgical treatment remains a challenge. However, some authors report that mortality is higher in the surgical technique with single retail. When the technique of one flap is replaced by the two flaps, AVSD repair is easier because it creates less distortion and facilitates obtaining a sufficient valve. Palliative treatment with pulmonary artery banding, which in the past had a mortality of about 50%, still today has a mortality of 5–10%, even in patients with mild impairment of atrioventricular valve. The combined mortality of palliative surgery with total correction makes early corrective surgery the best alternative.

Review About the Addressed Disease or Treatment

The AVSD is the most frequent congenital heart disease in patients with Down syndrome, corresponding to 40% of all heart disease in this group of patients [1]. The AVSD is classified as an acyanogenic congenital heart disease pulmonary blood flow, and therefore, patients in this risk group have more often a pulmonary hypertension frame (HP). The most common form, which causes greater comorbidity in patients with Down syndrome, is the complete form of AVSD. AVSD can be classified into three types: Rastelli types A, B, and C. The AVSD Rastelli type A is the most frequent in patients with Down syndrome and is characterized by the complete overlap of the upper left sheet on the left ventricle [2]. In the AVSD, there is the presence of an ASD, VSD, as well as a single atrioventricular valve. As a consequence of these findings, there is a progressive increase in volume of blood into the lung, causing, therefore, dyspnea and respiratory symptoms.

Preoperative assessment of pulmonary hypertension and operability in these cases is a hard choice. Complementary tests and clinical history provide primary data for surgery. The chest radiography shows signs of pulmonary blood flow, and when there is obstructive disease present, the exams demonstrate hypertranslucency and dilation of hilar vessels [3]. Angiography and cardiac catheterization are used for measurement of pulmonary vascular resistance.

This patient is a carrier of Down syndrome and presented ASVD type A of Rastelli with severe hypertension evidenced by echocardiography. Clinical studies have demonstrated the relationship between Down syndrome and pulmonary hypertension as the predominant clinical feature [4]. In addition, the chest radiography obtained by the patient showed significant cardiomegaly with dilatation fo the right cameras and of the pulmonary trunk. This radiographic finding demonstrates a volume overload in the right ventricle, probably due to the increased of pulmonary blood flow. Angiography performed by the patient had pulmonary vascular resistance index of 1 U/m^2, as important for surgery, since patients with pulmonary vascular resistance index less than 6 U/m^2 are eligible for correction surgery AVSD, even when they have pulmonary hypertension as a risk factor.

Surgical time is a key factor to increase the improvement rates of clinical and survival of patients with this pathology. The indicated age for total corrective surgery is from 4 to 6 months of life [5] and should not be delayed due to the risk of pulmonary occlusive vascular disease. Several authors [6–8] have suggested that children with Down syndrome develop changes in the pulmonary vasculature earlier and more progressively, compared with children not living with the syndrome. In addition, patients with pulmonary hypertension present a significant risk factor in the surgical time. It is known that patients with AVSD without surgical treatment evolve to worse prognostic.

Bibliography

1. Mahadevaiah G, Gupta M, Ashwath R. Down syndrome with complete atrioventricular septal defect, hypertrophic cardiomyopathy, and pulmonary vein stenosis. Tex Heart Inst J. 2015;42(5):458–61.
2. Saadi EK, Shore D, Lincoln C. Risk factors analysis in the surgical repair of complete atrioventricular septal defect. Rev Bras Cir Cardiovasc. 1993;2(8):136–51.
3. Huber J, Peres VC, Santos TJ, Beltrão LF, Baumont AC, Cañedo AD, Schaan BA, Pellanda LC. Congenital heart diseases in a reference service: clinical evolution and associated illnesses. Arq Bras Cardiol. 2010;94(3):333–8.
4. Mourato FA, Villachan LRR, Mattos SS. Prevalence and profile of congenital heart disease and pulmonary hypertension in Down syndrome in a pediatric cardiology service. Rev Paul Pediatr. 2014;32(2):159–63.
5. Ferrín LM, Atik E, Ikari NM, Martins TC, Marcial MB, Ebaid M. Complete atrioventricular canal. Clinical-anatomic correlations between patients with and without Down's syndrome. Arq Bras Cardiol. 1997;69(1):19–23.
6. Newfeld E, Sher M, Paul MH, Nikaidoh H. Pulmonary vascular disease in complete atrioventricular canal defects. Am J Cardiol. 1997;39(5):721–6.
7. Clapp S, Perry BL, Farooki ZQ. Down's syndrome, common atrioventricular canal, and pulmonary vascular obstructive disease. J Thorac Cardiovasc Surg. 1990;100(1):115–21.
8. Shaler R, Farina M, Porter I, Bishop M. Clinical aspects of congenital heart disease in mongolism. Am J Cardiol. 1972;29(4):497–503.

Surgical Treatment of Atrial Septal Defect by Occluder Device

Laura Gomes Flores, Cassiana Tomazoni, Patrícia Freitag, Evandro Luis Queiroz Flores, and Rui M. S. Almeida

Clinical Presentation

A 46-year-old patient, male, under cardiac evaluation. He claims palpitations and denies fatigue and dyspnea. He performs daily physical activity – walking 10 km/day. With a history of superior mesenteric venous thrombosis in January 2016, diagnosis of thrombophilia without other comorbidities. He takes rivaroxaban (20 mg 1×/day), losartan (50 mg), and HCTZ (12.5 mg in the mornings). He denies smoking and alcoholism. He has positive family history of coronary artery disease. On the physical examination, there were prominent and prominent systolic impulses in the chest region, palpable pulmonary artery pulsations in the second left intercostal space, mesodiastolic tinnitus in the lower left sternal margin, normal pulse, and wide and fixed division of the S2.

L. G. Flores (✉) · C. Tomazoni · P. Freitag · E. L. Q. Flores
Assis Gurgacz Foundation University (FAG), Cascavel, PR, Brazil

R. M. S. Almeida
Department of Cardiology and Cardiovascular Surgery, University Center Assis Gurgacz Foundation, Cascavel, PR, Brazil

R. M. S. Almeida, F. B. Jatene (eds.), *Cardiovascular Surgery*,
https://doi.org/10.1007/978-3-319-57084-6_18

Diagnosis, Assessment, and Treatment

First, electrocardiograms were requested, which showed sinus rhythm, frequency of 75 bpm, axis deviation to the right, rSr' pattern in right precordial leads (dilation of the right ventricular outflow tract), and chest X-ray, which revealed an increase in the right atrium and ventricle, pulmonary artery, and its branches. Due to the alterations found, uni-/bidimensional/Doppler echocardiography was requested, which showed increased LV parietal thickness, a slight increase in the LA cavity size, and mitral flow with increased A wave (E/A ratio < 1), indicating alteration of the diastolic relaxation of the LV and pulmonary flow with increased velocity (V = 1.52 m/s). Transesophageal echocardiography was then requested to investigate an anomaly that caused left-to-right shunt, which revealed an interatrial septum with a wide ostium secundum atrial septal defect (ASD) (D: 30 mm) (Fig. 18.1), with a bidirectional shunt, showing a bigger left-to-right shunt (Fig. 18.2). Thus, the diagnosis of ostium secundum ASD was confirmed. Due to its size and shape, significant left-to-right shunt (ratio of pulmonary to systemic flow> or = 2:1), and not having developed severe pulmonary hypertension, percutaneous closure of the ASD by occluder device was chosen.

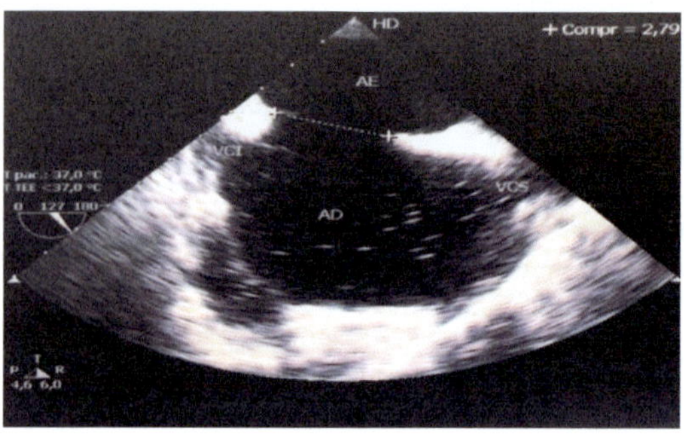

FIGURE 1 Echocardiography revealing interatrial septum with extensive ASD ostium secundum (D: 30 mm)

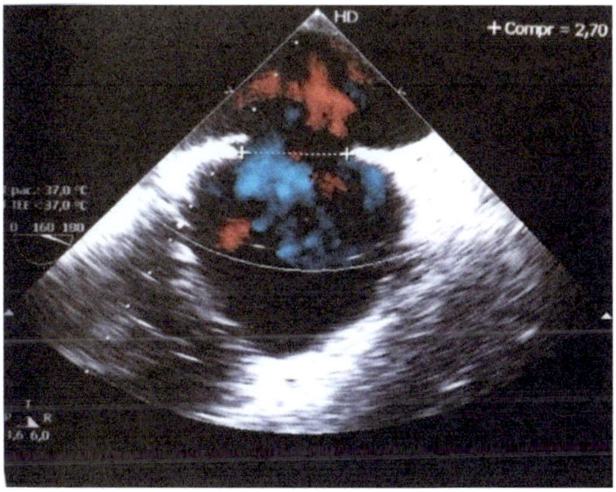

FIGURE 2 Echocardiography revealing atrial septal defect with a big left-to-right flow

The procedure is monitored by transesophageal echocardiography, and the access route is the femoral vein. Right and left catheterization is performed with pressure measurement in the various cavities, always taking care to identify pulmonary venous drainage. Next, a rigid guide, distally, is placed in the left superior pulmonary vein. On it, the measuring balloon is introduced, positioned through the defect, to obtain the stretched diameter (SD) (Fig. 18.3). The choice of prosthesis size obeys the standard criterion two to four millimeters above the SD. The occlusion device used was the Amplatzer prosthesis, with two self-expanding disks corresponding to the size of the atrial septal defect (ASD) (Fig. 18.4). A long sheath, of caliper compatible with the size of the prosthesis chosen, is positioned in the left atrium. Inside it, the Amplatzer prosthesis is carried and the distal disk is externalized. The prosthesis-sheath assembly is pulled toward the septum, and, by maintaining adequate tension in the system, the proximal disk is exteriorized in the right atrium. If the position is considered satisfactory and without periprosthetic residual flow, the device is detached from the release system, and the procedure is terminated [11]. After the procedure, the patient remained stable. The next morning, he was discharged, with instructions

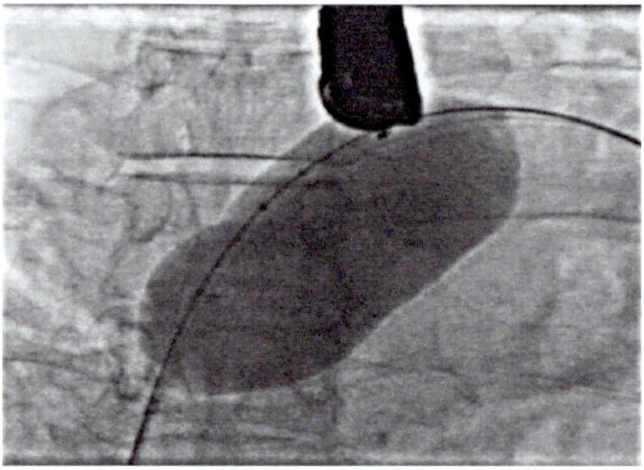

FIGURE 3 Preballoon implant for better accommodation and sizing of the prosthesis

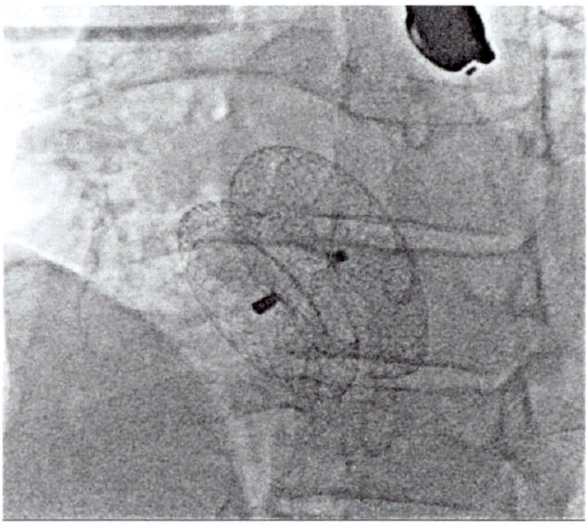

FIGURE 4 Occluder deployed

to use aspirin (200 mg) and to maintain the prophylactic antibiotic therapy, which began a few hours before the procedure, for 6 months. Clinical and echocardiographic evaluations were also requested – in which the patient reported complete remission of palpitation.

Questions

1. What are they, and how are different types of atrial septal defect distinguished?

We can distinguish different types of ASD by somatic embryogenesis mechanism presumably affected: persistent ostium primum ASD, ASD at the level of the oval fossa, and persistent ostium secundum ASD.

Persistent ostium primum ASD arises most often the abnormality of the atrioventricular cushions, which do not offer conditions for the grounding of atrial septa. The passage between the chambers will persist near the floor of the atria, truly representative of passage called ostium primum.

ASD within oval fossa, the most frequent type of ASDs, has one or more holes located within the limbo of the oval fossa.

Persistent ostium secundum ASD has passages between atria situated at the level of secundum ostium, being then a passage between the atria located in the cranial portion of the septum, near the mouth of the superior vena cava [7].

2. What factors influence the magnitude of the right-left shunt through the atrial septal defect?

The magnitude of the right-left shunt depends on the defect size, the relative compliance of the ventricles, and the relative resistance in the pulmonary and systemic circulations.

In patients with small atrial septal defects, left atrial pressure may exceed the right by several millimeters of mercury (mmHg), while, when the defect is large, the average pressure of both atria are almost identical.

During fetal life, the interatrial communication allows a right-to-left shunt. Soon after birth, the left-to-right blood flow is still limited by high pulmonary vascular resistance, low systemic vascular resistance, and reduced right ventricular compliance of the newborn. Over time, the pulmonary vascular resistance decreases and systemic vascular resistance increases, and then the interatrial communication allows shunting from left to right, which predominantly occurs at the end of ventricular systole and early diastole, with some increasing during atrial contraction. The shunt results in diastolic overload of the right ventricle and increased pulmonary blood flow [7].

3. What are the differences in cardiac auscultation of atrial septal defect compared to those found in acyanogenic congenital heart disease?

When the systolic murmur is characterized by its ejection, rude tone, being more audible in the upper left sternal border, and most of the time not accompanied by tremor, but by a second noise fixedly deployed and hyperphonetic, the diagnostic suspicion falls on atrial septal defect.

Holosystolic murmur, presenting variable tone, according to the degree of impact of the defect, with musical tone, the one with lesser magnitude and ruder the one with higher tone, usually accompanied by fremitus, low on the left sternal border and radiating to the right border, indicates diagnosis of ventricular septal defect (VSD).

Continuous murmur in the pulmonary area, with or without fremitus, with varying tones, is very suggestive of the ductus arteriosus.

In partial atrioventricular septal defect, the ejection systolic murmur, down the left sternal border, results from the discrete passage of blood from left to the right by the interventricular communication, due to the presence of reactive pulmonary hypertension, which limits and restricts the pulmonary flow and the impact of heart disease [5].

4. What is the natural history of this disease?

The cases where lung flow ratio divided by the systemic blood flow is less than 1.5 usually have important repercussions. In cases of moderate or large ASDs (with flow ratio above 1.5), patients usually remain asymptomatic until the third or fourth decade of life, when there is right ventricular dysfunction and patients begin to show signs and symptoms of right-sided heart failure. It rarely evolves to Eisenmenger syndrome.

Symptomatic patients often complain of dyspnea and fatigue. They may present symptoms related to right-sided heart failure, supraventricular arrhythmias, or embolization cases [3].

5. What are tests requested in the investigation of CIA?

Electrocardiogram typically has sinus rhythm and right ventricular overload. It is common to record complex QRS of rSr' morphology in the right precordial, generally of small scale; in the left precordial, the QRS complexes appear with thickened S waves. Only in the third or fourth decade atrial fibrillation may appear, atrial flutter or atrial tachycardia, especially in patients with severe left-to-right shunt.

Chest radiography is useful and presents increase in the pulmonary vasculature with bulging of the pulmonary trunk and increased heart area – by the increasing of RV and RA.

Echocardiography shows biatrial dilation and RV dilation; it usually identifies directly the location, size, and atrial septal flow. Transesophageal echocardiogram is indicated for the percutaneous closure; it determines the number and size of the defect, identifies the edges, shows the correct position of the prosthesis, and evaluates residual shunt, compromising the atrioventricular valves.

Cardiac catheterization is restricted to cases in which a study of pulmonary hypertension must be carried out in surgical patients over 40 years old, in situations where the echocardiogram shows no clear definition, mainly in the presence of associated injuries, and to guide percutaneous treatment [1, 4, 9].

6. In addition to percutaneous closure occluder device, to which other therapeutic modalities that patient could have been submitted?

The patient could have been subjected to surgical repair, usually accomplished with pericardial patch or prosthetic material, indicated as percutaneous occlusion in all patients with ostium secundum ASD, uncomplicated, with significant left-to-right shunt, that is, ratio between the pulmonary and systemic flows > or = 2:1.

If this patient had pulmonary hypertension, or some restriction to intervention treatment, the treatment of choice would be the clinical one, which is given for immediate eradication of respiratory infections, use of antiarrhythmic agents for atrial fibrillation or supraventricular tachycardia, usual measures to control high blood pressure, and treatment of any coronary artery disease or congestive heart failure [3].

7. What are the indications for percutaneous closure of atrial septal defect of the ostium secundum?

It is indicated for patients with clinical significance and flow ratio greater than 1.5:1, having diameters ranging from 6 to 34 mm. It is important that the edges of the ASD are consistent to support the prosthesis and that the defect has a distance of at least 5 mm from the right superior pulmonary vein, the mitral valve, and coronary sinus, so that these structures are not compromised by the occluder device. Patient selection is done by transesophageal echocardiography, which also serves as a guide for choosing the diameter of the prosthesis, proper positioning of it, and the presence or absence of residual shunt.

The percutaneous closure indication should be similar to the indications for surgery, with no justification for being performed, because it is a less invasive method, in very small ASDs or with no effects or complications [7, 10].

8. What is the echocardiogram most indicated for percutaneous closure of atrial septal defect? And what are the advantages of its use?

In closing ASD by devices introduced percutaneously, transesophageal echocardiography (TEE) is indispensable not only for the selection of candidates but especially in the hemodynamic room, for positioning and release of the prosthesis, besides the immediate evaluation of residual flows and the late follow-up. More specific information regarding the characteristics of defects, such as number of holes, their size, location in the septum, and characteristics of the edges that surround them, are better evaluated by transesophageal echocardiography, which can be performed on an outpatient basis or immediately before the procedure, in the hemodynamics room. Performing the transesophageal study prior to the catheterization day brings advantages concerning the procedure programming, device selection that will be used, and family counseling.

In percutaneous closure of ASD, echocardiography helps the orifice size and the choice of the device number to be used. It also monitors the positioning of guide wires, sheaths, and catheters within the heart and determines the arrangement of the left and right disks of the prosthesis before and after its release. It also constitutes fundamental role of echocardiography, careful analysis of the function of the aortic and tricuspid valves, and the detection and grading of possible residual flow [8].

9. What is the importance of having a trained team to percutaneous implant?

The echocardiographer-interventionist interaction is indispensable since the implantation of the prosthesis is guided by transesophageal echocardiography, and interventionist needs to be familiar with and master the echocardiographic images for correct opening and positioning of the prosthesis [6].

10. What are the major complications of percutaneous treatment of CIA compared with the complications of conventional surgical treatment?

Major complications of percutaneous procedure are very rare. Embolization cases occur infrequently (depending on the operator experience, type of prosthesis and defect size), and can be, in general, managed in the catheterization lab itself, with rescue devices. Late perforation with pericardial effusion and tamponade are exceptional. The occurrence of secondary stroke due to the detachment of a fragment of the platelet of white thrombus, occurred in the early stages immediately after device implantation, is rare, with rates of around 0.4%, corresponding to transient ischemic attacks without clinical sequelae. Late embolic episodes are exceptional, and there is virtually no risk after the endothelialization of the prosthesis (about 6–12 months). Moreover, surgery presents significant morbidity. The occurrence of pericardial effusion is relatively common, sometimes with cardiac tamponade and atelectasis in the postoperative infections (the wound, pneumonia), pain, stroke in older patients, and the need for blood products, among others [6].

Review About the Addressed Disease or Treatment

The atrial septum defect, an acyanotic heart disease with left-to-right shunt, occurs in a prevalence of 5–10% among all congenital heart defects; it is rarely diagnosed in childhood and is predominant in females [7].

Ostium secundum ASD, the most common form of this pathology, is located in the intermediate region of the septum and involves the oval fossa. The sinus venosus ASD occurs in the high atrial septum and is commonly associated with the anomalous connection of the pulmonary veins from the right lung with the junction of the superior vena cava or the right atrium. The ostium primum ASD is located in the lower atrial septum, adjacent to the atrioventricular valves, and is typical of Down syndrome [9].

The clinical manifestations usually begin between the third and fourth decades of life and consist of dyspnea, fatigue, and palpitation. Onset of symptoms is probably associated with the development of pulmonary hypertension [9].

Physical examination usually reveals prominent right ventricular impulse, palpable pulmonary arterial pulsation, the first sound of normal or unfolded heart auscultation with accentuation of tricuspid valve closure sound, second heart sound with wide and fixed unfolding, mesosystolic murmur in pulmonary focus, and loud mesodiastolic murmur, more audible in the fourth intercostal space and along the left sternal border, by hyperflow through the tricuspid valve.

The electrocardiogram of patients with ostium secundum ASD usually shows axis deviation to the right and rSr' pattern in the right precordial leads. In those with venous sinus ASD, the electrocardiogram pattern may be first-degree atrioventricular block, or atrial ectopic pacemaker, whereas ostium primum ASD usually has the conduction defect in the right ventricle accompanied by axis deviation to the left and orientation with counterclockwise QRS rotation in the frontal plane [9].

Chest X-ray shows enlargement of the right atrium and ventricle and pulmonary artery and its branches. Transthoracic echocardiography demonstrates dilation of the atrium and right ventricles and pulmonary artery with paradoxical movements of the interventricular septum in the presence of some volume overload of the right side of the heart. In addition, the ASD can be directly observed, by means of two-dimensional images with echo contrast or colored flow. Transesophageal echocardiography is indicated in cases in which transthoracic findings are inconclusive, or during catheterization, to close the communication. In case of inconsistencies in clinical data, suspicion of significant pulmonary hypertension, associated malformations, or possibility of coronary artery disease, cardiac catheterization should be performed [9].

In the absence of contraindications, such as significant pulmonary hypertension, the occlusion of atrial septal defects with significant pulmonary-systemic flow (greater than or equal to 1.5: 1) is recommended by surgical or endovascular procedure [9].

Bibliography

1. Braunwald E. Treaty of cardiovascular medicine, vol. 1. 6th ed. São Paulo: Roca; 2003. p. 198–200.
2. Humenberger M. Benefit of atrial septal defect closure in adults: impact of age. Eur Heart J. 2011;32:553–60.
3. Spina GS. Cardiology specialist title – study guide. 1st ed. São Paulo: nVersos; 2011. p. 616–9.
4. Macial BC, Marin JAN. Guide of cardiological clinical condutcs, vol. 3. São Paulo: Segmento Farma; 2005. p. 397–8.
5. Nobre F, Júnior CVS. Treaty of cardiology. 1st ed. São Paulo: Manole; 2005. p. 1326–7.
6. Pedra CAC, Pedra SRF, Fontes VF. Atrial septal defect of the ostium secundum type. Surgical treatment to percutaneous and the dinosaurs of the future. Braz Arch Cardiol. 2003;80(6):650–5.
7. Silveira AC, Rached EB, Campane FZ, Maielo JR. Atrial septal defect. J Sch Med Sci Sorocaba. 2008;10(2):7–11.
8. Barbosa MM, Nunes MCP, Campos FO, Camarozano A, Rabischoffsky A, Maciel BC, et al. Guidelines of echocardiography indications. Braz Arch Cardiol. 2009;93(6, supl. 3):294–6.

9. Longo DL, et al. Internal medicine Harrison, vol. 2. 18th ed. São Paulo: AMGH; 2013. p. 1921–2.
10. Oliveira EC, Paupério HM, Freitas IF, Adjuto GL, Katina T, Puerpério MM, Oliveira AAC. Atrial septal defect percutaneous closure with Amplatzer device. Braz J Cardiol Invasive. 2005;13(3):198–205.
11. Chamié F, Chamié D, Ramos S, Tress JC, Victer R. Percutaneous closure of complex atrial septal defects. Braz J Invasive Cardiol. 2006;14(1):47–55.

Percutaneous Occlusion of a Patent Foramen Ovale

Laura Gomes Flores, Cassiana Tomazoni, Patrícia Freitag, Evandro Luis Queiroz Flores, and Rui M. S. Almeida

Clinical Presentation

A 39-year-old white female with a complaint of migraine with aura, debilitating, recurrent, and refractory to medications from childhood, and dyspnea on exertion for 5 years, with no other concomitant symptoms. She reports that, at age 27, she suffered an ischemic stroke in the posterior cerebral artery with no thrombogenic focus found, which was diagnosed rapidly by acute ataxia and fugitive hemiplegia, being treated within the golden period, leaving no sequelae. She has a sedentary lifestyle and denies use of medication, smoking, and alcoholism. She presents positive family history for coronary artery disease. In physical examination, good general condition (stained, hydrated, anicteric, acyanotic); atypical and euphonic thorax, without respiratory effort (retractions or use of acces-

L. G. Flores (✉) · C. Tomazoni · P. Freitag · E. L. Q. Flores
Assis Gurgacz Foundation University (FAG), Cascavel, PR, Brazil

R. M. S. Almeida
Department of Cardiology and Cardiovascular Surgery,
University Center Assis Gurgacz Foundation, Cascavel, PR, Brazil

R. M. S. Almeida, F. B. Jatene (eds.), *Cardiovascular Surgery*,
https://doi.org/10.1007/978-3-319-57084-6_19

sory musculature); expandability preserved bilaterally; tactile vocal fremitus bilaterally performed; clear lung sounds to percussion; audible vesicular murmur without adventitious sounds; normodynamic precordium; invisible left ventricular (LV) stroke, palpable at fifth ICS at the left hemiclavicular line measuring about two finger pulps, not propulsive; absence of friction; normal heart sounds for S1 and S2; absence of murmurs or extrasystoles; absence of jugular vein distention (JVD); symmetrical, synchronous, and well-amplified peripheral arterial pulses; and absence of carotid murmurs.

Diagnosis, Assessment, and Treatment

A transesophageal echocardiography (TEE) was initially requested, which revealed the presence of patent foramen ovale (D = 18 mm), with a large right-to-left shunt, detected by the microbubble contrast of the agitated saline (even without Valsalva maneuver) (Fig. 1). Due to a history of stroke at 27 years with no identifiable cause and the result of TEE, percutaneous occlusion was chosen because it reduces the risk of recurrent embolic events.

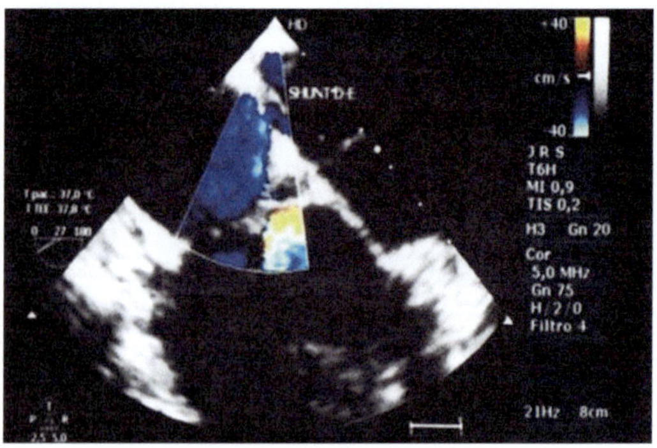

FIGURE 1 The observer point of view, to the superior and to the left structure, is the right atrium. Looking down to the right is the left atrium. Separating them there is the interatrial septum, where exists a patent oval foramen (POF) with a huge right-to-left shunt

Echocardiographic controls were used to guide the positioning of the occlusion device. Acetylsalicylic acid was prescribed to be started 5 days before the procedure and maintained for 6 months after implantation. The procedure is performed in a hemodynamic room and monitored by transesophageal echocardiography. Initially, the femoral vein was doubly punctured by placing two short sheaths and a right and left catheterization with pulmonary pressure recording. Then, an injection is made in the foramen itself so as to delineate the tunnel completely. The septum is crossed (using a hydrophilic guide, when necessary), placing the catheter in the left superior pulmonary vein. Inside it a rigid exchange guide is fixed, through which is inserted the long sheath, of a suitable size, to the prosthesis to be used, positioning it in LA. The occlusion device is chosen based on the length and unprovoked opening of the foramen, evaluated in the TEE and angiography. Among the available prostheses, such as Amplatzer, Cardio, Helex, CERA, and Occlutech, the chosen prosthesis for the patient was the Amplatzer PFO Occluder, available in three sizes: 18, 25, and 35 mm. The prosthesis, entangled around the release wire, is inserted in its own loader, from where it is transferred through the long sheath into the defect, into the left atrium. There, the distal disk is externalized. The prosthesis-sheath assembly is pulled toward the septum, and, by maintaining adequate tension in the system, the proximal disk is exteriorized in the right atrium. At this point, with the prosthesis still attached to the release wire, a bubble study is performed by the catheter placed in the other short sheath. If there is no bubble passage, the prosthesis is detached from the wire and new bubble study is performed. If negative persists, the procedure terminates [1].

The patient was advised to use aspirin and clopidogrel for 1 month, maintaining only aspirin until the sixth month post-procedure, when the prosthesis should be completely endothelialized. In the first and third months after closure, control was performed with transthoracic echocardiography. In the sixth month, a TEE was performed, which revealed preserved left ventricular (LV) global systolic function and normal relaxation, without detectable residual shunt. Due to the absence of residual shunt, aspirin was discontinued. The patient was instructed to maintain prophylaxis for infective endocarditis for the first 6 months after the procedure. The patient reported complete remission of migraine after percutaneous closure of the patent foramen ovale.

Questions

1. What is the definition of PFO, and in which population it is more prevalent?

During pregnancy, everything the fetus needs to receive from oxygen and nutrients is passed from the mother to the child through the umbilical cord. This blood reaches the heart of the fetus through the right atrium; however, as oxygenation does not occur in the lung, so that the blood circulates and passes to the left side, much of it does through a "tunnel" between the right and left atria called foramen ovale.

The foramen ovale, therefore, is a normal structure and is part of the life of the fetus. If it did not exist, there would be difficulty in blood circulation and the fetus probably would not survive.

Most children develop with natural ovale closure shortly after birth, but some of them grow and become adults while maintaining the patent foramen ovale. From statistical studies, it is known that approximately 25% of normal adults have foramen ovale, being considered relevant only when there is some complication due to their existence (fortunately, the minority of people).

Several studies with young people (<55 years) who had a non-determined ischemic stroke showed that, in this situation, the incidence of PFO rises from 25% in normal people to 40% [2, 3].

2. What are the main clinical implications in a patient with PFO?

They are stroke, migraine, platypnea-orthodeoxia, obstructive sleep apnea, decompression syndrome, surgical risk for major surgery, and persistent cyanosis [4].

3. What is the possible relationship between PFO and paradoxical embolism?

It is suggested that stress can induce episodic systemic platelet activation and hypercoagulability, which causes transient thrombus formation and subsequent embolization on both the arterial and venous sides of the circulation; the latter requires a PFO to cause a stroke (paradoxical embolism). The sum of these two mechanisms explains cryptogenic stroke.

Certain medical conditions should take into consideration a cryptogenic stroke, such as history of stroke <55 years of age, either TVP or PE, Valsalva maneuver preceding the neurological event, long journey in the previous 2 weeks, neurological deficit on awakening, and migraine history [5].

4. By what possible mechanisms PFO results in migraine? Is there remission just after occlusion?

One possible explanation for this would be the paradoxical passage of microemboli through the right-to-left shunt or direct passage of vasoactive substances (e.g., serotonin) that would normally be "filtered" by the lungs, from right-to-left movement. Furthermore, PFO and migraine could be reflecting manifestations of embryonic lateralization (pineal deviation caused by suboptimal levels of serotonin can promote migraine and incomplete closure of the oval fossa).

The patient, after occlusion, reported complete remission of migraine. Some retrospective studies suggest that the closure of the PFO plays a role in its improvement, such as Azarbal et al., who reported the presence of migraine in 42% (45% PFO/30% ASD) from 89 stroke patients (66 PFO/23 ASD). After 3 months of closure, migraine disappeared in 75% of MA+ patients and 31% of MA−, with significant improvement in symptoms of headache in others.

On the other hand, the MIST study [11] was a prospective, multicenter, double-blind, randomized, and controlled trial that evaluated the effect of closing PFO in migraine symptoms at the time of its oral presentation. At the time of his oral presentation, it was mentioned that the primary endpoint of complete resolution of migraine (healing) was not achieved, but the secondary endpoint planned 50% reduction in days of migraine; it was achieved in 42% of patients submitted to closure to 23% of the sham procedure ($p = 0.038$). Surprisingly, the published results of this study were totally negative.

Therefore, to establish the real benefits of PFO closure as a strategy in the treatment of migraine and multifactorial etiology of disease, more studies are necessary in a randomized and controlled nature [1, 6].

5. How is the diagnosis of PFO established?

The method of choice is transesophageal echocardiography sensitized by saline injection of microbubbles at the end of Valsalva maneuver performed. Transthoracic echocardiography can be used, but without the same sensitivity. Transcranial Doppler ultrasound has also been used along with other methods such as pulse oximetry, and indicator dilution, which are validated techniques, but less sensitive; they do not distinguish shunts from other regions nor inform morphology of the atrial septum [7].

6. Why was the interventional treatment chosen rather than clinical?

Currently, the evidence points that pharmacological treatment (antiplatelet agents and anticoagulants) and endovascular/surgical treatment are similar in most cases; they present results of similar recurring events – occurrence of new ischemic stroke. These first evidences came with the publication of two important clinical studies, PCI and RESPECT studies, both published in the medical journal *New England Journal of Medicine*.

However, the long-term results of follow-up patients in RESPECT trial showed that, in cases of younger people, with larger and more complex PFOs, the closure with the prosthesis was better.

Some anatomical factors such as the presence of concomitant atrial septal aneurysm, and detection of spontaneous shunt from right to left, through the transesophageal echocardiogram or transcranial Doppler study, are associated with increased risk of stroke in patients with PFO.

Therefore, once PFO is identified, it is important to analyze the presence of the situations mentioned above, to then assess whether it is a case with an indication of closure, or only to follow up with outpatients with oral medications.

Because the patient had a history of stroke at the age of 27 and presented spontaneous right-to-left shunt at the transesophageal echocardiogram, we opted for closure to reduce the risk of recurrence [8].

7. What are the advantages and disadvantages of ultrasound guidance during catheter-based PFO closure?

Among the advantages, there is less risk of misplacement or suboptimal placement if used in addition to fluoroscopy with contrast medium, less missing of residual or additional shunts, immediate information about tightness, and possibility of forgoing fluoroscopy altogether (pregnancy and sharing of responsibility – due to the work of two physicians).

Nevertheless, there are also some disadvantages, which include need for general anesthesia with intubation or, at least, a good sedation (risk of aspiration); in the case of transesophageal echocardiography, discomfort of transesophageal intubation and risk of aspiration (in case of sedation only); and cost and complications of echocardiography (second larger venous access required), in addition to at least the doubling of procedure duration.

By the way, the patient had no residual shunt, which was confirmed by a transesophageal echocardiogram performed later after the operation (Fig. 2) [9].

8. What reasons can lead to residual shunt after the closure?

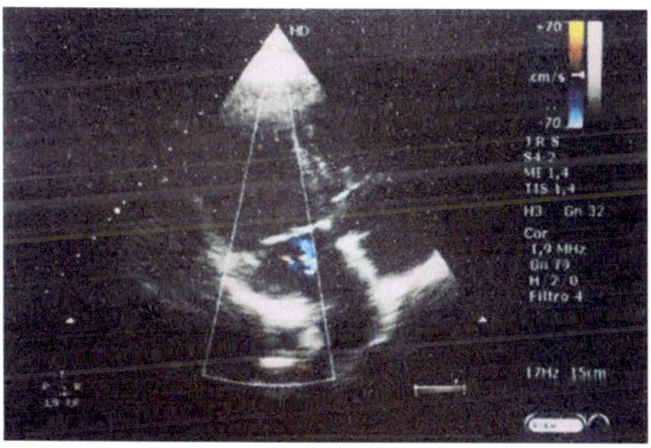

FIGURE 2 The POF is occluded by the prosthesis, with no shunt left

The most common reason is a device that is too small and that will not cover enough of the width of the PFO or a device that is too large that will stay at a distance from the septum rather than hugging it. A similar situation can be found in case of a partially fused PFO, with spaced apart residual shunts. There are multiple other morphological variations which may lead to incomplete closure. Fortunately, they are rather rare [3].

9. What are the major complications of percutaneous closure of PFO?

The two most frequent complications are an arteriovenous fistula at the puncture site in the groin (more common with simultaneous coronary angiography) and the creation of a new ASD because of an erosion of the thin septum primum at the lower rim of the device – the risk of further paradoxical embolism is smaller than the initial PFO because this new shunt is small and not in the direct shooting line of the inferior vena cava.

Besides these, there are also exceedingly rare complications as device thrombosis, erosion of a free wall of the atrium and erosion of valves, or blockages of inflow from pulmonary veins or the coronary sinus [10].

Review About the Addressed Disease or Treatment

Patent foramen ovale (PFO) is a small hole located in the middle of the wall of the muscle dividing the two atria, a normal structure during pregnancy that allows fetal blood flow between the right and left side of the heart. Most of the time, this hole closes at the date of birth or in the first months/years of life. However, it may not close and leave an opening between the atria. Its prevalence is 25% in normal adults and 40% in patients under 55 years of age with a history of cryptogenic stroke. Among the possible clinical implications, there are cryptogenic stroke, migraine, platypnea-orthodeoxia, obstructive sleep apnea, decompressive syndrome, increased risk for large surgeries, and persistent cyanosis.

The diagnostic method of choice is by transesophageal echocardiogram sensitized with saline injection of microbubbles at the end of Valsalva maneuver. Other tests for the diagnosis are the transthoracic echocardiography and skull echocardiography with pulse oximetry and indication of dilution; however, these present a lower sensitivity [7].

Treatment may be clinical (antiplatelet agents and anticoagulants) or interventional (surgery or endovascular therapy). The best therapeutic approach is defined according to the risk of stroke recurrence; an interventionist approach is preferred in patients and in those with the factors that increase the risk of stroke, such as the presence of concomitant septum aneurysm and the detection of spontaneous right-to-left shunt during transesophageal echocardiography or transcranial echocardiogram [8].

In addition, some studies indicate that interventional therapy also presents as an advantage a decrease in migraine after the procedure, allowing its use for patients with symptoms of PFO and severe migraine, persistent and refractory to intravenous therapy. However, further randomized trials are still necessary to definitively establish this benefit [1, 6].

Bibliography

1. Chamié F, Chamié D, Ramos S, Tress JC, Victer R. Patent foramen ovale percutaneous closure. Braz J Cardiol Invasive. 2005;3:185–97.
2. Miranda M. Patent foramen ovale and ischemic stroke. 2016. Available at: www.ineuro.com.br/para-os-pacientes/forame-oval patente-e-avc-isquemico/ (Accessed at 8 Aug 2016).
3. Nercolini D, Guérios EE, Selig FA. Questions about congenital heart defects. Center of Congenital and Structural Heart Diseases of Paraná website; 2010. Available at: www.centroconcept.com.br/faq1.php (Accessed at 8 Aug 2016).
4. Chamié FJA. Indications of patent foramen ovale closure. Paper presented at the annual course of revision in hemodynamic and interventional cardiology by Brazilian Society of Hemodynamics and Interventional Cardiology, November 5–6, São Paulo – BR; 2010.

5. Eggers AE. A new theory of cryptogenic stroke and its relationship to patent foramen ovale; or, the puzzle of the missing extra risk. Med Hypotheses J. 2006;67:1072–5.
6. Vigna C. Improvement of migraine after patent foramen ovale percutaneous closure in patients with subclinical brain lesions: a case-control study. J Am Coll Cardiol Intv. 2009;2:107–13.
7. Fukujima MM, Tatani SB, Prado GF. Patent foramen ovale and stroke – current trends. Neurosci Mag. 2004;12(4):209–11.
8. Abizaid A, Júnior JRC. Interventional cardiology guide of Dante Pazzanese Institute. 1st ed. Rio de Janeiro: Elsevier; 2013. p. 470–7.
9. Lavinsky M, Wolff FH, Polanczyk CA, Rohde LEP, Pagnoncelli A, Maulaz A. Summary of evidence and recommendations for percutaneous closure of patent foramen ovale in the secondary prevention of cerebrovascular events. 2007. Available at: www.unimed.coop.br/pct/servlet/ServletDownload?id=MjE0NzUxMTExMA== (Accessed at 28 Aug 2016).
10. Sabaté M. Percutaneous cardiac interventions – tips and tricks of new techniques beyond stenting. Toulouse: Europa Edition; 2010. p. 151–4.
11. Dowson A, Mullen MJ, Peatfield R, Muir K, Khan AA, Wells C, Lipscombe SL, Rees T, De Giovanni JV, Morrison WL, Hildick-Smith D, Elrington G, Hillis WS, Malik IS, Rickards A. Migraine Intervention With STARFlex Technology (MIST) Trial: A Prospective, Multicenter, Double-Blind, Sham-Controlled Trial to Evaluate the Effectiveness of Patent Foramen Ovale Closure With STARFlex Septal Repair Implant to Resolve Refractory Migraine Headache. Circulation. 2008;117(11):1397–404.

Transposition of Great Arteries with Pulmonary Valve Stenosis After Jatene Procedure

Camila Rocha Vieira Torres, Eugênio Patrício de Oliveira, Rayane da Silva Souza, Gabriel Pelegrineti Targueta, and Marisa Wanderley Casado

Clinical Presentation

Patient newborn, male, 28 days of life, was sent to our service because of the onset of vomiting after feeding followed recurrent blackouts 5 days ago, with the skin becoming increasingly cyanotic. The mother reports that pregnancy did not present any intercurrence and that she made adequate prenatal, with accomplishment of fetal echocardiograms in accordance with their own ranges of monitoring to low-risk pregnancy. She is not diabetic or had high blood glucose and had no infectious episode during the pregnancy. Gestational weeks were normal, and transvaginal parturition was at term. The newborn had birth weight of 3750 kg and birth length of 49 centimeters and head circumference at birth was not measured. They were discharged after a day of parturition. The child was asymptomatic in the first 2 weeks. On physical examination at the time of admission, the infant was moder-

C. R. V. Torres (✉) · E. P. de Oliveira · R. da Silva Souza
G. P. Targueta · M. W. Casado
Federal University of Paraíba (UFPB), João Pessoa, PB, Brazil

R. M. S. Almeida, F. B. Jatene (eds.), *Cardiovascular Surgery*,
https://doi.org/10.1007/978-3-319-57084-6_20

ately tachydyspneic, cyanotic, and on heart auscultation; an increased intensity of the second heart sound predominated.

Diagnosis, Assessment, and Treatment

As a first step therapy, the child was stabilized by receiving nasal oxygen catheter (2 L/min), but there was no improvement in cyanosis. Echocardiography was accomplished on the following day (Fig. 1a, b), showing transposition of great arteries (TGA) associated with atrial septal defect (ASD), patent ductus arteriosus, and ventricular septal defect (VSD), which kept the patient without symptoms in the first weeks after the birth. Then, the child received 240 mcg of prostaglandins IV every 24 h, to maintain the patent ductus arteriosus.

After we discovered the pathology, the patient was forwarded to a tertiary hospital, where he underwent Jatene procedure on the 15th day of diagnosis. After the surgical procedure, the patient remained for another fortnight admitted in use of antibiotic prophylaxis with cefuroxime 50 mg/kg IV every 12 h. In the first days after surgery, a new echocardiography was performed, showing the patient remained with a residual VSD type perimembranous, approximately 4 mm, with left-right shunt.

Posteriorly, the patient was referred to the pediatric intensive care unit, where he remained for 30 days until the end of

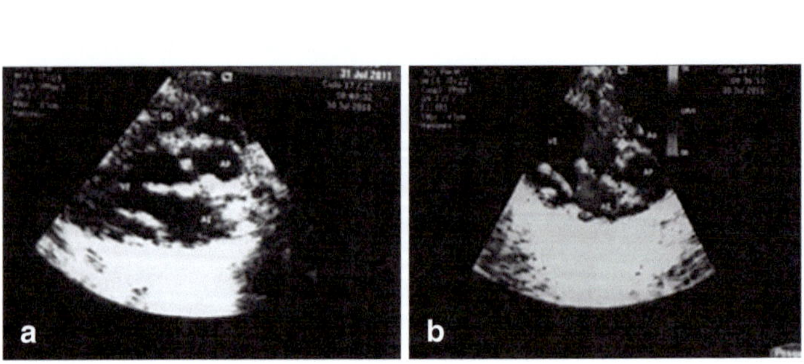

FIGURE 1 (**a**) Transthoracic echocardiography showing TGA. (**b**) Transthoracic echocardiography showing TGA with VSD

antibiotic prophylaxis. Progression cursed with the following immediate complications: low cardiac output, pulmonary atelectasis with respiratory failure, and fungal candida infection. Then, there was the need for high diuretic doses of dobutamine, prolonged intubation, and systemic antifungal as well as maintenance of antibiotic therapy. After this period, there was clinical improvement, and the patient was transferred to the infirmary and started oral feeding. Soon after, the patient was discharged without further complications. Five months after surgery, a new echocardiography was performed for clinical follow-up, being diagnosed a moderate pulmonary valve stenosis (Fig. 2) with peak systolic gradient between the right ventricle and the pulmonary trunk equal to 44 mmHg.

Despite such complications, the patient recovered well and progressed to a satisfactory psychomotor development until now, after 4 years of surgery. However, he presented, more recently, multiple clinical conditions of nonspecific febrile infection, in addition to referring a divergent squint in the right eye and bilateral cataracts, suggesting a possible relationship with neonatal infection TORCH (toxoplasma, rubella virus, cytomegalovirus, herpes simplex virus) group. However, there is no evidence of maternal infection before or during the pregnancy neither serology data of the patient.

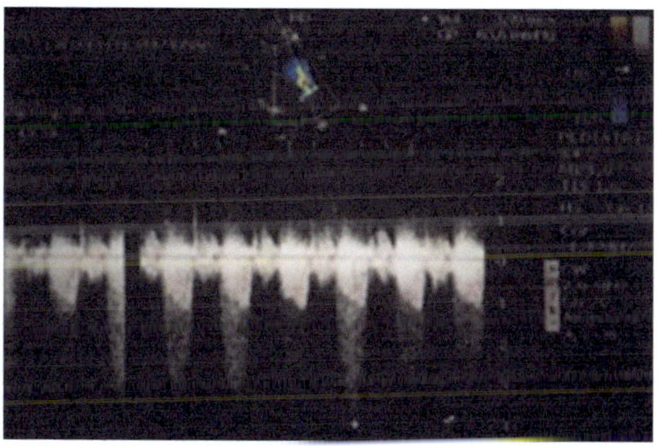

Figure 2 Transthoracic echocardiography with Doppler showing stenosis of the pulmonary valve

Questions

1. What is the pathophysiology of transposition of the great arteries?

The transposition of the great arteries (TGA) is a malformation that occurs with the inversion position between the two great vessels of the heart, the aorta and the pulmonary trunk. From the anatomically left ventricle leaves the pulmonary trunk and from the anatomically right ventricle the aorta. This description corresponds to most cases of TGA, called complete transposition of the great arteries [1].

2. What keeps alive the newborn after birth if two closed and parallel blood circulations are incompatible with life?

The two closed and parallel blood circulations are incompatible with life; therefore there must be some communication between them, either arterial, ventricular, or atrial. In the postnatal period, the pulmonary and systemic circulation maintained in parallel and systemic saturation depends exclusively on the degree of mixing between them. Therefore, the communication between the systemic and pulmonary circulation must remain in the postnatal period, through a patent foramen ovale, atrial septal defect (ASD), ventricular septal defect (VSD), or patent ductus arteriosus (PDA) [2].

3. How is the fetal circulation in intrauterine life?

In the intrauterine phase, the ventricles work in parallel and not in series because of these three essential paths, the ductus venosus, the foramen ovale, and the ductus arteriosus, which obliterate shortly after birth. This circulation allows the fetal heart to survive even with severe structural heart diseases such as transposition of the great arteries [3].

4. When is it recommended to do fetal echocardiography for the diagnosis of transposition of the great arteries in low-risk pregnancy?

In low-risk pregnancies, fetal echocardiography should be done preferably between 18 and 22 weeks of gestation. In this range of gestational age, fetal heart anatomy details can be well visualized and evaluated, as atrioventricular and ventriculoarterial connections [4].

5. What are the immediate complications of Jatene procedure?

The main immediate complications are transient left ventricular dysfunction, low cardiac output, respiratory failure requiring prolonged intubation, and infectious complications requiring the use of antibiotics [5].

6. What are the current surgical treatments recommended for transposition of the great arteries?

Currently, the surgical treatment of choice in newborns diagnosed with TGA is the Jatene procedure, which provides restoration of both heart anatomy and function. Complications in the respiratory tract may occur in the trunk or in the pulmonary arteries after bifurcation and are more related to the Lecompte maneuver that is the internalization of the pulmonary artery at the arteries' correct positioning [1].

7. What is the most frequent late complication in the postoperative period of Jatene procedure?

Belatedly, the most common complication of Jatene procedure is pulmonary supravalvular stenosis. The incidence may range from 3% to 30% [1].

8. What is the importance of fetal echocardiography in the diagnosis of transposition of the great arteries?

Fetal echocardiography importance of is due to be the gold standard exam for prenatal diagnosis of congenital heart disease and is a precise and safe tool used as a means of screening and helping in counseling legal guardians about the prognosis and treatment options for children. Some studies show better results after birth when the diagnosis of congenital heart disease is carried in the prenatal period, with decreased preoperative morbidity, less chance of acidosis, lower risk of hemodynamic disturbances, and improvement of perfusion to tissues. Therefore, it is important the screening fetuses for congenital heart disease requiring specific early postnatal therapy, in particular the transposition of the great arteries [6].

9. What are the limitations of fetal echocardiography in medical routine of some health services?

Fetal echocardiography is an operator-dependent examination, which requires good experience, caution, and technique described in the literature, which unfortunately is not yet available in all prenatal services [7].

10. What are the main indications of fetal echocardiography?

Fetal echocardiography indications should be if there is always be indicated if there is maternal history of gestational diabetes mellitus, rubella, lupus, and phenylketonuria, if the mother is exposed to teratogenic drugs, and if the mother has past history of alcoholism. Fetal echocardiography indications should be if there is also be indicated in the fetus with polyhydramnios; non-immune hydrops fetalis; arrhythmia; chromosomal abnormalities (trisomies, microdeletions); symmetrical intrauterine growth restriction (IUGR); cardiac morphological abnormalities detected during routine obstetrical examination, which increased in the first quarter in nuchal translucency measurement; and multiple extracardiac anomalies (omphalocele, duodenal atresia, spina bifida). Besides that, is indicated in mothers with any family history of congenital heart disease [8].

Review About the Addressed Disease or Treatment

Transposition of the great arteries (TGA) is the most common cyanotic congenital heart lesion that presents in neonates. It is a malformation that was occurred with an inversion of position between the two great vessels at the base of heart, such as aorta and pulmonary arteries [1].

The hallmark of TGA is ventriculoarterial discordance, in which the aorta arises from the morphologic right ventricle and the pulmonary artery arises from the morphologic left ventricle [1]. It changes the way blood circulates through the body, leaving a shortage of oxygen in blood flowing from the heart to the rest of the body. Without an adequate supply of oxygen-rich blood, the body can't function properly [3].

Transposition of the great arteries is usually detected either prenatally or within the first hours to weeks of life. It may be detected as a heart murmur, the baby's mouth and skin will be cyanotic, and the tests include ECG, pulse oximetry, echocardiogram, or fetal echocardiogram [9].

In nearly a fourth of children with transposition will also have a ventricular septal defect (VSD). Others may also have patent foramen ovale, atrial septal defect (ASD), and patent ductus arteriosus (PDA) [8]. Besides that, infants may have narrowing below the pulmonary valve that blocks blood flow from the left ventricle to the lungs [1].

The usual treatment for TGA is a corrective surgery soon after birth. The most famous operation is Jatene procedure. Adib Jatene, a Brazilian surgeon, performed successfully for the first time a truly anatomical correction in the form of an ASO in 1975 at the University of São Paulo Heart Institute, São Paulo, Brazil [1].

The first two patients were operated using profound hypothermia and total circulatory arrest. Coronary buttons were excised and the openings created were closed using homologous dura mater. After completing coronary transfer to the new site, the great vessels were transected; the ventricular septal defect was closed with a Dacron patch through a right ventriculotomy [10].

In 1981, Lecompte from Paris, France, described a technically important modification of surgically translocating the great vessels, thereby avoiding the use of prosthetic conduit. He has anteriorized the pulmonary artery at the moment of correct repositioning of the arteries. This is now popularly called the "Lecompte maneuver." This greatly simplified the method of right ventricular outflow tract reconstruction during the ASO, besides providing a better anatomical lie for the coronary arteries and the newly reconstructed aortic anastomosis [1].

This was a near revolution, and nearly all surgeons around the world routinely perform this maneuver during the ASO [1]. Today, infants who undergo palliative or corrective procedures have a dramatic 90% rate of survival [9].

In postoperative period of Jatene procedure, the main complications are related to vascular suture plan, in which the arterial exchange was performed, and in coronary reimplantation. Intercurrences in pulmonary territory can occur in the trunk or after bifurcation of pulmonary arteries, being more related to the Lecompte maneuver [10].

Bibliography

1. Jatene IB, Jatene MB. Transposição das Grandes Artérias. In: Croti UA, Mattos SS, Pinto Jr VC, Aiello VD, Moreira VM, editors. Cardiologia e cirurgia cardiovascular pediátrica. 2nd ed. São Paulo: Roca; 2012. p. 529–60.
2. Zipes DP, et al. Braunwald's heart disease. In: A textbook of cardiovascular medicine. 8th ed. St. Louis: Saunders, EUA; 2007.
3. Charpie JR, Maher K. Transposition of the great vessels. Atlanta: E Medicine Cardiology, EUA; 2009.
4. SBC-Sociedade Brasileira de Cardiologia. II Diretriz Brasileira de Cardiopatia Grave. Arq Bras Cardiol, Rio de Janeiro, RJ, Brazil. 2006;87(2):223–32.
5. Brooks P, Penny DJ. Management of the sick neonate with suspected heart disease. In: Early human development, vol. 84. Melbourne: Elsevier; 2008. p. 155–9.
6. Jone PN, Schowengerdt KO. Prenatal diagnosis of congenital heart disease. Pediatric Clinics of North America. Adv Neonatol, Colorado, EUA. 2009;56(3):709–15.
7. Zielinsky P. Malformações cardíacas fetais. Diagnóstico e Conduta. Arq Bras Cardiol. 1997;69(3):209–18. São Paulo, SP, Brazil.
8. Barbosa MM, Nunes MCP, Campos FO, Camarozano A, Rabischoffsky A, Maciel BC. Sociedade Brasileira de Cardiologia. Diretrizes das Indicações da Ecocardiografia. Arq Bras Cardiol. 2009;93(6 supl. 3):265–302.
9. Mayo Clinic. Transposition of the great arteries. 2016. Available at: http://www.mayoclinic.org/diseases-conditions/transposition-of-the-great-arteries/home (Accessed 12 Oct 2016).
10. Jatene MB, et al. Prevalência e abordagem cirúrgica da estenose supravalvular pulmonar pós-operação de Jatene para transposição das grandes artérias. Arq Bras Cardiol, Rio de Janeiro, RJ, Brazil. 2008;91(1):18–24.

Part VI
Endovascular Therapies

Transcatheter Aortic Valve Replacement (TAVR) and Angioplasty in a High-Risk Patient

Flávia Cristina Kufner, Carlos Henrique Romancini, Caroline Kelli Domingues dos Santos, Evandro Luis Queiroz Flores, and Rui M. S. Almeida

Clinical Presentation

ZVB, a male, 60-year-old, white, businessman, was admitted to the hospital with a clinical condition of dyspnea on exertion with progressive worsening, reporting orthopnea and dyspnea at rest. The patient was hospitalized in the city of origin for 4 days, where he began using oxygen therapy and a wheelchair, without reversal of the situation with clinical treatment. Patient reports prior hypertension, type II diabetes and severe chronic obstructive pulmonary disease (COPD). He is in use of metformin, carvedilol, furosemide,

F. C. Kufner (✉) · C. H. Romancini · C. K. D. dos Santos
State University of Western Paraná (UNIOESTE), Cascavel, PR, Brazil

E. L. Q. Flores
Assis Gurgacz Foundation University (FAG), Cascavel, PR, Brazil

R. M. S. Almeida
Department of Cardiology and Cardiovascular Surgery, University Center Assis Gurgacz Foundation, Cascavel, PR, Brazil

R. M. S. Almeida, F. B. Jatene (eds.), *Cardiovascular Surgery*, https://doi.org/10.1007/978-3-319-57084-6_21

spironolactone, aspirin, omeprazole, and clonazepam. No history of surgery and allergies were noted. The patient reported cigarette smoking, 40 pack-years, and sedentarism.

On physical examination, the patient was in mild general condition, lucid and oriented in time and space, and hydrated, with cyanosis and global plethora and dyspnea to the supine position in 45°.

Arterial pressure, 130 × 90 mmHg; heart rate, 68 bpm; respiratory frequency, 27 rpm; height, 1.70 m; weight, 87kg; BMI, 30.1 kg/m^2.

Respiratory system: Symmetrical vesicular murmur, globally decreased, with snores scattered across the chest.

Cardiovascular system: Rhythmic heart sounds and hypophonic, in two stages, with pancardiac systolic murmur, 3+/6, without irradiation. There is resence of bilateral jugular engorgement.

Abdomen: Globular, flaccid, normoactive bowel sounds, painless to palpation, without visceromegaly

Lower limbs: Palpable and symmetrical foot pulses, no edema

Diagnosis, Assessment, and Treatment

Patient was admitted from the city of origin with dyspnea upon exertion without compensation with clinical treatment, diagnosed by echocardiography with aortic stenosis and coronary artery disease, and sent to our clinic for surgical evaluation.

On admission was continued on the previous pharmacological treatment and requested laboratory tests and electrocardiogram (ECG), which were within the normal range. Then, a transthoracic echocardiography was performed to confirm the diagnosis, with the following conclusion:

"Left ventricle (LV) contractile pattern with important diffuse hypokinesia, LV wall thickness with a slight increase (discrete LV symmetric hypertrophy) and LV cavity dimension with a large increase (LV end diastolic diameter of 6.9 cm and end systolic diameter of 6.1 cm). Heavily calcified aortic valve, with valve dynamics greatly reduced. Maximum aortic systolic gradient of 31.1 mmHg and average of 18.4 mmHg. Aortic valve area of 0.96 cm^2. Mild mitral regurgitation. Ejection fraction of 23%."

Thus, given the clinical condition of frank cor pulmonale by aortic stenosis, aggravated by severe COPD, the family was advised about the surgical possibilities, explaining the patient's high surgical risk due to the comorbidities. A transcatheter approach procedure was indicated, considering that's a possible longer stay in the intensive care unit (ICU) due to the patient's lung disease.

After the patient's and family consent, a CT angiography (Fig. 1) for surgical planning was performed, which presented:

"Atherosclerotic disease predominantly involving the abdominal aorta, iliac and femoral arteries with stenosis of moderate to severe degree of distal segments of the superficial femoral artery and moderate stenosis in the right external iliac artery. Diameter of the aortic annulus of 3.0 × 3.5 cm; right common iliac of 0.8 cm; left common iliac of 10 cm; right external iliac of 0.5 cm; left external iliac of 0.61 cm; right femoral of 0.6 cm; left femoral of 0.8 cm. Coronary atherosclerosis with signs of important left anterior descending artery injury."

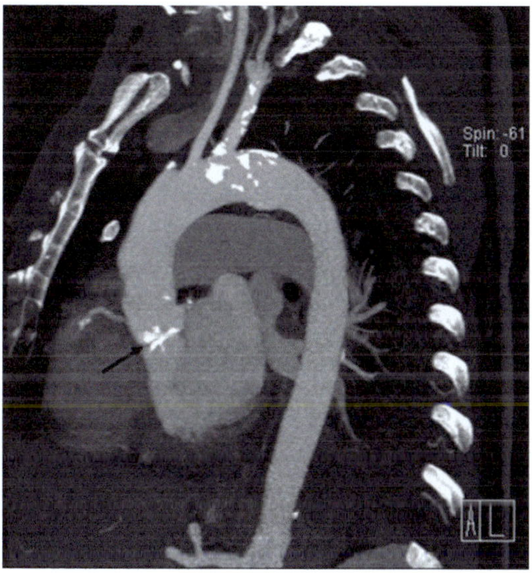

Figure 1 Preoperative chest tomography in sagittal section. Hyperattenuating regions in the aortic valve, aorta, and its branches showing calcifications. Black arrow: calcified aortic valve

From this, the possibility of transfemoral procedure requiring the coronary disease treatment was discussed.

During the days of hospitalization preceding the procedure, the patient had periods of improvement but with repeated need for oxygen use.

Six days after admission, with the due preparation of the patient, we performed left anterior descending artery angioplasty and a transcatheter aortic valve replacement (TAVR), using CoreValve (# 31), two pharmacological coronary stents, and a temporary pacemaker.

The procedure started with the placement of a temporary pacemaker through right subclavian vein puncture, and the electrode was positioned in the right ventricle (RV). A femoral artery puncture for endovascular procedures was performed. Coronary angiography showed partial stenosis of the left anterior descending artery (Fig. 2), in which angioplasty was performed in proximal and middle-distal thirds using drug-eluting stents, expanded with a balloon catheter. It was then introduced a catheter to implant the aortic valve (Fig. 3). After the procedure, the Perclose method was used to perform femoral artery suture.

The patient was taken to the ICU, hemodynamically compensated with low doses of vasoactive drugs, keeping blood pressure at an average of 86 mmHg, and extubation was performed soon after the procedure. On the same day, laboratory tests and ECG had no abnormalities. The pacemaker was removed with no episodes recorded of abnormal rhythms. The patient received ICU discharge on the same day.

In the infirmary, the antihypertensive drugs previously used were reintroduced with the maintenance of aspirin and metformin and the addition of clopidogrel and rosuvastatin.

With hemodynamic and respiratory stability, the patient was discharged 6 days after surgery.

One week later, the patient required readmission for pulmonary decompensation, medically treated. A first-degree atrioventricular block was diagnosed, with biventricular overload, without clinical repercussions.

The follow-up happened in 3, 6, and 12 months, with the echocardiogram results presented in Table 1.

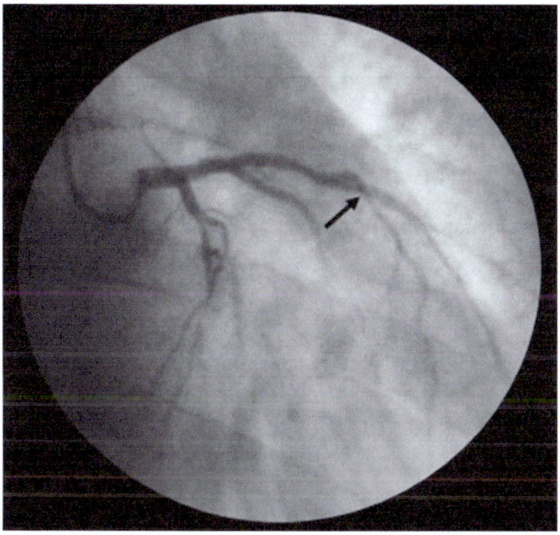

FIGURE 2 Pre-TAVR coronary angiography. Black arrow showing left anterior descending artery stenosis

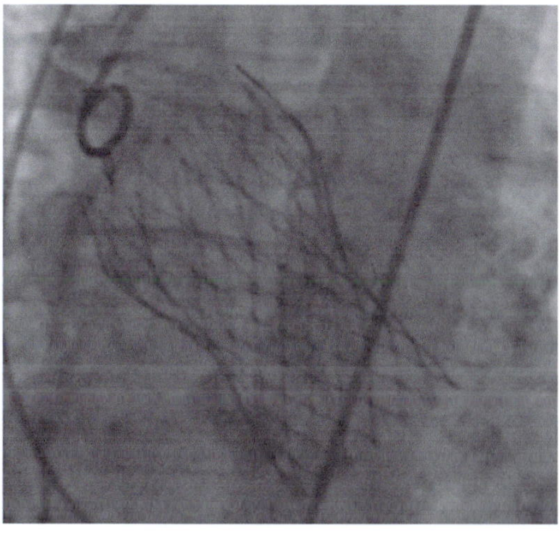

FIGURE 3 Radioscopic image showing positioned aortic valve prosthesis

Table 1 Evolution of hemodynamic measurements of transthoracic echocardiograms

Transthoracic echocardiography	Ejection fraction (%)	Maximum aortic valve systolic gradient (mmHg)	Mean aortic valve systolic gradient (mmHg)
Preoperative	23	31.1	18.4
Postoperative	31	16.4	8.8
One month after procedure	43	14.6	9.2
Four months after procedure	45	15.6	10

The patient had no new symptoms, and the control echocardiograms showed a well-positioned prosthesis free of dense echoes inside, with internal diameter of 2.0 cm without paravalvular regurgitation. The patient showed significant clinical improvement. Patient reports, in the 1-year return, ability to walk up three blocks without symptoms (NYHA II), the lung condition being an important confusing factor for this assessment.

It is planned to follow the patient every 6 months, with periodic transthoracic echocardiography, maintaining clopidogrel and aspirin during the first 6 months, due to the TARV procedure. The aspirin will be kept indefinitely due to coronary stents.

Questions

1. Discuss the clinical diagnosis and the tests that should be ordered.

The clinical condition presented by the patient is compatible with cor pulmonale triggered by decompensation of one or more of the comorbidities previously presented: DM, CAD, aortic stenosis, and COPD. Thus, it is demonstrated the need to request tests to rule out lung diseases and acute myocardial infarction, such as chest X-ray, electrocardiogram, and myocardial necrosis enzymes. Then the transthoracic echocardiography was requested to reevaluate aortic stenosis with symptoms and signs (IA Evidence, [8]), which confirmed moderate aortic stenosis [8], with a valve area of 0.96 cm^2, systolic gradient of 31.1 mmHg, severe calcification, and significant ventricular dysfunction with an ejection fraction of 23%. In addition, to surgical planning, coronary angiography (IA Evidence, [8]), and CT angiography of the thoracic aorta, abdominal, iliac, and femoral arteries were requested.

2. What are the possible etiologies of the aortic stenosis?

In adults, there are three possible etiologies for aortic stenosis: degeneration of congenitally abnormal aortic valve, rheumatic valvular fibrosis, and senile calcific aortic stenosis. In aortic stenosis by congenitally abnormal valve, the most commonly found abnormality is a bicuspid aortic valve, which, over the years, becomes rigid and calcified, being considered stenotic in the sixth decade of life.

The rheumatic etiology generates commissural fusion coupled with valve calcification, which may cause shrinkage and anterior shortening of the margins of the leaflets, leading to some degree of aortic regurgitation associated with the stenosis.

Senile calcific stenosis is fairly common in elderly patients. In this type of stenosis, early degenerative changes occur through deposition of calcium on the leaflets and collagen fragmentation, leading to obstruction in variable time intervals, being possible to occur in only 2 years, as evidenced in the literature.

3. Discuss the pathophysiology of the disease.

The aortic valve stenosis may be asymptomatic, even in patients with severe stenosis. However, most patients with moderate stenosis already show symptoms.

The classic symptoms of this disease can be explained from the pathophysiology. The narrowed valve leads to obstruction of the outflow of the left ventricle, which increases the intracavitary pressure. This increase in systolic LV pressure, coupled with the higher ejection period, culminates in increased ventricular function and therefore the O_2 consumption by the myocardium.

If the patient performs physical exertion or is in a period of excitement, ventricular work previously increased by the aortic stenosis further rise and may precipitate angina and syncope, since there is no increase in cardiac output in response to the increased demand.

Systolic overload of the LV results in left ventricular hypertrophy of concentric nature. As ventricular ejection is prolonged and low, there is an increase in the duration of systemic arterial pulses.

In addition, the increase in LV diastolic pressure caused by aortic stenosis can produce increased pressure in the left atrium and symptoms of left heart failure, due to reduced LV compliance by hypertrophy or reduced ejection fraction, featuring another symptom of the aortic stenosis triad.

4. What are the indications for aortic valve replacement?

Aortic valve replacement is recommended in symptomatic patients with severe aortic stenosis (Class I, level of evidence B, AHA), D1 stage with (a) decreased systolic opening of a calcified aortic valve or congenitally stenotic, (b) aortic flow of 4 m/s or greater or medium pressure gradient of 40 mmHg or greater, and (C) symptoms of heart failure, syncope, dyspnea on exertion, angina, or reported pre-syncope or in exercise stress test.

It is also indicated for asymptomatic patients with severe aortic stenosis, C2 stage, and an ejection fraction less than 50%, with reduced systolic opening of a calcified aortic valve with increased aortic flow of 4 m/s or greater or medium pressure gradient of 40 mmHg or greater.

It is still indicated for patients with severe aortic stenosis, stage C or D, when undergoing cardiac surgery for other indications and has systolic opening reduced by a calcified aortic valve with increased aortic flow of 4 m/s or higher or medium pressure gradient of 40 mmHg or greater.

5. What is the indication for TAVR?

The choice of whether to proceed with TAVR versus surgery is based on various parameters, including surgical risk, patient frailty, and comorbidities. TAVR is recommended for patients who reach the indications for aortic valve replacement and have a prohibitive risk for surgical exchange and a post-TAVR expected survival greater than 12 months (Class I, Level of Evidence B, AHA), although study PARTNER has demonstrated the noninferiority of TAVR regarding heart surgery for high-risk patients with conditions for surgical valve replacement.

6. What was the indication for the revascularization of the left anterior descending artery through angioplasty?

According to the I Inter-American Guideline in Valvulopathy of 2011, coronary angiography before intervention with transcatheter aortic valve replacement in patients with risk factors for CAD have Class I recommendation, with level of evidence C. Therefore, although the evidence come from reports cases, there is consensus for the indication in these cases, as the patient in question.

7. The surgical risk varies according to the patient and the type of desired procedure. How is the surgical and mortality risk calculated to indicate a safer option for the patient?

There are two scores worldwide used to estimate mortality risk according to the surgical procedure planned, as well as to predict possible complications, such as stroke and wound infection, the EuroSCORE and the STS score. According to the patient in question, estimates, considering two surgical procedures, are:

EuroSCORE: 12–14. 26.77%
STS:
Mortality risk: 4.715%
Morbidity or mortality: 34.704%
Stroke: 0.719%
Prolonged ventilation: 20.145%
Reoperation: 13.572%
Wound infection (sternum): 0.871%

8. How to proceed with anticoagulation in TAVR?

Heparin must be used during the TAVR procedure coupled with dual antiplatelet therapy with aspirin and thienopyridines for 6–12 months, depending on the clinical case. Concerning drug-eluting stents, patients should use dual antiplatelet therapy indefinitely.

9. How are we going to choose the best access of TAVR? Are there differences between them?

There are several access methods to perform TAVR; the two most common are:

(a) Via the femoral artery called transfemoral approach, which does not require a surgical incision or a minimal one
(b) Transapical approach, in which a small incision in the chest is made to reach the site of the aortic valve through the left ventricle apex

Generally, the transfemoral approach is preferred because it is less invasive and allows using lower profile delivery systems. This approach has the disadvantage of being impossible to perform in patients with small diameter vessels (<6 mm) and in patients with occlusive disease in the aortoiliac arteries. Extreme tortuosity of vessels can also compromise the technique. Because of these method limitations, a plan to assess the luminal diameter of the arteries and their level of calcification and tortuosity should be made, requesting a CT scan with contrast, which can be associated with angiography or intravascular ultrasound.

The transapical approach is the second most used method, having as an advantage the fact that virtually all patients are candidates for this strategy. It should also be considered an advantage the small distance between the incision and the aortic valve, which is in a straight line, allowing the use of a more rigid equipment, which facilitates a correct valve placement. As a disadvantage, the method is more invasive, with the need to perform a surgical thoracotomy, endangering especially the elderly, debilitated patients and those with significant lung disease.

There are other methods, such as the direct aortic approach and the subclavian approach.

10. How is the follow-up after TAVR?

Follow-up (FU) post-TAVR presents various aspects to be analyzed, including multiple comorbidities and complications inherent in the implant of any valve provided specifically for

TAVR. The Mauriziano TAVR follow-up program proposed the following flowchart:

- First scheduled visit in 3 months or more: analysis of clinical status, ECG, blood tests, major adverse cardiovascular and cerebrovascular events and other adverse events, adherence to prescriptions, and associated with the review of prosthesis performance and heart dynamics by the echocardiography
- Second visit in 6 months or more: clinical and echocardiographic review
- Final TAVR-FU in 12 months after TAVR: clinical and echocardiographic review

After these, it is possible to continue the Follow-up by new clinical and echo reviews at the cardiologic center or by local physicians with periodic contacts between them and the cardiologists of the center where the procedure was done.

Bibliography

1. American Heart Association and American College of Cardiology. Guideline for the management of patients with valvular heart disease. J Am Coll Cardiol. 2014;63:57–185.
2. Aranzulla TC, Benedictis M, Asteggiano R. Follow-up management after transcatheter aortic valve implantation (TAVI). E-J Cardiol Pract. 2016;14. Available at: https://www.escardio.org/Journals/E-Journal-of-Cardiology-Practice/Volume-14/Follow-up-management after transcatheter-aortic-valve-implantation-TAVI (Accessed 20 Aug 2016).
3. EuroSCORE Study Group. 2011. EuroSCORE. Available at: www.euroscore.org/calc.html (Accessed 20 Aug 2016).
4. Mack MJ. Access for transcatheter aortic valve replacement - which is the preferred route. J Am Coll Cardiol Cardiovasc Interv. 2012;5:477–8.
5. Piérard L. Transcatheter aortic valve implantation: indications. E-J Cardiol Pract. 2016;14. Available at: www.escardio.org/Journals/E-

Journal-of-Cardiology-Practice/Volume-14/transcatheter-aortic-valve-implantation-indications (Accessed 20 Aug 2016).

6. Ramlawi B, Anaya-Ayala JE, Reardon MJ. Transcatheter aortic valve replacement (TAVR): access planning and strategies. Methodist DeBakey Cardiovasc J. 2012;8(2):22–5.
7. Smith CR, et al. Transcatheter versus surgical aortic-valve replacement in high-risk patients. New Engl J Med. 2011;364:2187–98.
8. Sociedade Brasileira de Cardiologia and Sociedade Interamericana de Cardiologia. Diretriz Brasileira de Valvopatias/I Diretriz Interamericana de Valvopatias. Arq Bras Cardiol. 2011;97:1–67.
9. Society of Thoracic Surgeons. STS adult cardiac surgery database risk Model Variables. 2014. Available at: http://riskcalc.sts.org/stswebriskcalc/#/ (Accessed 20 Aug 2016).
10. Thibault GE, DeSanctis RW, Buckley MJ. Estenose Aórtica. In: Eagle KA, DeSanctis EHRW, Austen G, editors. Cardiologia. Vol. 1, 2ª edição, Medsi Editora Médica e Científica Ltda; 1993.

Aortic Coarctation

Laura Gomes Flores, Luana Luiza Vieira, Heloísa Guedes Andrade, Fábio Selig, and Rui M. S. Almeida

Clinical Presentation

An 11-year-old, white patient was admitted to the hospital with severe headache. After physical examination, he was overweight and had high blood pressure. Blood pressure was discrepant between upper and lower limbs, presenting a pressure gradient of 50 mmHg. At the vascular physical examination, arterial pulses of the lower limbs were reduced. Patient did not present comorbidities or changes in physical examination.

Diagnosis, Assessment, and Treatment

Initially, an electrocardiogram was performed. It showed sinus rhythm, heart rate of 75 beats per minute, and left ventricular cardiac axis, suggesting left ventricular hypertrophy.

L. G. Flores (✉) · L. L. Vieira · H. G. Andrade · F. Selig
Assis Gurgacz Foundation University (FAG), Cascavel, PR, Brazil

R. M. S. Almeida
Department of Cardiology and Cardiovascular Surgery, University Center Assis Gurgacz Foundation, Cascavel, PR, Brazil

R. M. S. Almeida, F. B. Jatene (eds.), *Cardiovascular Surgery*,
https://doi.org/10.1007/978-3-319-57084-6_22

After the electrocardiogram, angiotomography of the thoracic aorta was requested, which identified coarctation area of the descending thoracic artery near the ascendance of the subclavian artery on the left. The aortic arch had preserved caliber (20.1 cm × 18.8 mm). At coarctation level, the aorta had approximately 12.3 × 8.5 mm and posterior to the coarctation area had 17.7 × 17.2 mm, evidencing the diagnosis of coarctation of the aorta (Fig. 1).

After the diagnostic confirmation, the need for interventional therapy was defined because the patient had a pressure gradient greater than 20 mmHg between the upper and lower limbs (Fig. 2).

The therapeutic options available to the patient were balloon angioplasty, balloon angioplasty and stenting, and cardiac surgery. Because it is a less invasive procedure and has good long-term results, initially the therapeutic option chosen was balloon angioplasty associated with stenting. However, in the service in which the procedure was performed, there was no stent with optimal measurements for the patient's aorta,

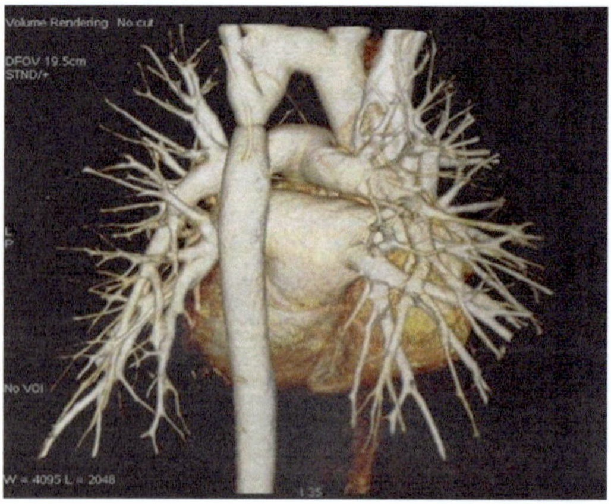

FIGURE 1 CT angiography of the thoracic aorta, showing coarctation area of the descending thoracic artery next to the emergence of the subclavian artery to the left

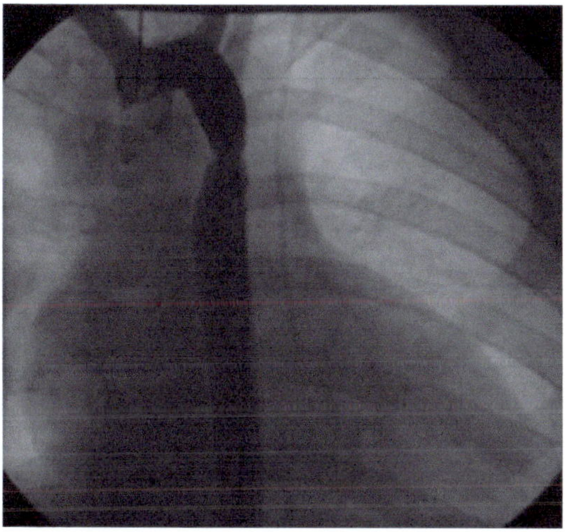

FIGURE 2 Aortography prior to the procedure

and *balloon angioplasty* was then chosen. This procedure was performed under general anesthesia and administration of heparin 100–150 U/kg and antibiotic for prophylaxis of infective endocarditis. From this, the right radial artery was punctured for manometry and angiography to guide the positioning of the balloon. After being well positioned, the balloon was inflated, dilating the constriction site. This mechanism always results in rupture of the inner layer of the vessel and, in this case, also resulted in rupture of the middle tunica at the base of the left subclavian artery, which favored the immediate onset of aneurysm (Fig. 3). Due to the fact that the bulging formed was greater than 50% of the vessel diameter, it was opted for its immediate exclusion with the placement of a stent. For this, radial access continued to be used to obtain images and pressure measurements and, because of the size of the introducer measuring 12 French, the femoral artery had to be dissected for its introduction. Although the femoral artery of the patient is overweight and hipodeveloped, his dissection was performed, and the correction of the aneurysm was successfully obtained (Fig. 4).

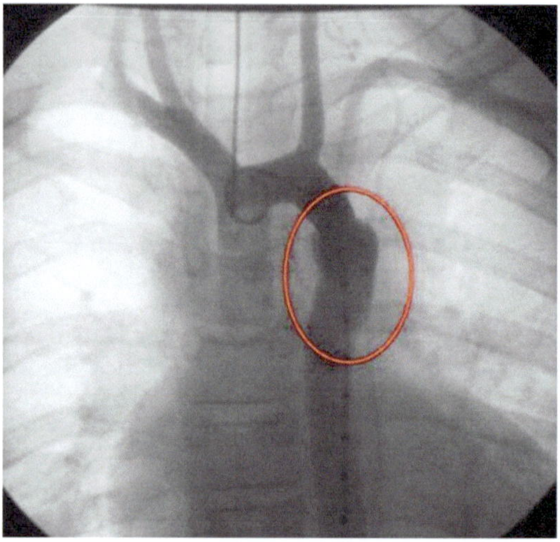

Figure 3 Aortography showing the aneurysm formed immediately after the procedure, with bulging greater than 50%

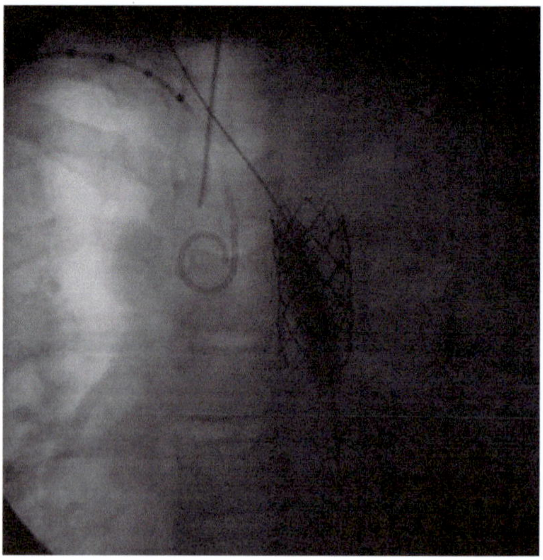

Figure 4 Exclusion of the aneurysm with covered stent

After angioplasty, the patient remained stable, with normalization of blood pressure and absence of gradient. He was discharged within 2 days and continued to use ASA and clopidogrel.

Questions

1. What complementary tests can be ordered on suspicion of coarctation of the aorta, and what are the suggestive findings of the pathology?

Chest X-ray, electrocardiogram, echocardiogram, aortic angiotomography, and aortography may be ordered.

Bilateral erosions in the posterior portion of the lower edge of the costal arches can be found from the chest radiograph. On the electrocardiogram, there are signs of left ventricular hypertrophy.

It is possible to visualize the coarctation zone and the presence of cardiac anomalies and to calculate the transcoarctation gradient from the bidimensional echocardiography associated with the Doppler.

Aortography and angiotomography define the location and extent of the obstruction and evaluate its severity and the presence and extent of collateral circulation [1].

2. What is the relationship between the pathophysiology of aortic coarctation and its clinical implications?

Obstruction of blood flow through the narrowing present in coarctation of the aorta causes different clinical manifestations that depend on the location and extent of the obstruction [1].

Generally in children, adolescents, and adults, left ventricular hypertrophy develops as a mechanism of progressive adaptation in order to maintain systolic performance in response to pressure overload. Thus, with the development of compensatory mechanisms, coarctation is rarely associated with exuberant symptoms after the first year of life. Patients in these age groups may complain of fatigue, headache, visual changes, and cramps in the lower limbs [2].

In neonates and infants up to 1 year, the left ventricular ejection fraction is reduced due to the intense and abrupt increase of the afterload and the nondevelopment of compensatory mechanisms, resulting in heart failure or cardiogenic shock [2]: approximately half of the newborns develop heart failure in the first months of life and may be fatal in 5–10% of cases [1].

3. What are the differential diagnoses of aortic coarctation?

Diseases that lead to heart failure and shock are differential diagnoses of aortic coarctation in neonates. Defects in the atrioventricular septum, aortic stenosis, mitral stenosis, and left heart hypoplastic syndrome are congenital heart diseases that also constitute differential diagnosis of coarctation [3].

In older children, diseases that cause changes in the peripheral pulses and other causes of hypertension and primary or secondary ventricular hypertrophy or dilatation are differential diagnoses [3].

There are several causes of secondary hypertension, such as renal artery stenosis or thrombosis, renal failure, congenital adrenal hyperplasia, acute glomerulonephritis, pheochromocytoma, and use of corticosteroids [3].

Ventricular hypertrophy may occur in aortic stenosis, aortic coarctation, and in cases of arterial hypertension [3].

Takayasu's arteritis – vasculitis that affects the aorta and its primary branches – leads to coarctation in the thoracic or abdominal aorta [3].

4. When should surgical treatment and endovascular treatment be performed?

In the first year of life, the surgical approach is the treatment of choice. The most commonly used operative techniques consist of an end-to-end anastomosis and subclavian flap, which, by using autologous tissue, allow the vessel to grow in accordance with the patient's overall growth. Between the two techniques, the end-to-end anastomosis is mainly used, since the subclavian flap is associated with higher rates of complications, such as aortic aneurysm development and recoarctation. Balloon angioplasty has very high rates of restenosis in patients of this age group and is considered an alternative only in unstable newborns with high surgical risk, providing hemodynamic relief for elective posterior repair surgery [4].

Between the first year of life and 8–10 years, surgery remains the therapeutic approach of choice, since, despite the effectiveness of angioplasty in reducing the aortic gradient in children, there is a high risk of recoarctation, rupture, and formation of aneurysms. From this age group, balloon angioplasty becomes a viable option, with good long-term results. It is recommended that stent placement be associated with this procedure, since it avoids elastic retraction of the vessel wall, allowing the stabilization and fixation of the intima, which reduces the risk of aortic rupture and formation of aneurysms [4].

There is still much discussion about the best therapeutic option for adults, but several authors advocate the use of stents as the most effective and safe option.

This is due to the fact that the surgical approach, either by the end-to-end anastomosis operative technique or by graft interposition in the primary coarctation, presents a mortality of 31% for 40 years – mainly due to significant consequences of the disease in the long term, such as heart insufficiency – and be associated with renal insufficiency and postoperative paraplegia, results of unsafe organ perfusion. And due to balloon angioplasty, despite having an initial success rate of 80–90%, a post-optimal procedure result is presented, with a residual gradient greater than or equal to 20 mmHg in more than 90% of the cases [4].

5. What are the most common complications of a balloon angioplasty procedure?

Complications of balloon angioplasty can be classified into technical ones, related to the aortic wall or peripheral vascular, and occur in up to 14% of cases. Stent migration or fracture, balloon rupture, and unintentional stent placement covering the vessels of the aortic arch are technical complications. Complications related to the aortic wall include dissection, flap formation, or aneurysms. Cerebral stroke, peripheral embolism, and femoral artery injury are peripheral vascular complications [5].

6. The procedure performed resulted in the formation of an aneurysm. What mechanism could have caused it, and what conduct could be taken?

There was immediate aneurysm formation in the patient's procedure, a fact that reflects the mechanism of action of this technique: angioplasty acts by causing a lesion in the vessel wall because of the radial forces of the balloon with rupture of the intima layer and part of the middle layer. Consequently, healing occurs in the vessel wall with increased intraluminal diameter. The improvement of local flow promotes remodeling and development of the aortic arch and isthmus. However, the rupture may extend through the middle tunic, sparing only the adventitia, which favors the appearance of an aneurysm, probably in areas with the appearance of cystic necrosis. If the patient has bulging greater than 50% of the diameter of the vessel and is adult or weighs more than 30 kg, as in this case, its exclusion is indicated, by means of covered stents, in order to avoid possible vascular rupture [5].

7. How is the follow-up of the patients who underwent the therapeutic intervention?

Patients with repaired or unrepaired coarctation must be followed by a cardiologist throughout their lifetime. For those who have undergone repair, this follow-up should be at least annually, with specific attention paid to baseline or exercise-induced hypertension. Patients with parietal irregularities or bulges smaller than 50% of the vessel diameter should be monitored clinically, with strict control of blood pressure, and should perform control tests periodically (MRI and spiral CT). By the 2007 American Heart Association guidelines, endocarditis prophylaxis is not routinely recommended beyond the first 6 months after surgical or transcatheter intervention, barring a previous history of infectious endocarditis [6].

8. What is the prognosis of patients with aortic coarctation?

Patients with coarctation of the aorta have survival below the general population [1]: the mean survival time of nonoperated patients is 35 years. Frequent complications in patients are hypertension, acute myocardial infarction, accelerated coronary heart disease, and congestive heart failure: the main cause of death in patients with coarctation is acute coronary disease [4].

Patients undergoing successful repair before the age of 5 remain with a lower survival rate than the general population – 91% of operated patients remain alive at age 20 and 80% at 40–50 years. The age of the repair is a determinant factor in the survival of the patients, so that the late diagnosis negatively influences the survival and the early treatment is recommended. However, patients with late diagnosis are candidates for repair since they benefit from reduced risk of cardiovascular events and increased survival [4].

Review About the Addressed Disease or Treatment

Coarctation of the aorta consists of a narrowing of the aorta. The most common localization is in the distal segment to the origin of the left subclavian artery, close to the insertion of the arterial ligament, but may occur in any region along the aorta [7]. Coarctation of the aorta is the sixth most common congenital heart disease: 6–8% of congenital heart diseases [2]. It is more frequent in males, and in about 30% of cases, it occurs concomitantly with other malformations [4]. Clinical manifestations depend on the location and severity of the obstruction and may present asymptomatically or with the presence of symptoms such as headache, epistaxis, cold extremities, and claudication to the efforts [7]. The presence of adaptive mechanisms, such as left ventricular hypertrophy and the development of collateral circulation in response to obstruction and pressure overload, may mask the severity of coarctation and reduce the gradient present through obstruction [4]. At physical examination, the classic manifestations are the difference in blood pressure and pulse amplitude between the upper and lower limbs. The lower limb pulses may be absent, markedly reduced or retarded [7].

Complementary examinations such as electrocardiogram, chest X-ray, echocardiogram, and magnetic resonance imaging or computed tomography can be performed [7].

The electrocardiogram may show signs of left ventricular hypertrophy. The location of the narrowing can be evidenced by bidirectional echocardiogram (suprasternal window), and the pressure gradient can be measured with Doppler echocardiography. The severity and length of the obstruction and the presence of collateral arteries can be evaluated by magnetic resonance imaging or three-dimensional computed tomography [7].

Catheterization in adults is indicated primarily for evaluation of coronary arteries prior to therapeutic procedures [6] or for catheter interventions [7].

The therapeutic options for coarctation of the aorta are surgical treatment, balloon angioplasty, or stenting. Surgery is the therapy of choice until around 8–10 years of age. In older children and adolescents, balloon angioplasty or stent placement becomes a viable option because it is less invasive and has good long-term results [4].

The survival of patients with coarctation of the aorta is inferior to the survival of the general population. The age of the repair is a determinant factor in the survival of patients, so early treatment is recommended. However, patients with late diagnosis also benefit from repair because of reduced risk of cardiovascular events and increased survival [4].

Bibliography

1. Souza G, et al. Coarctação de aorta: uma causa rara de hipertensão arterial. Med Int. 2001;6(2):7–9.
2. Pedra CAC. Análise dos resultados imediatos e tardios do tratamento percutâneo da coarctação da aorta em adolescentes e adultos: comparação entre balões e stents, Tese de Doutorado da Faculdade de Medicina da Universidade de São Paulo. 2004.
3. Horta da Silva J. Tratamento endovascular em criança portadora de coarctação da aorta: relato de caso clínico. Programa de Residência Médica em Pediatria – Secretaria de Estado de Saúde do Governo do Distrito Federal. 2008.
4. Clare Sousa Ennis G. Tratamento da coarctação da aorta: Revisão da literatura nos últimos cinco anos. Mestrado integrado em medicina – Faculdade de Medicina Universidade do Porto. 2014.

5. Costa RC, Fontcs VM, Pedra CAC. Intervenções percutâneas nas principais cardiopatias congênitas obstrutivas. In: Abizaid A, Costa Jr JR, editors. Manual de Cardiologia Intervencionista do Istituto Dante Pazzanese. 1° ed. Rio de Janeiro: Elsevier Editora Ltda; 2013.
6. Torok RD, Campbell MJ, Fleming GA, Hill KD. Coarctation of the aorta: management from infancy to adulthood. World J Cardiol. 2015;7(11):765–75.
7. Longo DL, et al. Internal medicine Harrison, vol. 2. 18th ed. São Paulo: AMGH; 2013. p. 1925–6.

Endovascular Treatment for Abdominal Aortic Aneurysm

Rômulo Martins de Camargo, Rodrigo Mendes, Nelson Américo Hossne Junior, Eduardo Gregório Chamlian, and Fabiano André Pereira

Clinical Presentation

A 58-year-old female patient presented at São Paulo Hospital with intense abdominal pain in epigastric region, for 2 weeks. She related the pain had a sudden onset, with irradiation to the back, on the last days. She denied any other associated symptoms. The patient was born in Mandaguaçu and lives in São Paulo. She is widow, catholic and has three children (G3P3A0). She also reported to be a smoker, 40 packs-year, and takes captopril 25 mg 12/12 h. Her medical history is significant for systemic arterial hypertension (SAH), and she had a tubal ligation 36 years ago. Her family history revealed her mother was hypertensive and had diabetes mellitus type 2. Both her mother and father died of unknown cause.

At physical examination, she was flushed, hydrated, acyanotic, anicteric, feverless, eupneic in rest, and neurologically oriented. Her blood pressure was 130/80 mmHg, pulse rate 80

R. M. de Camargo (✉) · R. Mendes · N. A. H. Junior
E. G. Chamlian · F. A. Pereira
Federal University of São Paulo (UNIFESP), São Paulo, SP, Brazil

R. M. S. Almeida, F. B. Jatene (eds.), *Cardiovascular Surgery*,
https://doi.org/10.1007/978-3-319-57084-6_23

beats/min, oxygen saturation 96%, and respiration rate 14 breaths/min. There were no carotid bruits and no jugular stasis. Pulmonary and cardiac auscultations were normal, there was good expansiveness when breathing, and ictus cordis was palpable at the fifth intercostal space. The abdomen was normotensive and painless to palpation with liver and spleen not palpable. It also presented a large pulsatile mass with imprecise limits in the mesogastric region. Furthermore, limbs had no edema, and symmetrical palpable pulses were noted.

The patient possesses two risk factors for atherosclerosis (smoker and SAH). The presence of pain and a pulsatile mass, added to the risk factors, suggested an aneurysm as possible diagnostic. Considering the imprecise limits of the pulsatile mass on abdominal palpation, it could be a thoracoabdominal aortic aneurysm, with a supradiaphragmatic proximal neck. For complementary investigation of this patient, laboratory tests for hematological and biochemical evaluation, chest X-rays, electrocardiogram, transthoracic echocardiogram, coronary angiography, due to risk factors for atherosclerosis, and tomography of descending aorta with intravenous contrast were demanded.

Diagnosis, Assessment, and Treatment

Laboratory results are the following: hemoglobin, 12.5 g/dL; hematocrit, 35.7%; leukocytes, 9120/mm^3; platelets, 227000/mm^3; Na, 139 mmol/L; K, 5.1 mmol/L; urea, 136 mg/dL; creatinine, 1.65 mg/dL; thromboplastin partial activated time, 35.6 s/1.24; prothrombin activity, 100%/0.97; C-reactive protein (CRP), 19 mg/L; and erythrocyte sedimentation rate (ESR), 93 mm/h. An increased level of creatinine indicates chronic kidney disease, justified by SAH. It also can be noted an elevation in markers of inflammation (CRP and ESR), which suggests, with a normal leukogram and absence of fever, inflammatory activity of atherosclerotic disease.

Electrocardiogram (Fig. 1) showed normal sinus rhythm with a rate of 65 beats/min, left ventricle overload, and normal heart axis. The left ventricle overload denotes the long-standing and poorly controlled SAH.

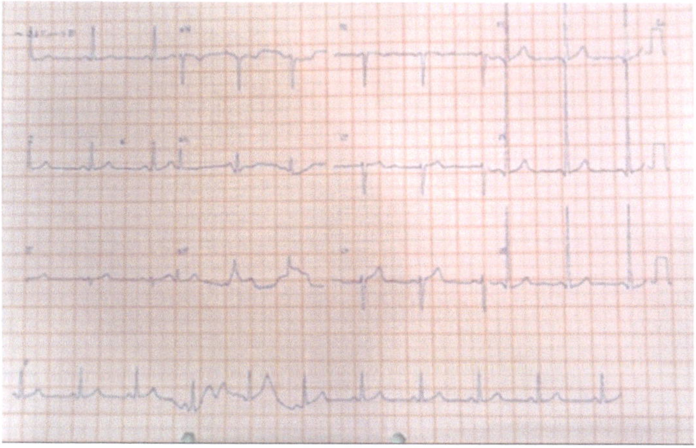

FIGURE 1 Electrocardiogram showing a left ventricle overcharge

Echocardiogram revealed concentric remodeling of the left ventricle, ventricular septum in sigmoid format (10 mm), mild to moderate tricuspid regurgitation, PASP (pulmonary artery systolic pressure) (25 mmHg), mild ectasia of the aortic root (40 mm), and LVEF (left ventricular ejection fraction) (60%). The concentric remodeling of the left ventricle reinforces the diagnosis of poorly controlled SAH, with consequent hypertrophy. It is also noticed mild ectasia in the aortic root.

In the X-rays (Fig. 2), cardiac silhouette is normal in size, and it can be observed presence of aortic knob calcifications, secondary to the atherosclerosis.

Tomography (Fig. 3) evidences an abdominal aortic aneurysm (AAA), infra diaphragmatic, with a proximal neck below the emergence of the superior mesenteric artery; sparing the bifurcation of iliac arteries.

Coronary Angiography showed right dominant coronary circulation, 30% stenosis of the left coronary trunk ostium, left anterior descending artery with severe calcification in the proximal third, 70% stenosis of the diagonal branch, left circumflex artery with parietal irregularities, marginal branch with parietal irregularities, 30% stenosis

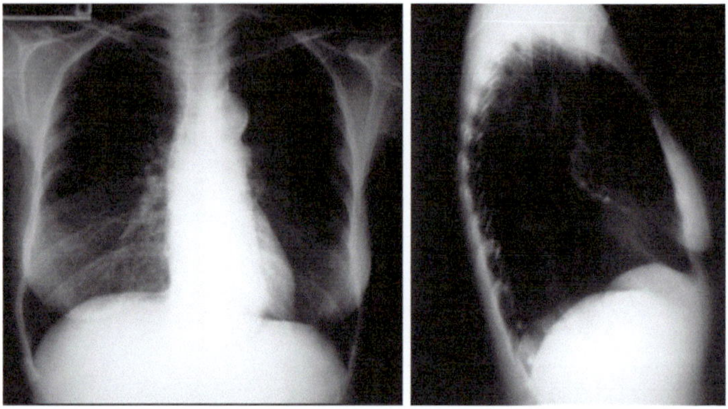

FIGURE 2 X-rays – presence of aortic knob calcifications

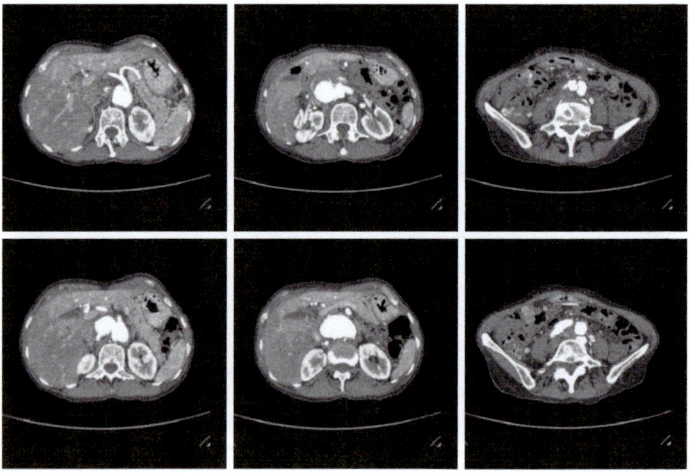

FIGURE 3 Tomography revealing an abdominal aortic aneurysm and its limits

of right coronary artery in the middle third. Posterior ventricular branch and posterior descending with parietal irregularities. These results demonstrate the systemic nature of atherosclerotic disease, with presence of coronary lesions in the left coronary artery (30%), diagonal artery (70%), and right coronary artery (30%).

According to the exams, she was diagnosed with an abdominal aortic aneurysm (infra-mesenteric), systemic arterial hypertension, and chronic coronary insufficiency. Considering that the aneurysm of this patient has a good proximal neck, without aortic dilatation at the level of renal arteries and superior mesenteric artery, it was proposed the endovascular stent-graft treatment with bifurcated aortic endoprosthesis implantation through femoral artery puncture, with both iliac arteries covered with isolated stent grafts. Regarding the chronic coronary insufficiency, this patient has no indication of a revascularization procedure for the present lesions. In addition, as she is an asymptomatic patient, with no angina or dyspnea, it was opted for clinical treatment.

The AAA was successfully repaired (Fig. 4), and the patient made a good recovery, being discharged home after 7 days in hospital.

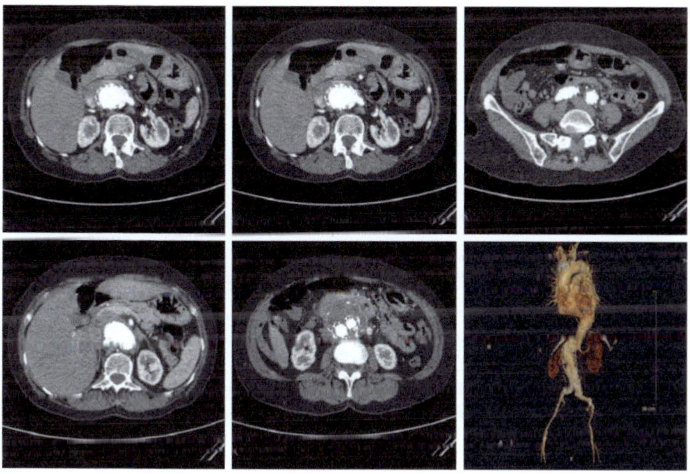

FIGURE 4 Postoperative tomography showing the successful AAA's endovascular repair

Questions

1. What are the normal dimensions of the thoracic aorta?

The normal dimensions of the thoracic aorta are the following: aortic annulus, 2–3 cm; sinuses of Valsalva, 2.5–3.5 cm; sinotubular junction, 2–3 cm; ascending aorta, 2.5–3.5 cm; aortic arch, 2.5–3 cm; descending aorta, 2–3 cm; diaphragmatic aorta, 2–2.5 cm; and infrarenal aorta 1.5–2 cm.

2. Why in this particular case the correct diagnosis is abdominal aortic aneurysm and not abdominal aortic dilatation?

Because an aneurysm is defined as a permanent localized dilatation of an artery (≥150% diameter of the normal caliber).

3. What is the pathologic classification of the aortic aneurysms?

There are two types of aneurysms: a true aneurysm, in which the dilated segment involves all three layers of the vessel, and a false or pseudoaneurysm, which is a contained hematoma outlined by adventitia or surrounding tissues.

4. What are the predisposing factors for a thoracic aortic aneurysm?

The predisposing factors for the aneurysm are age, atherosclerosis, bicuspid aortic valve (associated with fibrillin deficiency), blood pressure (hypertension), connective tissue disorders (Marfan syndrome, Ehlers-Danlos Syndrome), dissection, degenerative (cystic medial degeneration), trauma, aortitis, infection, and syphilis.

5. What are the clinical features of patients with thoracic aortic aneurysms?

Many patients are asymptomatic and discover the aneurysm by incidental finding on imaging exams. For symptomatic patients, clinical features are pain – anterior chest pain or back pain (typically interscapular), with sudden onset of the pain suggesting dissection or impending rupture; compression of nearby structures resulting in hoarseness (recurrent laryngeal nerve), dysphagia (esophagus), and stridor and dyspnea (trachea); and fistula resulting in hematemesis (esophagus) or hemoptysis (lung, bronchi).

6. How are thoracic aortic dissections classified?

There are two widely known classifications of dissections, Stanford and DeBakey. Stanford type A includes dissections that involve the ascending aorta, whereas type B dissections do not involve the ascending aorta. DeBakey type 1 dissections involve the whole aorta, type 2 dissections involve only the ascending aorta, type 3a dissection involves the descending aorta, and type 3b involves the descending and the abdominal aorta. Aortic dissections can also be classified by timing: acute (<14 days), subacute (14 days–2 months), and chronic (>2 month).

7. What is acute aortic syndrome?

Acute aortic syndrome is defined as a group of life-threatening thoracic pathologies that includes aortic dissection, penetrating aortic ulcer, intramural hematoma, and leaking aortic aneurysm.

Review About the Addressed Disease or Treatment

The term aortic aneurysm refers to a pathological dilatation of the normal aortic lumen involving one or several segments. Although perhaps no definition is universally accepted, an aortic aneurysm is best described as a permanent localized dilatation of the aorta having a diameter at least 1.5 times that of the expected normal diameter of that given aortic segment ([9], p. 1424). Aneurysms are usually described in terms of their location, size, morphology, and etiology.

Abdominal aortic aneurysms (AAA) are much more common than thoracic aortic aneurysms, and its annual incidence in western populations is approximately 2.5–6.5 cases in 1000 people [7]. AAAs occur four to five times more frequently in men than women, being age as an important risk factor inasmuch as the incidence rises rapidly after 55 years of age in men and 70 years of age in women ([9], p. 1424).

Many aneurysms can be detected on physical examination, although even large aneurysms may be difficult or impossible to detect in obese individuals. When palpable, a pulsatile mass extending variably from the xiphoid process to the umbilicus may be appreciated. Because of difficulty distinguishing the abdominal aorta from surrounding structures by palpation, the size of an aneurysm tends to be overestimated on physical examination ([9], p. 1425). The diagnosis is usually based on imaging exams, which is why major parts of aneurysms are incidentally found. Computed tomography is the best method to diagnose aortic aneurysms and sizing them.

The pathogenesis of AAA is a multifactorial process, with underlying genetic, inflammatory, infectious, and autoimmune components. After an aneurysm is formed, its risk of rupture is related to a series of factors, including maximum diameter, rate of expansion, hypertension, and age, among others. The natural history of AAA is progressive expansion, subsequent increased aneurysm wall stress, and eventual rupture. AAA rupture has a mortality rate of 81% ([8], p. 1407), which shows how important it is to predict this risk and to perform an intervention, such as an endovascular repair or open surgery, when the risk of rupture is significant. Among the factors above, size remains the most suitable criterion to predict the risk of rupture of an aneurysm, although other factors such as rate of expansion and wall stress also play an important role. This way, even asymptomatic aneurysms, larger than 5.0 cm of diameter, are referred to repair, if surgical risk is acceptable ([9], p. 1426).

The choice of surgical technique depends on each pathophysiology. The endovascular technique consists in a femoral artery puncture, through which a catheter is inserted and advanced to the aneurysm site. A guide wire and an expandable stent graft are advanced through the catheter. When positioned correctly, the stent graft is allowed to expand within the artery. The wire frame pushes against healthy portion of the aorta to seal the device in place. Once in place, the blood flows through the stent graft and cannot enter the aneurysm. This technique is usually preferred for unruptured AAAs because of its greater speed, less exposure (less invasive procedure), shorter postoperative recovery time, fewer pain complaints, and less risk of ischemia (due to constant flow in the aorta). However, it cannot be performed in all patients, since in some cases, the aortic aneurysm may not have an anatomic favorable to the endovascular treatment, or it may be very close to other organs, not having sufficient space for the "landing zone," which is the place of support and fixation of the prosthesis, thus requiring a traditional open surgery.

Endovascular surgery to repair aortic aneurysm is not free of complications, which may appear during or after the procedure. Batt et al. ([6], p. 339) classify postoperative complications in both early and late stages. The most common are related to the surgical procedure, such as persistent bleeding with consumption of coagulation factors, vascular lesions, parenchymal organ damage, ureter injury, embolisms, hypothermia, and thrombosis. Late complications are anastomotic pseudoaneurysms, aorto-enteric fistulas, thrombosis, and graft infection. Patients with a history of smoking and chronic obstructive pulmonary disease have a risk factor for the development of failure. Other complications associated with this method include endoleak (persistent blood flow within the aneurysm sac), which may cause prosthesis thrombosis; blockage of blood flow through the stent graft, movement of the stent graft out of the original positioning site, fracture of the stent graft, and aortic aneurysm during the placement of the stent due to dilatation caused by the angioplasty balloon; and possibility of occlusion of any major artery (e.g., renal artery).

The increased morbidity and mortality of patients who underwent surgery for correction of endovascular aneurysm of the aorta is not defined, not yet knowing whether or not it is related to the surgical technique ([2], p. 14).

Bibliography

1. Bastos RM, Filho AR, Blasbalg R, Caffaro RA, Karakhanian WK, Esteves FP, et al. Trombose na endoprótese do aneurisma da aorta: avaliação por TC multidetector. Rev Assoc Med Bras. 2011;57:31–4.

2. Koning GG, Vallabhneni SR, Marrewijk CJV, Leurs LJ, Laheij RJF, Buth J. Mortalidade relacionada ao tratamento endovascular do aneurisma da aorta abdominal com o uso dos modelos revisados. Rev Bras Cir Cardiovasc. 2007;22:7–14.
3. Parodi JC, Palmaz JC, Barone HD. Transfemoral intraluminal graft implantation for abdominal aortic aneurysms. Ann Vasc Surg. 1991;5:491–9.
4. Silvestre JMS, Motta F, Sardinha WE, et al. Endovascular treatment of infrarenal abdominal aortic aneurysm in patients with favorable anatomy for the repair - initial experience in a university hospital. J Vasc Bras. 2011;10:31–9.
5. Prinssen M, Verhoeven EL, Buth J, et al. A randomized trial comparing conventional and endovascular repair of abdominal aortic aneurysms. N Engl J Med. 2004;351:1607–18.
6. Batt M, Staccini P, Pittaluga P, Ferrari E, Hassen-Khodja R, Declemy S. Late survival after abdominal aortic aneurysm repair. Eur J Vasc Endovasc Surg. 1999;17:338–42.
7. Forsdahl SH, Singh K, Solberg S, Jacobsen BK. Risk factors for abdominal aortic aneurysms: a 7-year prospective study: the TromsoStudy 1994–2001. Institution: Institute of Community Medicine, University of Tromso; 2009.
8. Reimerink JJ, van der Laan MJ, Koelemay MJ, Balm R, Legemate DA. Systematic review and meta-analysis of population-based mortality from ruptured abdominal aortic aneurysm. Br J Surg. 2013;100:1405–13.
9. Braunwald E, Zipes D, Libby P. Herat disease: a textbook of cardiovascular medicine. 6th ed. Philadelphia: W. B. Saunders Company; 2001.
10. Patel MR, Dehmer GJ, Hirshfeld JW, Smith PK, Spertus JA. ACCF/SCAI/STS/AATS/AHA/ASNC/HFSA/SCCT appropriate use criteria for coronary revascularization focused update: a report of the American College of Cardiology Foundation Appropriate Use Criteria Task Force, Society for Cardiovascular Angiography and Interventions, Society of Thoracic Surgeons, American Association for Thoracic Surgery, American Heart Association, American Society of Nuclear Cardiology, and the Society of Cardiovascular Computed Tomography. J Am Coll Cardiol. 2012;59:857–81.

Part VII
Heart Failure

Acute Heart Failure Without Prior History of Myocardial Dysfunction

Felipe Bruno Santos da Cunha, Diogo Assis Souza, Henrique Louzan Machado, and Helmgton José Brito de Souza

Clinical Presentation

M.C.O.M., female, 62 years old, admitted in the emergency room with sudden and progressive onset of dyspnea for about an hour before admission. Refers rheumatoid arthritis and upper airways infection (UAI) for about a week. On examination, the patient was tachycardic, tachypneic, and hypotensive (96 × 60 mmHg), presenting jugular venous distention and plethora in the face, neck, and upper chest. Cardiac auscultation showed hypophonic sounds.

Diagnosis, Assessment, and Treatment

The patient was intubated in the emergency room, being placed on mechanical ventilation and initiated continuous infusion of noradrenaline (0.2 mcg/kg/min). Electrocardiogram (ECG)

F. B. S. da Cunha (✉) · D. A. Souza · H. L. Machado
H. J. B. de Souza
Unified School of Brasília (UNICEUB), Brasília, DF, Brazil

R. M. S. Almeida, F. B. Jatene (eds.), *Cardiovascular Surgery*,
https://doi.org/10.1007/978-3-319-57084-6_24

at admission showed atrial fibrillation (AF) and arterial blood gas values for PCO_2, 54 mmHg; pH, 6.58; PO_2, 52 mmHg; HCO_3, 9.9 mEq/L; and SO_2, 54%. Still had WBC, 14,350/mm^3; band cells, 4%; platelet, 130,000/mm^3; C-reactive protein (CRP), 1.07 mg/dL (Reference Value – RV, 0.5 mg/dL); troponin, 0.846 ng/ml (RV < 0.016); and CK mass, 17.9 ng/mL (RV < 3.4).

Transthoracic echocardiogram showed severe left ventricular dysfunction and mild to moderate pericardial effusion with the collapse of the right ventricle. The patient was subjected to pericardiocentesis with removal of a small amount of liquid (130 ml) and transferred to intensive care unit (ICU), where a catheter was inserted for invasive hemodynamic monitoring (Swan-Ganz) in the left subclavian vein and continuous blood pressure (BP) in MSE.

Another echocardiogram showed severe biventricular dysfunction (EF 15%) (Fig. 1, ECO transthoracic). A progressive increase of noradrenaline (01 mcg/kg/min), associated with dobutamine (08 mcg/kg/min) and vasopressin (0.04 U/min), was necessary. Held chemical cardioversion of AF with amiodarone and electrical cardioversion. Intra-aortic balloon was installed without significant improvement in hemodynamic

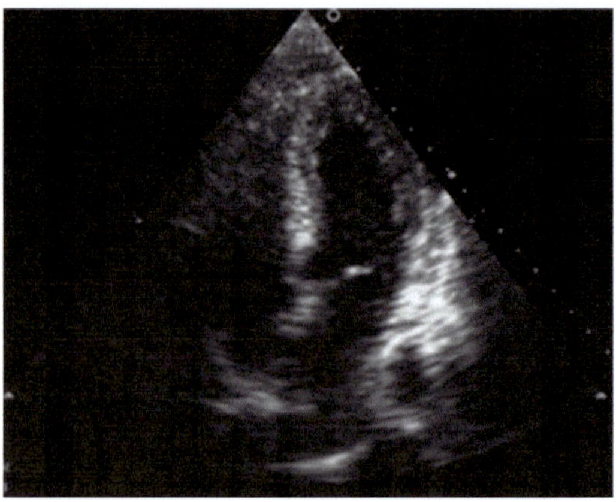

FIGURE 1 ECO transthoracic (EF, 15%)

condition. Arterial blood gas analysis showed severe respiratory acidosis with pH, 7.2 (RV = 7,35–7,45); blood lactate, 28 mg/dL (RV = 4,5–14,4 mg/dL); PCO_2, 58 mmHg (RV = 35–45 mmHg); PO_2, 68 mmHg (RV = 80–100 mmHg); HCO_{3-}, 29 mmHg (RV = 22–36 mmHg); SpO_2, 83% (RV = 95–100%); SVO_2, 65% (RV = 68–77%).

Considering the refractory cardiogenic shock and clinical progression with multiple organ failure, it was decided by the installation of circulatory assist device – extracorporeal membrane oxygenation (ECMO) in venoarterial mode with right femoral vein (23F Maquet cannula) and femoral artery (17F Maquet cannula) cannulation by the Seldinger technique. Patient progressed after 6 h of ECMO installation with hemodynamic improvement, being possible to reduce vasoactive amines (noradrenaline, 0.5 mcg/kg/min; dobutamine, 8 mcg/kg/min; vasopressin, 0.02 U/min) and improvement of metabolic acidosis, with blood gas pH, 7.3; PO_2, 105 mmHg; PCO_2, 45 mmHg; HCO_3, 20 mEq/L; and SpO_2, 94%. Echocardiogram after installation of ECMO showed moderate decompression of the heart chambers but maintenance of biventricular dysfunction (ejection fraction, 15%).

By completing 24 h of circulatory assistance, continuous infusion of heparin (10 U/kg/h) was started. Patient presented bleeding puncture and melena, and endoscopy showed gastric ulcer. After 48 h of circulatory assistance, she returned to present AF, despite of the continued use of amiodarone and multiple electrical cardioversion, requiring increased vasoactive amines. There was the need for blood transfusions with packed red blood cells (04 IU) and platelets (15 IU). Another echocardiography showed biventricular asystole and strain of the cardiac chambers. Exams on the second day of circulatory support showed arterial gasometry – pH, 7.38 (RV = 7,35–7,45); pCO_2, 58 mmHg (RV = 35–45 mmHg); PO_2, 71 mmHg (RV = 80–100 mmHg); HCO_3, 34 mEq/L (RV = 22–26 mEq/L); SpO_2, 94% (RV = 95–100%); SVO_2, 77% (RV = 68–77%); WBC,12,000/ mm^3 (RV = 5.000–10.000/mm^3); band cells, 10% (RV = 2–6%); platelet, 74.000/mm^3 (RV = 150–400/mm^3); PCR, 144 mg/dL (RV = 0,4–0,5 mg/dL); troponin, 0.705 ng/ml (RV = < 0,030 ng/ mL); CK mass, 2.10 ng/ml (RV = < 4,94 ng/mL); fibrinogen, 230 mg/dL (RV = 150–370 mg/dL); Hb, 10,6g/dL (RV = 12–16 g/dL); Ht, 32% (RV = 35 a 45%); lactate, 25 mg/dL (RV = 4,5-19,8 mg/dL); albumin, 3.5 g/dl (RV = 3,5 a 5,2 g/dL); urea, 81 mg/dL (RV = 16–40 mg/dL); creatinine, 0.98 mg/dL (RV = 0,6–1,2 mg/dL); and Na+, 150 mmol/L (RV = 135–145 mmol/L); K+, 3.5 mmol/L (RV = 3,5–5,5 mmol/L). Research for rheumatic disease and autoimmune were negative: CH50 < 60 U/CAE (RV = 60–144 U/CAE); C3, 35 mg/dL (RV = 84–193 mg/dL); C4, 9 mg/dL (RV = 16–47 mg/dL); negative anti-CCP; anti-DNA < 1.0 U/mL (RV = < 68, 6 U/mL); FAN, nonreactive (RV = nonreactive); ANCA C and P, nonreactive (RV = nonreactive); and FR, < 9.3 UI/mL (RV = < 14,0 UI/mL).

Hemodynamic instability, due to the persistence of atrial arrhythmia (atrial fibrillation), is not responsive to electrical cardioversion therapy coupled with the strain of the cardiac chambers and reduced urine output with increased slag, determining the replacement of ECMO to paracorporeal biventricular circulatory support device (CentriMag). The procedure was performed in the operating room under general anesthesia by median thoracotomy and extracorporeal circulate. Two drainage cannulas were installed, one in the right atrium and the other in the left atrium, the last positioned in the left ventricle under the guidance of transesophageal echocardiography. Two return cannulas were installed in the main pulmonary artery and the ascending aorta (Fig. 2).

Upon returning to the ICU, the patient developed hemodynamic instability in the early hours of biventricular assistance, managing to restart weaning amines 24 h after installation of the devices, and maintained only dobutamine (8 mcg/kg/min). There was improvement in urine output due to the diuretic stimulus. Patient needed another transfusion (CH, 03 IU) due to the worsening of the white blood cell count (23,200 with 19% rods), and Vancomycin was started. Sedation was suspended to assess the level of consciousness. As the service protocol, daily echocardiography was performed to evaluate ventricular function, which showed progressive improvement. Patient maintained minor bleeding through mediastinal drain and puncture sites, and anticoagulation control was done by tempo de coagulação ativado activated coagulation time

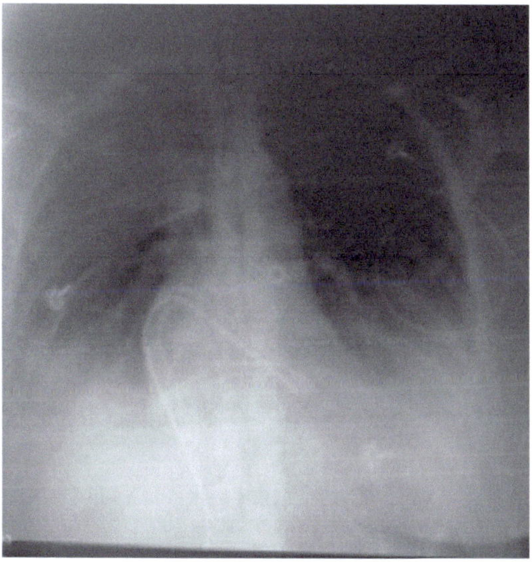

FIGURE 2 XR after installation of biventricular CentriMag

(ACT) every 2 h (within the range therapy). There was the need for blood transfusion. Considering the positive accumulation of fluid balance, dialysis was started from the fifth day of circulatory support with good tolerance.

By completing 9 days of circulatory assistance, there was full recovery of biventricular function (CentriMag Biventricular®), being decided by the weaning and explantation of the devices. Procedure was performed in the operating room under general anesthesia. In the ICU, tracheostomy was done to facilitate weaning, which was achieved 13 days after explantation of the devices.

She was discharged from ICU 31 days after explant of circulatory assist devices.

Questions

1. How is the cardiogenic shock diagnosis done?

According to the 2016 ESC Guidelines for the Diagnosis and Treatment of Acute and Chronic Heart Failure, cardiogenic shock (CS) is characterized by marked persistent (>30 min) hypotension with signs of hypoperfusion, blood pressure (BP) <90 mmHg, decrease in cardiac index < 2.2 L/min/m^2, and elevated ventricular filling pressure (pulmonary capillary wedge pressure > 18 mmHg/central venous pressure > 20 mmHg). Other markers of metabolic and invasive hemodynamic monitoring in CS are also mentioned, such as systemic vascular resistance > 2000 dines/s/cm^3/m^2 and increased arteriovenous difference of O_2 > 5.5 ml/dl. The identification of the shock etiology is crucial in order to establish the appropriate treatment and the consequent hemodynamic stabilization and/or reversal of dysfunction.

2. What is the best treatment choice for the cardiogenic shock?

For the patient with suspected cardiogenic shock, the initial workup includes chest X-ray, electrocardiogram, and echocardiogram.

The pharmacological management is the use of inotropic and vasopressor agents. There is a constant monitoring of hemodynamic perfusion. In this case, the pulmonary artery catheterism should be considered. Dobutamine is the most constant inotropic. Norepinephrine is an important vasopressor. The use of intra-aortic balloon, although questionable, as the latest guideline of heart failure of the European Society of Cardiology (ESC 2016) and other publications, can be used, especially if there are no more effective devices. However, often the use of circulatory assist devices should be considered when there is not an adequate response [1].

3. What is myocarditis?

Myocarditis corresponds to the inflammation of the heart muscle due to exposure to external antigens such as viruses, bacteria, parasites, drugs, or internal trigger such as autoimmune activation against autoantigens. This inflammation is also associated with any form of injury to the heart, including ischemia, by mechanical trauma and genetic conditions.

The pathological diagnosis according to the Dallas criteria calls for the presence of inflammatory cells simultaneously with myocyte necrosis in the same microscopic preparation. However, the criteria have become very criticized for being too narrow and difficult to apply. Thus, myocarditis became an exclusion diagnosis. The own diagnostic definition has become broader, including the presence of viral genome or molecular markers of immune activation, in agreement with the advent of new techniques of molecular diagnosis.

This existing failure in accurate diagnosis or the failure to detect subclinical cases is reflected in the difficult affirmation of the true incidence of myocarditis, always depending on the inclusion and applied diagnostic criteria. In young adults who had sudden death, it was suggested a higher incidence of myocarditis up to 8.6%. This shows that myocarditis is not clinically suspected, leading to death or severe heart failure [5].

4. What is the pathophysiology of viral myocarditis?

According to the 2013 Brazilian guidelines on myocarditis and pericarditis, the pathophysiology of viral myocarditis can be divided into acute, subacute, and chronic phases.

The acute phase is characterized by the presence of viremia. The virus reaches the myocardium through hematogenous or lymphatic dissemination. There is loss of myocytes by necrosis due to direct action of the virus, cytotoxic effects of inflammatory mediators, and oxidative stress products associated with endothelial dysfunction and ischemia. The direct action occurs by the entry of the virus into the cell, through membrane receptors such as CAR (coxsackie-adenovirus receptor) and cytoplasmic and nuclear injuries. As the viral aggression progress, there is an activation of a mechanism from the immune system with important inflammatory infiltrate with natural killer cells and macrophages. The production of cytokines (interleukin 1 and 2, interferon γ and tumor necrosis factor) is part of this inflammatory response, which can damage myocytes depending on the time and exposure levels of these cells.

The subacute phase starts from the 4th day of inoculation and extends until the 14th day. The T lymphocyte infiltrate continues in myocardial invasion, peaking 7–14 days after viral inoculation. In this phase occurs the main myocardial cell damage. There is also B lymphocytes infiltration, and the proportion increases gradually during the first to the third month. The humoral immune response has an important role in myocardial injury and dysfunction. The direct or indirect myocyte injury releases myosin into the circulation, and the presence of this protein promotes the release of antibodies against the myosin heavy chain and stimulates CD4 + T lymphocytes, which can perpetuate and amplify the lesion of cardiac cells. This amplification stimulated by CD4 T lymphocytes occurs by stimulating B lymphocytes in the production of anti-myosin antibodies and by stimulating the cytotoxic presence of CD8 T lymphocytes. Cross-reaction of antibodies between viral antigens and myocardial cells also provides damage to myocytes.

The third phase begins on the 15th day and continues until the 90th day after viral inoculation and is characterized by the intense deposition of collagen in the myocardial interstitium with myocardial fibrosis evolving to dilation, dysfunction, and heart failure.

5. What are the indications for mechanical circulatory support in cardiogenic shock?

According to the Guideline of Mechanical Circulatory Assistance from the Brazilian Society of Cardiology (2016), the following considered indications for implantation of mechanical circulatory assist devices (MCAD) in cardiogenic shock, in the context of acute insult: post-acute myocardial infarction cardiogenic shock, acute fulminant myocarditis, peripartum, exogenous intoxication, Takotsubo, postcardiotomy, cardiac allograft dysfunction, right ventricular dysfunction post-implant of left MCAD, acute heart valve disease, pulmonary embolism, and sepsis.

In the case of cardiogenic shock in acute chronic patients, the following are considered indications for implantation of mechanical circulatory assist devices (MCAD): chronic cardiomyopathy with indication for heart transplantation, eligible cardiomyopathies for long-term devices, and congenital cardiopathies.

According to the Guidelines of the European Society of Cardiology – ESC 2016 – the use of mechanical circulatory support, including heart percutaneous support equipment, extracorporeal life support (ECLS), and extracorporeal membrane oxygenation (ECMO), attends in life support of patients with left ventricular or biventricular failure, until heart and other organ functions return. The use of this equipment is restricted to a few days and weeks. The score of survival after venoarterial ECMO use can help in predicting survival in patients receiving ECMO to contain refractory cardiogenic shock.

The ECLS and ECMO can be used as a bridge to decision in patients with acute and rapid deterioration in heart failure or cardiogenic shock, serving for hemodynamic stabilization and clinical evaluation for possible heart transplant procedure or a more durable mechanical circulatory support.

Regarding the guidelines from the International Society for Heart and Lung Transplantation (2013), the extended use of mechanical circulatory assistance (MCS) in patients with acute cardiogenic shock is indicated as these evidence levels:

- Evidence level B, inotropic dependent patients, representing a high mortality group even in continuous medical treatment.
- Evidence Level C, patients with ventricular function considered unrecoverable, patients with hemodynamics and vital organ function maintenance difficulties, patients with a significant capacity for recovery quality of life and organ dysfunction, and patients with irreversible organ damage.
- Evidence level C, patients with end-stage systolic heart failure, being necessary to calculate the risk and cardiopulmonary stress test.
- Evidence level C, heart failure patients at high risk of death for a year, using prognostic models, with indication for heart transplantation or MCS, as a bridge to transplantation or destination therapy.

6. How to manage a patient in use of mechanical circulatory support?

According to the Guideline of Mechanical Circulatory Assistance from the Brazilian Society of Cardiology (2016), the following actions should be taken during mechanical circulatory support:

- Monitoring of the perfusion status through continuous cardiac monitoring, pulse oximetry, invasive measurements of blood pressure, central venous pressure, and diuresis control.
- Monitoring of renal and liver function, tissue perfusion (lactate), and venous oxygen saturation index measures should be made by laboratory tests.
- Routine inspection (every 6 h) of the whole circuit with special attention to the puncture site and membrane oxygenation, measuring the drainage pressures before and after the membrane.
- Strict gasometric control, from the patient and from the circuit (pre and post membrane).
- Blood pressure control, arrhythmias, and collateral effects by use of vasoactive drugs.
- Monitoring of coagulation tests by measuring the activated partial thromboplastin time (APTT) every 6 h or thromboelastogram daily with adjustment of the heparin infusion dose and replacement of clotting factors, primarily platelets (preventing reduction to less than 60,000/mm^3).
- Hematimetric control with maintenance of hemoglobin levels above 12 mg/dL.
- Chest X-ray and daily transthoracic echocardiography, with evaluation of the positioning of the cannulas, decompression of the heart chambers, the opening of the aortic valve, myocardial contractility, and measures of the filling pressure (PASP and PVC).

The levels of renal dysfunction are high mortality factors after mechanical circulatory support implantation, as well as hepatic dysfunction. Elevated bilirubin, INR and transaminases, ascites presence and hepatic encephalopathy, hypoalbuminemia, Model for End-Stage Liver Disease (MELD), and Child-Pugh high scores are the main hepatic alterations related with this worse prognosis.

7. What are the criteria for weaning and explant of circulatory assistance device?

According to the Guideline of Mechanical Circulatory Assistance from the Brazilian Society of Cardiology (2016) the explant or MCAD weaning should occur under the following conditions: when in minimal assistance condition (flows from 1.5 to 1.0 L/min) check the opening of the aortic valve associated with improved left ventricular function (LVEF 40–45%), cardiac chambers decrease and maintenance of adequate hemodynamic parameters.

In cases of severe complications related to the device, such as bleeding and hemolytic, thrombotic and embolic complications, it's indicated the explant [2].

8. What are the main complications in circulatory assistance?

The main complications of circulatory assistance involve problems arising from the need for continuous anticoagulation, mainly bleeding in puncture and digestive sites, as well as pericardial effusion and infection.

Hemorrhagic complications should be promptly evaluated with the objective of reversing the effects of anticoagulants and antiplatelet agents and exploration for bleeding, if necessary.

Hemolysis is associated with negative pressure elevations in the venous line, persistent maintenance of high blood flow, or inappropriate choice of drainage and infusion cannulas.

Thrombus formation in the circuit and embolic events are mainly caused by the difficulty of modulating the necessary coagulation target.

The increase in complications after mechanical circulatory assist devices (MCAD) implant is directly related to assistance time. In this way we should take into consideration the migration to other devices or assistance mode whenever there are signal of inappropriate response to therapy.

Review About the Addressed Disease or Treatment

Heart failure (HF) represents the common pathway of most heart diseases, being a growing epidemic problem. As for definition, Ponikowski et al. [1] characterize HF as an abnormality of cardiac function or structure that progresses to failure in the delivery of commensurate levels of oxygen and are determinants for tissue metabolic needs. In addition, there are hemodynamic changes involving inadequate cardiac output responses and elevated pulmonary and systemic venous pressures. This reduction in cardiac output contributes to a state of inappropriate tissue perfusion [7].

Another necessary point is the correlation of the diagnosis of HF and the initial symptoms, such as cardiogenic shock (CS), identifying details that may conclude in the diagnostic description. The CS relates to the inability of the cardiac muscle to provide adequate output to the needs of the organism, which generates signs and symptoms of low cardiac output associated with degrees of pulmonary congestion. Persistence of the shock frame results in the onset and worsening of hypoxia, with accumulation of metabolites, acidosis, and endothelial and cellular damage. As a consequence, there are interferences on inotropism and/or cardiac chronotropism, which decreases cardiac work, contributing to the onset of arrhythmias, inflammation, and myocardial ischemia, among other complications [6].

All this dysfunction of the heart muscle may also be associated with the so-called myocarditis, which indicates the classic paradigm of cardiac injury: the pathogenesis of myocarditis followed by an inflammatory immune response of the host, such as cardiac inflammation. The consequences of this intense immune response, as in the case of viral myocarditis, may be dilated cardiomyopathy and acute heart failure with refractory cardiogenic shock.

Bibliography

1. Ponikowski P, Voors AA, Anker SD, Bueno H, Cleland JGF, et al. 2016 ESC guidelines for the diagnosis and treatment of acute and chronic heart failure. Eur Heart J. 2016;18:891.
2. Ayub-Ferreira SM, Souza Neto JD, Almeida DR, Biselli B. Diretriz de Assistência Circulatória Mecânica da Sociedade Brasileira de Cardiologia, Sociedade Brasileira de Cardiologia. Arq Bras Cardiol. 2016;107:1–33.
3. Feldman D, Pamboukian SV, Teuteberg JJ. The 2013 International Society for Heart and Lung Transplantation Guidelines for mechanical circulatory support: EXECUTIVE summary. J Heart Lung Transplant. 2013;32:157.
4. Montera MW, Mesquita ET, Colafranceschi AS, Oliveira Junior AM, Rabischoffsky A, Ianni BM, et al. I Diretriz Brasileira de Miocardites e Pericardites, Sociedade Brasileira de Cardiologia. Arq Bras Cardiol. 2013;100:1.
5. Libby P, Bonow R, Mann D, Zipes D. Braunwald – Tratado de doenças cardiovasculares. Rio de Janeiro: Editora Elsevier; 2010.
6. Knobel E. Choque Cardiogênico. Arq Bras Cardiol. 1999;72:405–13.
7. Cowie MR. The epidemiology of heart failure – an epidemic in progress. In: Coats A, Cleland JGF, editors. Controversies in the management of heart failure. Edinburgh: Churchill Livingstone; 1997. p. 11–23.

Part VIII
Heart Transplantation

Cardiac Transplantation in Situs Inversus Totalis: A Surgical Challenge

Vanessa Lopes Vieira, Guilherme Henrique Ribeiro de Carvalho, Leandro Pedro Goloni Bertollo, Fabio Biscegli Jatene, and Fabio Antonio Gaiotto

Clinical Presentation

A 45-year-old male patient presented a 6-month report of fatigue on moderate exertion, dyspnea at rest, and paroxysmal nocturnal dyspnea. He searched for medical care in his hometown and was diagnosed with non-compacted right ventricle, situs inversus totalis, dilated cardiomyopathy, and decompensated congestive heart failure. After being hospitalized for 1 month, he was discharged with prescriptions of carvedilol, captopril, furosemide, acetylsalicylic acid, spironolactone, omeprazole, and marcoumar (Phenprocoumon), with important clinical improvement. He stopped using medication due to gastric intolerance, and his decompensation worsened. In this period he also presented an episode of arterial thrombosis, with cyanosis in lower limbs and local pain, requiring surgical intervention (embolectomy) and oral anticoagulation. The patient underwent a new hospitalization as his condition deteriorated, and he started to feel discomfort when carrying any physical activity, in addition to dyspnea

V. L. Vieira (✉) · G. H. R. de Carvalho · L. P. G. Bertollo
F. B. Jatene · F. A. Gaiotto
Faculty of Medicine of University of São Paulo (FMUSP),
São Paulo, SP, Brazil
e-mail: vanessa.vieira@fm.usp.br

R. M. S. Almeida, F. B. Jatene (eds.), *Cardiovascular Surgery*,
https://doi.org/10.1007/978-3-319-57084-6_25

at rest. Following this change of heart failure functional classification (NYHA III to IV), he was finally transferred to our service due to refractoriness to clinical treatment, in use of intravenous inotropic medication (Dobutamine 6 mcg/kg/min). On his admission physical examination at our service, the patient presented a significantly compromised general health, as well as cachexia and adynamia, although his vital signs were good (pulse 60 bpm, blood pressure 116 × 74 mmHg). His lungs were clear to auscultation, and the cardiac examination presented normal S1 and S2, with regular rate and rhythm. No edema or cyanosis was noted on his extremities.

Diagnosis, Assessment, and Treatment

An initial chest radiography showed cardiomegaly and dextrocardia (Fig. 1). The measurements of his cardiac chambers verified on the echocardiography were as follows: left atrium, 43 mm (reference ranges, 20–40 mm); right ventricle, 25 mm (20–40 mm); interventricular septum, 8 mm (6–11 mm); and left ventricle posterior wall, 8 mm (6–11 mm). There was an important diffuse hypokinesia, and the ejection fraction was 24%. The LV diastolic diameter was 71 mm (37–55 mm), and the LV systolic diameter was 63 mm (20–40 mm).

A gallium scintigraphy requested in the patient's hometown presented scintigraphic signs of discrete myocarditis.

The patient had negative serologies for Chagas disease, cytomegalovirus (IgG and IgM), syphilis (negative VDRL and FTA-ABS), hepatitis C, and hepatitis B surface antigen; he also had negative anti-HBe and anti-HBc; serology for toxoplasmosis was IgM-negative and IgG-positive.

The coronary arteries did not present any obstructive lesions in the coronary angiography; pulmonary artery pressure was 25 × 11 mmHg, and its mean pressure was 16 mmHg (reference ranges, 12–16 mmHg).

An abdominal USG confirmed situs inversus totalis, without other abnormalities.

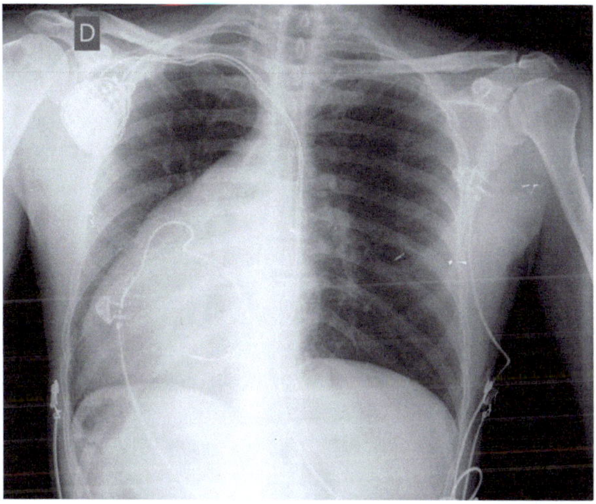

FIGURE 1 Initial chest radiography showing an enlarged cardiac silhouette, with the base-apex axis pointing to the right (dextrocardia). The aortic arch and the gastric bubble are seen on the right as well

His immune panel showed absent response to class I and class II HLA molecules (both had a reactivity of 0%).

The highly decompensated heart failure demanded the maintained use of intravenous inotropic medication (Dobutamine 6 mcg/kg/min). The patient evolved with heart failure compensation, and dobutamine was then suspended. Investigation for thrombophilia (Factor V Leiden, prothrombin mutant, antithrombin 3, lupus anticoagulant, and anticardiolipin) was negative. Oral anticoagulation was adjusted (enoxaparin 40 mg SC 12/12, warfarin 5 mg/d). He was discharged with dyspnea on mild exertion, INR 1,1, and prescriptions of captopril, carvedilol, spironolactone, and hydralazine. The patient was also included in heart transplant queue.

He underwent further hospitalizations for low cardiac output symptoms (dizziness, asthenia) and for a complaint of intermittent claudication to short distances due to right lower limb pain; arterial Doppler of this limb presented signs of occlusion/subocclusion in popliteal, peroneal, and tibial anterior arteries, requiring a new embolectomy.

The patient was subjected to bicaval orthotopic heart transplant with a normal heart donor who was a 38-year-old man, smoker, and a victim of traumatic brain injury. Donor myocardial was protected with a single dose of Custodiol. The total ischemia time was 3 h 40 min, and extracorporeal circulation lasted 1 h 25 min (Fig. 2). The implant was made with ¼ h counterclockwise rotation (Fig. 3), bringing the left auricle to medial position and the right chambers to a posterior position (retroaortic superior vena cava and posterior inferior vena cava). Left ventricle was anteriorized; the isotopic pulmonary trunk and the aorta were both in end-to-end anastomosis. The cardiac beating recovery was good.

Immunosuppression was held with corticotherapy, mycophenolate, and cyclosporine, and an endomyocardial biopsy was performed 16 days after surgery, with no signs of rejection.

Postoperative transthoracic echocardiograms showed important ventricular function improvement, with absence of blood flow obstruction in venoatrial and ventriculoarterial

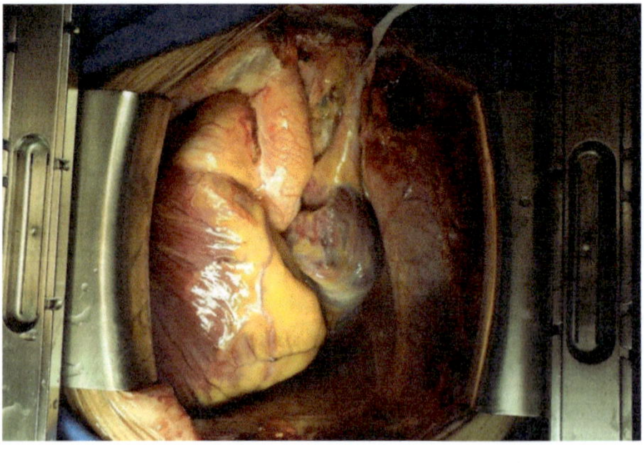

Figure 2 Picture taken immediately after sternotomy and opening of the pericardium sac showing recipient heart with its axis directed to the right and mirrored-positioned vascular pathways

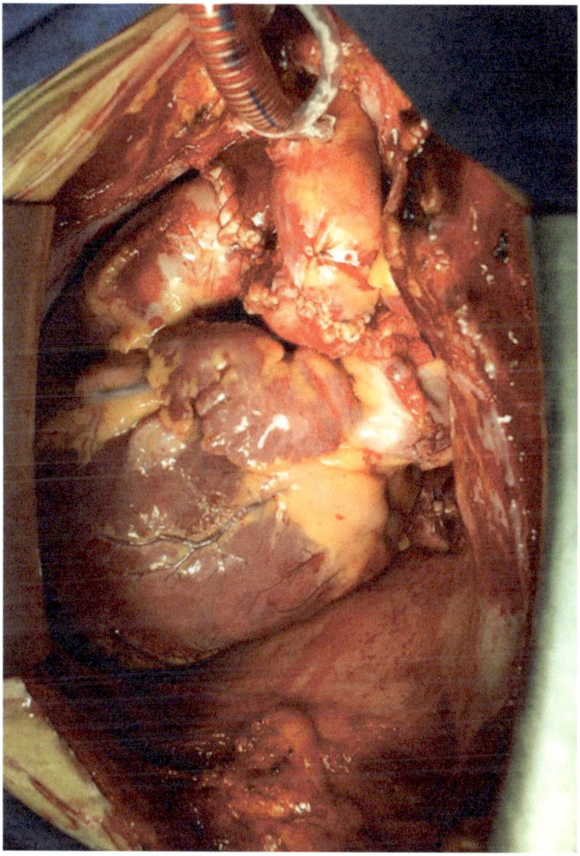

FIGURE 3 Normal donor heart implanted with ¼ h counterclockwise rotation, with the left ventricle in medial position and the right chambers and inferior vena cava in posterior position. The aorta and pulmonary trunk were both in end-to-end anastomosis

connections, preserved left ventricular function, ejection fraction of 60%, and discrete right ventricular diffuse hypokinesia.

In the first postoperative days, the patient presented catheter-related infection and urinary tract infection, both resolved with tazocin and vancomycin. Two weeks after surgery, he had as complications a left phrenic palsy, an esophageal candidiasis (managed with fluconazole), an esophageal ulcer with a biopsy suggestive of herpes simplex virus infection, and a mild cyclosporine-induced hyperkalemia.

The patient evolved well and was discharged on the 28th postoperative day. Ten months after surgery, he is still hemodynamically stable and without any signs of rejection.

Questions

1. What is non-compacted cardiomyopathy, how is it manifested, and how to make this diagnosis?

Noncompaction cardiomyopathy is a rare congenital disease characterized by the presence of prominent trabeculae with intertrabecular recesses which penetrate deeply through the ventricular myocardium, forming a loose network of intertwined muscle fibers with communications between the non-compacted myocardial layer and the ventricular cavity [1]. Patients may remain asymptomatic or develop symptoms of heart failure, ventricular tachycardia, or thromboembolic events due to thrombus in the atria or in the intertrabecular recesses. The diagnosis is made through image exams, with Doppler echocardiography being the procedure of choice [1]. It is also recommended the support of other images, such as cardiovascular magnetic resonance, since echo has several limitations, including high operator dependence and misdiagnosis of non-compacted cardiomyopathy in normal individuals with fine trabeculations [1].

2. Is the thromboembolic event related to the initial diagnoses?

There is a possible cardioembolic origin for these events, with support by the fact that investigation for thrombophilic syndromes turned out to be negative. As mentioned above, some of the symptoms that might develop from noncompaction cardiomyopathy are thromboembolic events, since the multiple ventricular trabeculations are believed to be an important anatomic substrate to form thrombi (prophylactic anticoagulation may be indicated) [1]. There may be also a contribution from the component of blood stasis resulting from ventricular hypokinesia.

3. Would heart transplantation be indicated in this case?

Considering the presence of persistent functional class III heart failure and refractoriness to clinical management, with dependence on inotropic drugs, and the recurrent hospitalization history, the heart transplant is indicated in this case [2]. Besides, to be on the heart transplant waiting list, other criteria need to be accomplished: negative serologies, not using drugs or smoking for at least 6 months, and absence of severe lung disease and pulmonary hypertension [3]. The priority is established by analyzing factors as dependence on inotropic drugs, use of intra-aortic balloon pump or other ventricular assist devices, and dependence on mechanical ventilation [3].

4. How to evaluate a candidate to heart transplant?

Evaluation of cardiac transplant candidates aims to identify comorbidities and contraindications that would have a negative impact on the surgery or that might decrease short- or long-time survival. It involves a series of prognostic criteria, such as, according to the II Brazilian Guidelines for Cardiac Transplantation [2], complete history taking and physical examination, immunocompatibility tests (ABO, HLA typing, panel reactive antibody (PRA)), assessment of heart failure severity (cardiopulmonary test, Doppler echocardiography, pulmonary hemodynamic assessment, resting ECG), functional assessment of multiple organs (biochemistry of blood, urinalysis, glomerular filtration rate, 24-h proteinuria, blood gas analysis, chest X-ray, abdominal ultrasound), serologies for infections and vaccination (HbsAg, anti-Hbc, anti-Hbs, anti HCV, HIV, HTLV, CMV, toxoplasmosis, EBV, varicella, antipneumococcal vaccine, influenza vaccine, hepatitis B vaccine, anti-Hbs, prophylaxis for verminosis), screening for malignancies according to age range and indication (fecal occult blood, colonoscopy, mammography, cervical cytology, PSA), and multidisciplinary assessment (nutritional, social, and nursing evaluation, other specialties if indicated).

5. Would it be possible to find a donor heart with dextrocardia?

From the technical perspective, it would be ideal to find a donor with dextrocardia and with the vascular roots compatible with those of the recipient, but this is virtually impossible given the very low incidence of dextrocardia (1:12000) [4].

6. What are the possible surgical techniques for an orthotopic heart transplant?

There are two techniques for orthotopic heart transplant: classic and bicaval. The difference between them relies on atrial resection. In the classic technique, the right atrium is opened in its anterior face, while in the bicaval technique, a section is made in the superior atriocaval junction, removing a bigger part of the receptor right atrium and preserving the donor sinoatrial node; the left atrium is completely removed except for the segment where pulmonary veins are inserted, which is maintained for suture of the left atrium [2]. Bicaval technique utilization led to a decrease in complications often seen in patients who underwent classic orthotopic cardiac transplant, such as insufficient atrioventricular valves, arrhythmias, and intracardiac thrombi [2].

7. What is the importance of endomyocardial biopsy for assessing rejection?

Endomyocardial biopsy is the gold-standard procedure for assessing rejection and is required whenever rejection is suspected, being used with frequency in the first postoperative phases [2]. It is a percutaneous procedure that consists of removing fragments from the interventricular septum, guided by fluoroscopy or echocardiography; access pathways include femoral and jugular veins [2].

8. What are the possible posttransplant complications?

Important posttransplant complications are infections (with special attention to toxoplasmosis and cytomegalovirus), Chagas disease reactivation, neoplasias, retransplant (usually for early failure or for allograft vasculopathy), and comorbidities such as hypertension (associated to certain immunosuppressants like corticosteroids and calcineurin inhibitors) and diabetes mellitus (negative impact of cyclosporine and tacrolimus on pancreatic function) [2].

Review About the Addressed Disease or Treatment

Heart transplant is a well-established, gold-standard therapy for refractory end-stage heart failure. Brazil has had increasing participation on the global account of procedures, with the rise of important transplant centers; a great challenge remains the lack of effective donors. The surgical techniques involved have suffered few changes along the years, with the major revolution on patient survival remaining discovery of cyclosporine in the late 1970s, allowing a superior rejection control. Orthotopic cardiac transplantation is often associated with tricuspid insufficiency (besides other complications already mentioned above such as arrhythmias and intracardiac thrombi), especially the classic technique, which involves bigger geometric changes of the right atrium tricuspid valve, due to donor and recipient atrium anastomosis [2]. Heterotopic transplant is an option to the orthotopic technique that may be considered in patients unable to use mechanical circulatory assistance devices and in other situations that include pulmonary vascular resistance >5 uW after use of vasodilators and disproportion between recipient and donor weight [2].

There are few scientific reports of cardiac transplantation in patients with situs inversus totalis. Situs inversus can be classified further into situs inversus with levocardia or situs inversus with dextrocardia [5]. It is a condition transmitted through autosomal recessive genes in which the atrial chambers and the viscera are in a mirrored position when compared to normal (normal viscera positioning is named situs solitus) [5]. Dextrocardia is a term that applies specifically to the cardiac apex direction, which in this case is directed to the right, not implying a morphologic inversion. In situs totalis with dextrocardia, however, the morphologic right atrium is on the left and the morphologic left atrium is on the right. Situs inversus with dextrocardia is also termed situs inversus totalis because the cardiac position, as well as the atrial chambers and abdominal viscera, is a mirror image of the normal anatomy [5]. It is a rare condition (less rare than situs inversus with levocardia, though), specially to be found in an adult. The late diagnosis in this patient may be explained by the relative lack of associated cardiovascular malformations, except for the noncompaction cardiomyopathy, whose association with situs inversus and dextrocardia is extremely rare and almost inexistent in the literature [1]. Even though situs abnormalities may be first recognized by using radiography and ultrasonography, computed tomography scanning is the preferred examination for the definitive diagnosis of situs inversus with dextrocardia, providing good anatomic detail for confirming visceral organ position, cardiac apical position, and great vessel branching [5].

The greatest difficulty of heart transplant in patients with situs inversus totalis is the reconstruction of the systemic and pulmonary venous pathways [6–8]. The first techniques described to resolve this problem were the removal of extra length of the donor's veins and confection of conduits to connect recipient and donor vessels. Doty et al. [9] used a conduit made of pericardium connecting both the inferior vena cavas (IVC), while Rubay et al. [7] used a piece of aortic homograft and a conduit made of recipient right atrium and pericardium. Chang et al. [6] used a conduit made of right atrium free wall. The vascular endothelial surface of the right atrium free wall was superior to a prosthetic graft [6]. Cooper et al. [8] attempted to eliminate the necessity of managing the roots of superior and inferior vena cavas through artificial or autogenous conduits. His group developed a method in which the heart receives slight counterclockwise rotation, allowing to connect donor and recipient IVCs directly. A patient operated under such method by Chang's team, though, presented a sudden collapse on the 8th postoperative day that was attributed to a heart twist possibly secondary to the rotation [6].

However, besides the alignment of the IVCs, seating the normal donor heart in dextrocardia allows a better accom-

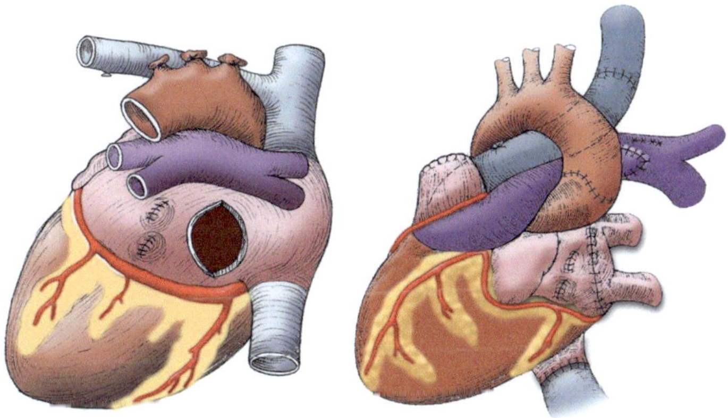

FIGURE 4 Donor cardiectomy was accomplished with en bloc removal of the superior vena cava and innominate vein and extra length removal of the inferior vena cava, aorta, and pulmonary artery. The donor graft was then prepared by oversewing the left pulmonary vein orifices and by opening the left atrium between the right pulmonary veins. (Adapted from Deuse and Reitz [10])

modation of the organ in the recipient pericardial cavity; it avoids ventricular compression from the three-lobed left lung, which would simulate a tamponade [10]. These were the reasons which led to the choice for this surgical technique in our case (Fig. 4).

Bibliography

1. Gonçalves LFG, Souto FMS, Faro FN, Mendonça RC, Oliveira JLM, Sousa ACS. Dextrocardia with situs inversus associated with non-compaction cardiomyopathy. Arq Bras Cardiol. 2013;101(2):e33–6. https://doi.org/10.5935/abc.20130158.
2. Bacal F, Souza-Neto JD, Fiorelli AI, Mejia J, Marcondes-Braga FG, Mangini S, et al. II Diretriz Brasileira de Transplante Cardíaco. Arq Bras Cardiol. 2009;94(1 supl.1):e16–73.
3. Pereira WA. Diretrizes básicas para a captação de múltiplos órgãos da Associação Brasileira de Transplante de Órgãos. São Paulo: ABTO; 2009.

4. Uoc NH, Quan PT. Heart transplant for dextrocardia situs inversus with very complex congenital lesions a challenge of cardiac surgery. Int J Clin Cardiol. 2015;2:049.
5. Wilhelm A, Holbert JM. Situs inversus imaging. Medscape. 2016; n.d. Available at: http://emedicine.medscape.com/article/413679-overview?pa=fdlomegjfp19yx1cjsrxyzoy5eys2/o60o2vskngm5k/hfgkrfndfm+98n7yw1xqa57m2kvf/ddbsmwljcqitrgdh0iyuyergfy/yxjhzue= (Accessed 27 Sept 2016).
6. Chang YL, Wei J, Chang CY, Chuang YC, Sue SH. Cardiac transplantation in situs inversus: two cases reports. Transplant Proc. 2008;40(8):2848–51. https://doi.org/10.1016/j.transproceed.2008.07.115.
7. Rubay JE, d'Udekem Y, Sluysmans T, Ponlot R, Jacquet L, de Leval MR. Orthotopic heart transplantation in situs inversus. Ann Thorac Surg. 1995;60(2):460–2.
8. Cooper DK, Ye Y, Chaffin JS, Zuhdi N. A suggested technique for "orthotopic" heart transplantation in a patient with situs inversus. Tex Heart Inst J. 1993;20:281–4.
9. Doty DB, Renlund DG, Caputo GR, et al. Cardiac transplantation in situs inversus. J Thorac Cardiovasc Surg. 1990;99:493.
10. Deuse T, Reitz BA. Heart transplantation in situs inversus totalis. J Thorac Cardiovasc Surg. 2010;139(2):501–3.

Part IX
Mechanical Circulatory Support

Mechanical Circulatory Support in Patient with Pulmonary Dysfunction

Amanda Dorighetto Tomazelli, Matheus Ramos Dal Piaz, Nathalia Spandl Falqueto, and Melchior Luiz Lima

Clinical Presentation

Patient WCV, masculine, 51 years old, without comorbidities, went to the hospital complaining of a sore throat, fever (38.5 °C), and nonproductive cough. There were no alterations at the chest radiography and sinus radiograph, and the patient was discharged. Three days later, the patient returned with the same symptoms, and the chest radiography revealed a discrete pulmonary infiltration at the right lung base. Therapy was initiated with levofloxacin 750 mg once a day, for 3 days. However, even after the proposed treatment, the patient continued with a fever and dry cough, presenting malaise in the morning, cold extremities, fatigue, and SpO_2 70%. Treatment with oseltamivir, ceftriaxone, and clarithromycin was started, but the patient remained with intermittent noninvasive ventilation with SaO_2 96%. When using high-flow oxygen mask, the SaO_2 dropped down to less than 90%.

After 3 days, the patient was admitted to the ICU with the diagnosis of severe acute respiratory syndrome and severe community-acquired pneumonia caused by H1N1. The next day, the patient was in refractory hypoxemia despite the

A. D. Tomazelli · M. R. D. Piaz · N. S. Falqueto (✉) · M. L. Lima
School of Sciences of Santa Casa de Misericórdia de Vitória (EMESCAM), Vitória, ES, Brazil

R. M. S. Almeida, F. B. Jatene (eds.), *Cardiovascular Surgery*,
https://doi.org/10.1007/978-3-319-57084-6_26

mechanical ventilation with SaO_2 80% and FiO_2 100%, using a low dose of norepinephrine and presenting asynchronous breathing. Doctors increased the sedation and performed three alveolar recruitments with good results, getting SaO_2 92%, and maintaining minimum PEEP (11 cmH2O) to keep a SaO_2 of at least 90%. After 2 days, the patient was still in refractory hypoxemia, so the doctors decided to start the ARDS (acute respiratory distress syndrome) protocol, with volume control and FiO_2 50%. Five days after, the patient developed pneumomediastinum, cervical emphysema, and progressive subcutaneous emphysema with decreased ventilation and laminated pneumothorax on the left side (Fig. 1). Besides that, the doctors decreased the PEEP and increased the FiO_2. A thoracic drainage catheter at the left side, beneath the lung, to drain the serous liquid from the thorax was installed, and cervical tracheostomy was performed.

The next day, the patient's hypoxemia worsened, also developing a pulmonary dysfunction with high ventilatory parameters installed (PEEP 18, FiO_2 100%, PaO_2/FiO_2 ratio 66) besides taking methylprednisolone.

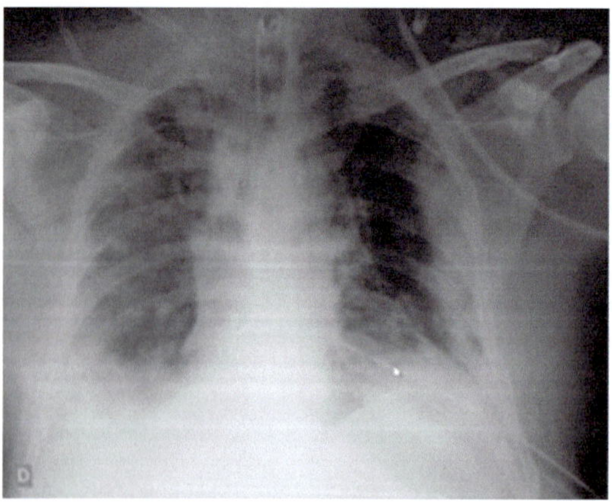

Figure 1 Posteroanterior chest X-ray showing subcutaneous emphysema and pneumomediastinum

Diagnosis, Assessment, and Treatment

After several conventional interventions like antibiotics and antiviral drugs to control the causal factor, noninvasive ventilation, mechanic ventilation, sedation, the use of corticosteroid, and other interventions, the patient remained in refractory hypoxemia. Therefore, doctors decided to install the veno-venous ECMO (extracorporeal membrane oxygenation), by puncturing the right femoral vein and right jugular internal vein, to begin with a membrane oxygenation support, using a blood and oxygen flow of 6 liters per minute and FiO_2 94%. Right after the support installation, the parameters improved (Table 1).

Table 1 Arterial blood gas values before and after ECMO installation

	Before ECMO		**After ECMO**	
	06:39 AM	**09:16 PM**	**Pre-membrane 11:00 PM**	**Post-membrane 11:03 PM**
pH (7.35–7.45)	7.35	7.48	7.53	7.59
PaO_2 (80–95 mmHg)	63	337	38	358
$PaCO_2$ (35–45 mmHg)	57	43	37	30
HCO_3 (21 28 mmol/L)	31.5	32	30.9	28.8
CO_2 total (24–31 mmol/L)	33.2	33.3	32	29.7
Base excess (−3 to +3)	4.7	7.7	7.6	7.3
$SatO_2$ (95–99%)	91	100	80	100

At the next day, there was a significant improvement of hypoxemia, with pH of 7.56 (range 7.35–7.45), PaO_2 96 mmHg (range 80–95 mmHg), $PaCO_2$ 31 mmHg (range 35–45 mmHg), and $SatO_2$ 98% (range 95–99%). Weaning VV-ECMO attempt was performed on the sixth day under circulatory support with good evolution, returning to the protection parameters and re-evaluating in 24 h. One day later, the patient showed an increase of urea, with hemodialysis without loss being indicated. Three days later, there was another attempt to weaning VV-ECMO, but the patient presented hypercapnia and acidosis, and only after 24 h it was possible to start weaning by reducing the blood flow and the gas to 2 L/min with FiO_2 30% and mechanical ventilation with a respiratory rate of 26 breaths/min and FiO_2 50%. The patient maintained $PaO_2 > 60$ and $PaCO_2 > 45$ without acidosis. However, hypoxia detected and hemodynamic instability led to the need to increase the parameters of VV-ECMO. The patient was responding unsatisfactorily to weaning VV-ECMO, and during this period, there were five bleeding events, at the drain and venipuncture sites.

Five days later, left anisocoria was noted, and a computed tomography (CT) was performed with the patient heparinized. There was no answer to nociceptive stimuli, mydriatic pupils, corneal reflex absent bilaterally, Glasgow 3 and Ramsay 6. They turned off sedation. In the CT scan, right massive temporal-parietal bleeding associated with hemoventricle, Duret hemorrhage, diffuse brain swelling, and a great deviation from the midline structures were noted (Fig. 2). There was no indication of surgical treatment; therefore ECMO veno-venous weaning and blood replacement were made. The next day the protocol of brain death secondary to severe intracerebral hemorrhage with tetraventricular flood was started, with confirmation of brain death by cerebral arteriography.

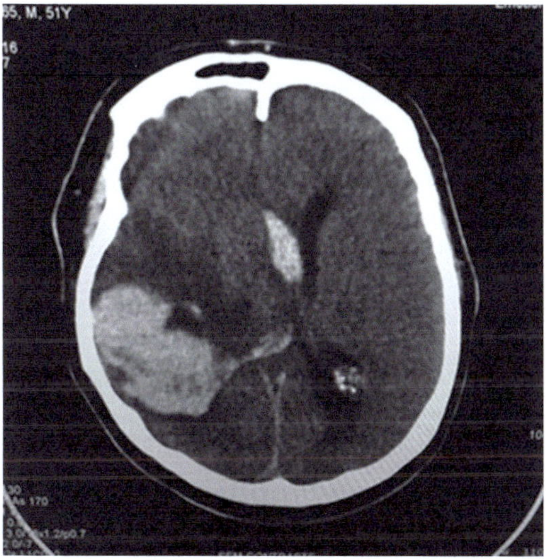

FIGURE 2 CT scan showing cerebral hemorrhage

Questions

1. What is ECMO?

The *extra corporeal membrane oxygenation* system (ECMO) – a set of cannulae, an artificial oxygenation membrane, and a pump – is an extracorporeal circulation closed circuit. It provides pulmonary, heart, or cardiorespiratory support. When used for cardiorespiratory assistance, it is in the occurrence of heart failure, pulmonary failure, or both. Deoxygenated, carbon dioxide-rich blood is drained from the venous system and pumped through an artificial oxygenation membrane, to then return to the arterial system after oxygenation. It is a continuous flow. The aim is to keep tissue perfusion with oxygenated blood while waiting for the recovery of an impaired organ: the heart, lungs, or both.

2. What are the criteria for ECMO installation statement? Does patient in question had these criteria?

The mandatory criteria are:

- Tracheal intubation and mechanical ventilation
- Acute onset lung disease
- Bilateral pulmonary infiltrate
- PaO_2/FiO_2 ratio < 200 with positive end-expiratory pressure ≥ 10 cmH2O
- Reversible lung injury

And the complementary criteria are (at least one must be met):

- PaO_2/FiO_2 ratio ≤ 50 with a $FiO_2 = 1$, for at least 1 h, with or without the use of rescue therapies (alveolar recruitment, inhaled NO, and prone position)
- Hypercapnia with pH remaining ≤ 7.20 using an RR ≥ 35 breaths/min (whenever possible), a tidal volume = 4–6 mL/Kg, and a plateau pressure ≤ 30 cmH2O
- Murray lung injury score > 3, with worsening of the clinical status
- PaO_2/FiO_2 ratio ≤ 50 with a $FiO_2 \geq 0.8$ for at least 3 h, despite the use of rescue therapies

It is important to remember that there are contraindications: mechanical ventilation for more than 7 days with plateau pressures > 30 and FiO_2 > 90%, severe immunosuppression, and recent brain hemorrhage.

The patient had all mandatory criteria and one complementary criterion (PaO_2/FiO_2 ratio ≤ 50 with a $FiO_2 \geq 0.8$ for at least 3 h, despite the use of rescue therapies).

3. What benefits ECMO brings to the patient?

The circulatory support made by VV-ECMO promotes appropriate oxygenation of the blood, as the patient cannot do this due to severe lung injury. Thus, membrane oxygenation improves tissue perfusion, significantly reducing the ventilatory parameters, which saves work for the lungs and allowing their recovery.

If the patient had a heart failure (e.g., due to congenital diaphragmatic hernia, pulmonary hypertension refractory, cardiomyopathy, or heart failure), instead of respiratory failure, ECMO-VA would be the best intervention option because it provides cardiac support, promotes excellent oxygen delivery, and allows rapid stabilization.

The benefits of ECMO in adult patients with cardiac failure or refractory acute respiratory distress syndrome (ARDS) are still debated; ECMO was initially associated with poor survival rates. However, recent technological advances in the ECMO circuit have led to a reduction in the rate of technical issues and complications. Moreover, improved understanding of the benefits of ECMO has emerged from its widespread use as a rescue therapy for ARDS and refractory hypoxemia associated with H1N1/2009 infection ("swine flu").

4. In which other situations was the use of mechanical circulatory assist devices considered/indicated?

Circulatory assist devices can be used in patients with terminal heart failure since the heart transplant is a limited option for the insufficient number of donors to meet the demand of patients with terminal heart failure. The devices can also be used as a bridge to recovery, bridge to decision (when it is not yet clear whether the patient is or is not eligible for transplant), bridge to transplantation, or destination therapy.

5. What are the possible complications of implanted ECMO?

Hemorrhage and infection are the two main complications related to ECMO. Most patients require continuous anticoagulation, and more than 50% of them will suffer at least one hemorrhagic complication. Hemorrhage can occur in any organ, with intracranial bleeding being the most devastating. Other complications such as multiple transfusions, thromboembolism, limb ischemia, per-ECMO hemodialysis, and right ventricular dysfunction are also common.

ECMO circuit failure or breakage may lead to catastrophic failure, but this is unusual as long as all components are secure. Bedside staffs are trained to check the circuit integrity regularly to prevent problems and to react promptly in the case of acute failure. Cannula displacement or malposition is a major issue as this affects blood flow and ECMO efficiency.

6. When should we start the mechanical assistance weaning?

It is not recommended that the patient remains supported by more than 8–10 days. However, to start weaning it is necessary to meet the following criteria:

- pH – 7,5
- PaO_2 – 136 mmHg
- $PaCO_2$ – 57 mmHg
- PaO_2/FiO_2 – 388
- PEEP – 6 cmH2O
- FiO_2 – 35%
- Respiratory rate – 15 breaths/min
- Tidal volume/ideal weight – 5.8 mL/Kg
- Plateau pressure – 22 cmH2O
- Peak inspiratory pressure – 26 cmH2O
- Static lung compliance – 20 mL/cmH2O
- Norepinephrine – 0,00 μg/kg.min
- Mean arterial pressure – 90 mmHg
- Heart rate – 80 bpm
- Lactate – 0,9 mmol/L
- Base excess – 17 mmol/L
- C-reactive protein – 17 mg/L
- Hemoglobin – 9 g/dL
- Midazolam – 0,00 mg/kg.h
- Fentanyl – 2 μg/kg.h
- Atracurium – 0,00 mg/kg.h
- Sequential Organ Failure Assessment Score – 7
- Murray score – 1,2

7. What are the types of ECMO?

There are three ways to set up an ECMO circuit: venoarterial ECMO (VA-ECMO), veno-venous ECMO (VV-ECMO), and arteriovenous ECMO (AV-ECMO). The VA-ECMO allows gas exchange and hemodynamic support while blood is pumped from the venous to the arterial side. VV-ECMO facilitates gas exchange removing the blood from the venous side and then pumping back into it, but without providing hemodynamic support. AV-ECMO facilitates gas exchange by using the patient's own arterial pressure to pump the blood from the arterial to the venous side.

8. Why was it chosen VV-ECMO in this patient?

When the cardiac function is preserved, VV-ECMO is the best option to improve gas exchange. The patient did not need any hemodynamic support because his cardiac function was preserved. The only dysfunction was a respiratory one; he had a severe lung injury, which was caused by ARDS, making a poor oxygenation. Therefore, VV-ECMO was the best choice and assistance for this patient.

Review About the Addressed Disease or Treatment

As seen in the case, H1N1 infection can generate severe inflammation in the body, thereby compromising the respiratory function of the patient. This inflammatory process generated by this infection caused serious damage to the patient progressively, reaching a point where refractory hypoxemia remained even after several interventions, making ECMO an option.

In order to recover the organ, it is recommended to use ECMO as therapy, since it maintains a good tissue perfusion in a patient in whom this function is being prevented due to some lung injury, which was the case. This process is performed by oxygenating the venous blood through the artificial oxygenation membrane present in the system, and since the patient in the case had preserved cardiac function, VV-ECMO was the best choice.

Bibliography

1. Roncon Albuquerque R Jr. ECMO (extracorporeal membrane oxygenation) como opção terapêutica no ARDS grave. Rev Port Med Intensiva. 2010;17(1):43–6.
2. Martinez G, Vuylsteke A. Extracorporeal membrane oxygenation in adults. BJA Educ. 2012;12(2):57–61.

3. Saueressig MG, Schwarz P, Schlatter R, Moreschi AH, Wender OCB, Macedo-Neto AV. Extracorporeal membrane oxygenation for postpneumonectomy ARDS. Braz J Pulmonol. 2014;40(2):203–6.
4. Azevedo LCP, Park M, Costa ELV, Santos EV, Hirota A, Taniguchi LU, Schettino GPP, Amato MBP, Carvalho CRR. Extracorporeal membrane oxygenation in severe hypoxemia: time for reappraisal? Braz J Pulmonol. 2012;38(1):7–12.
5. Colafranceschini AS, Monteiro AJO, Canale LS, Campos LAA, Montera MW, Silva PRD, Fernandes MR, Pinto AA, Molas SM, Mesquita ET. Adult extracorporeal life support: a failed or forgotten concept? Arq Bras Cardiol. 2008;91(1):36–41.
6. Peura JL, Colvin-Adams M, Francis GS, Grady KL, Hoffman TM, Jessup M, John R, Kiernan MS, Mitchell JE, O'Connell JB, Pagani FD, Petty M, Ravichandran P, Rogers JG, Semigran MJ, Toole JM. Recommendations for the use of mechanical circulatory support: device strategies and patient selection: a scientific statement from the American Heart Association. Circulation. 2012;126(22):2648–67.

Pediatric Ventricular Assist Device (VAD) as Successful Bridge to Heart Transplantation

Guilherme Henrique Ribeiro de Carvalho, Vanessa Lopes Vieira, Leandro Pedro Goloni Bertollo, Fabio Biscegli Jatene, and Luiz Fernando Caneo

Clinical Presentation

A 1-year-old male infant presented flu symptoms when he was 30 days old, with evolving low cardiac output and cardiorespiratory arrest. He was admitted *for* 15 days in another hospital and, after discharge, referred to our outpatient facilities, where he received prescriptions of carvedilol, furosemide, spironolactone, and captopril. In his last appointment, when he was 7 months old, cardiac transplantation was indicated, but he wasn't listed. One month later, he was admitted in another service for fever, loss of appetite, and vomiting, associated with progressive respiratory discomfort, and had another cardiorespiratory arrest for 5 min during a diaper change. He started to need increased doses of vasoactive drugs and was then transferred again to our service, where he was diagnosed with dilated cardiomyopathy (Fig. 1), important left ventricular dysfunction of unknown etiology, left

G. H. R. de Carvalho (✉) · V. L. Vieira · L. P. G. Bertollo
F. B. Jatene · L. F. Caneo
Faculty of Medicine of University of São Paulo (FMUSP), São Paulo, SP, Brazil
e-mail: guilherme.carvalho@fm.usp.br

R. M. S. Almeida, F. B. Jatene (eds.), *Cardiovascular Surgery*,
https://doi.org/10.1007/978-3-319-57084-6_27

ventricular ejection fraction of 24%, mild right ventricular dysfunction, and septic/cardiogenic shock, and put on mechanical ventilation.

He was stabilized with three cycles of levosimendan, intubated, progressively discontinued from vasoactive drugs, and, finally, listed for heart transplantation. A few days later, the boy presented an acute lung edema followed by bradycardia and decreased saturation. He had an important worsening of hemodynamic parameters and was referred to our pediatric cardiovascular surgery team.

Diagnosis, Assessment, and Treatment

The patient presented a difficult ventilation and important desaturation, requiring manual ventilation and higher infusion rates of vasoactive drugs. He was evaluated for surgery and ECMO was indicated as an emergency procedure. Cannulation through the right internal jugular vein was initially attempted unsuccessfully since the vein was apparently obstructed; as the femoral vein was very thin to be cannu-

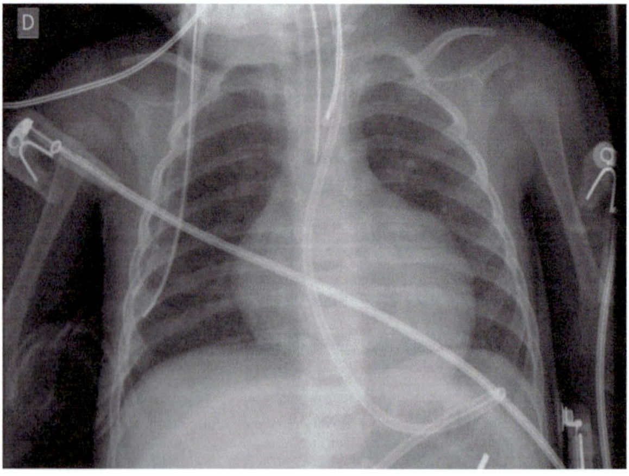

FIGURE 1 Initial chest radiograph showing cardiomegaly due to dilatation of the heart chambers

lated, it was decided to cannulate the right atrium directly through a small right anterior thoracotomy. Eight days after, since he presented important pulmonary improvement, VAD implant was indicated as a bridge to transplantation; the infant then underwent a new surgery for implantation of a 10 mL left ventricular assistance device (Berlin Heart EXCOR® – Fig. 2), with apical cannulation, and was temporarily removed from the transplant list. The procedure was guided through transesophageal echocardiography. Since he became hemodynamically stable, was extubated, and both his hepatic and kidney functions were normal, he was listed for transplantation again 10 days after the VAD implantation.

The infant had a good evaluation in the months that followed, with preserved hepatic and kidney functions and weight gain of 2 kilograms. His right ventricular function was also normal. He suffered an embolic cerebrovascular accident but had complete recovery. After 11 months, he finally underwent cardiac transplantation and is currently stable.

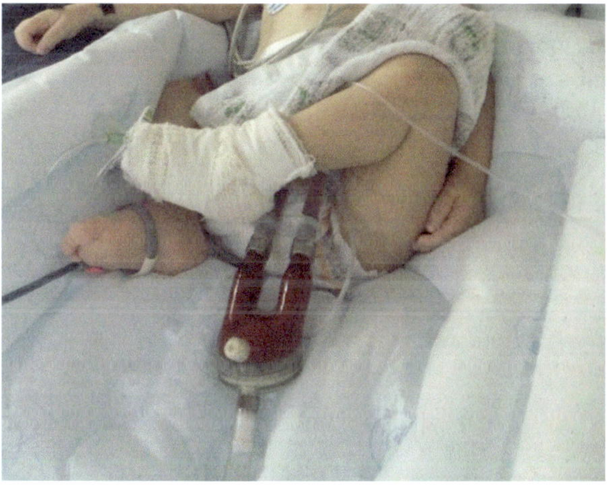

FIGURE 2 The implanted VAD Berlin Heart Excor and its cannulas positioned into the left ventricle apex and into the aorta

Questions

1. How is the clinical presentation of congestive heart failure in children? Which were the signs and symptoms presented in this patient that suggested the diagnosis?

Pediatric heart failure is a relatively uncommon condition leading to little practical experience with its presentation and management. The clinical manifestations might be dissimilar to those of adults and quite variable. Eighty-seven percent of cases of new-onset heart failure in children only reach a diagnosis when the patient is in a state of severe decompensation [1]. In infants and young children, the main symptoms that should draw the attention of the pediatrician or cardiologist are tachypnea, feeding difficulty (reflux, vomiting, and feeding refusal – that can lead to poor weight gain and failure in linear growth), diaphoresis, and pallor. Less frequently these can be present: cyanosis, palpitations, syncope, facial edema, dependent edema, and ascites [1]. Specifically for dilated cardiomyopathy, they are frequently encountered for the first time as acute decompensated heart failure, manifesting most commonly in the first year of life. Irritability, abdominal distress and feeding intolerance are typical symptoms, with sudden or aborted sudden death occurring less commonly. Signs of hypoperfusion and respiratory distress frequently herald an impending collapse [1]. Our patient started with an acute decompensated heart failure, being held in the hospital for 15 days for stabilization. The symptoms started really early, during the first year of life. He then presented loss of appetite, vomiting, and progressive respiratory discomfort, followed by a new decompensation. His clinical picture is compatible with dilated cardiomyopathy.

2. What are the main causes of congestive heart failure in children?

Heart failure in pediatric patients has many different etiologies. These include congenital heart disease, cardiomyopathies, rhythm disorders, as well as acquired heart disease, due to myocarditis, Kawasaki disease, or secondary to chemotherapies for oncological processes [2]. Regarding congenital heart disease, it is the predominant underlying etiology of heart failure in children worldwide [2]. Cardiomyopathies are another diverse category of possible etiology for heart failure. It is categorized as primary or acquired, with dilated or hypertrophic cardiomyopathies as examples of primary etiology and myocarditis, anthracycline exposure, and arrhythmia for secondary. The prevalence of heart failure can range significantly – 71% of children with dilated cardiomyopathy compared with only 13% of those with hypertrophic cardiomyopathy [2]. Dilated cardiomyopathy is the most common one diagnosed in childhood and the leading indication for pediatric heart transplantation [2]. In addition, certain systemic processes such as inflammatory diseases, metabolic disorders, endocrine derangements, and kidney disease result in an unknown number of cases. On a global scale, parasitic infection, nutritional deficit, and rheumatic heart disease are the likely predominant causes of heart failure in childhood [1].

3. How to classify the congestive heart failure severity in the pediatric population? Which would be this patient classification?

The Ross classification has been applied to younger children to quantify changes in functional capacity in established chronic heart failure [1]. The Ross classification is divided in four classes, according to symptom severity. Class I means an asymptomatic patient. Class II refers to mild tachypnea or diaphoresis with feeding but no growth failure. Class III refers to marked tachypnea or diaphoresis with feeding and growth failure. Class IV refers to tachypnea, diaphoresis, or respiratory distress at rest [1]. A more recent guideline for the management of heart failure in children has categorized the evolution and progression of the heart failure into four stages. Stage A (at-risk stage) includes patients born with congenital heart defects, a family history of cardiomyopathy, or exposure to a cardiotoxic agent such as anthracyclines. Stage B (preclinical stage) includes patients with abnormalities of ventricular size, shape, and/or function with no past or present symptoms of heart failure. An example of such patients would include those with cardiomyopathies with asymptomatic left ventricular dysfunction. Stage C (present or past history of heart failure) represents a progression of stage B patients to overt symptoms of heart failure. Stage D (end stage) includes patients with persistent symptoms at rest who require continuous infusion of intravenous inotropic agents, mechanical ventilatory support, and/or mechanical circulatory support [3]. Our patient would be classified in the Ross scale as Class IV and as Stage D.

4. What is the INTERMACS score and how is it utilized? Which would be our patient classification?

The Pediatric Interagency Registry for Mechanical Circulatory Support (PediMACS) is a national registry for US Food and Drug Administration (FDA)-approved VADs in patients <19 years of age. Patients undergoing placement of durable continuous flow (CF) VADs between September 2012 and June 2015 were included, and outcomes were compared with those of adults from the Interagency Registry for Mechanically Assisted Circulatory Support (INTERMACS). The INTERMACS score for advanced heart failure was proven to be useful also for pediatric population to access the use of MCS outcomes since 2010, and its particular levels are shown in Table 1 [4].

Observing the hemodynamic parameters, our patient was then classified as INTERMACS level 1.

5. What are the general indications for the use of mechanical circulatory support (MCS) in children?

There is proven benefit for the use of MCS in INTERMACS levels 1–4 [4]. The use of ventricular assist devices (VADs) in children has increased dramatically over the past decade, with multiple single-center and device-specific reports demonstrating overall improvement in outcomes for children bridged to transplant or recovery with a VAD [5]. Although ECMO has become a standard of care in many pediatric cardiac centers, its use is limited to short-term support in INTERMACS level 1, as a rescue for other long-term device.

Since the mid-1990s in the United States, more than a half of all children supported with ECMO as a bridge to heart

TABLE 1 INTERMACS profiles of advanced heart failure

Profile	Hemodynamic conditions
1	*Critical cardiogenic shock*: persistent hypotension despite rapidly escalating vasoactive drugs, critical organ hypoperfusion
2	*Progressive decline*: intravenous inotropic support, maintaining acceptable pressure levels, progressive nutritional depletion, worsening renal function, or fluid retention
3	*Stable but inotrope dependent*: stable blood pressure dependent on inotropic support, unable to wean due to hypotension, renal dysfunction, or worsening of symptoms
4	*Resting symptoms*: without use of inotropes but recurring symptoms and fluid retention. Worsening is "recurrent"
5	*Exertion intolerant*: severe limitations to physical activity, comfortable at rest, little fluid retention, and at times some renal dysfunction. Living predominantly within the home and neighborhood
6	*Exertion limited*: capable of some activity but fatigues easily, intolerance to fluid overload
7	*Advanced NYHA class III*: clinically stable, reasonably comfortable with activities despite previous history of recent worsening

Adapted from Caneo et al. [4]

transplantation failed to survive to hospital discharge. The majority of deaths occurred while they were on the waiting list, but children who were successfully bridged to transplantation also had high posttransplantation mortality. Patient factors predicting non-survival were a cardiac diagnosis, renal dysfunction, and duration of ECMO for more than 14 days. That's why more effective modalities for chronic circulatory support in children, such as VADs, are needed, and the use of ECMO alone is not a good option as a bridge to transplantation [6].

6. What are the MCS available for the pediatric patients and the indications of each one? Which one would be indicated for our patient?

There are specific MCS to be used for short- and long-term support. ECMO and centrifugal pumps are the most commonly used devices in the pediatric population to provide support for acute cardiac failure patients, but not as good options for bridging to transplantation. On the other hand, the Berlin Heart EXCOR® pediatric ventricular assist device (VAD) represents the most important tool for long-term support to help pediatric patients of all age groups, from newborns to teenagers, to survive until a donor heart can be identified. The VAD system is designed for isolated left ventricular or right ventricular support, but with two pumps connected in series, it can also be modified to provide biventricular support. This approach is, however, rather complex and demanding in terms of pump regulation [7]. If all intensive pharmacologic treatment fails, the patient should be supported with a VAD suitable for long-term implantation, since heart transplantation is the primary goal and the waiting time is unpredictable. Besides, acute viral myocarditis comprises the group most likely to benefit from VAD use [7]. After all of these reasons, the most indicated to our patient would be the VAD, like the Berlin Heart EXCOR® (Table 2).

7. What and how is the surgical procedure done to install the ECMO (extracorporeal membrane oxygenation) and VAD (ventricular assist device – Berlin Heart EXCOR®)?

The standard ECMO procedure for cardiac support in pediatric patients is venoarterial bypass, in which a cannula is placed through the jugular vein toward the right atrium; blood is drained to a reservoir and pumped by a centrifugal pump through an oxygenator before being heated and pumped back to the circulation through a cannula on the right carotid artery [7]. The surgical access for the ECMO cannula implantation in children is usually done by direct cannulation of the jugular vein or the carotid artery. Another option is direct cannulation of the right atrium and aorta through a median sternotomy. In this case, due to his clinical

TABLE 2 Selecting a type of MCS

Device selection criteria	ECMO	Centrifugal pump	Pulsatile VAD
Membrane oxygenator	Yes	No	No
Thoracotomy necessary	No/ optional	Yes	Yes
Support time	1–2 weeks	1–3 weeks	Several months
Area of support	Heart and lung	Right or left ventricle	Right, left, or both ventricles
Anticoagulation	Extensive	Less than ECMO	Less than with all other devices
Complications	Moderate	Few	Few
Mobility to the child	No	No	Yes

Adapted from Hetzer and Stiller [8]

condition, we choose the peripheral cannulation using the neck vessels. Unfortunately, the jugular vein was occluded, and we made an unusual approach for the right atrium cannulation using an anterior thoracotomy.

The Berlin Heart® implantation is made using a cardiopulmonary support and normothermia. Implantation of VAD cannulas begins with the insertion of the LVAD inflow cannula, which is placed in the left ventricular apex. This portion of the procedure can be done with the heart beating or with the heart arrested. The aortic cannula is placed in the aorta, using a longitudinal aortotomy and anastomosed to the aortotomy with a continuous monofilament suture. After completion of the attachment of the cannula to the aorta, the cross-clamp (or partial occlusion clamp) is removed, and the ascending aorta is vented into the cannula. The next step is to attach the cannulas to the blood pump and begin de-airing the system. With completion of de-airing confirmed by transesophageal echocardiography, as well as meticulous inspection of the VAD chamber and cannulas, LVAD pumping is commenced. Full ventilation is initiated, and cardiopulmonary bypass is slowly weaned, continuing echocardiographic visualization to detect residual intracardiac air. Continuous direct inspection of the transparent blood pump chamber is also mandatory to be certain of the adequacy of de-airing [9].

8. Does the use of MCS pretransplantation change the mortality rates and long-term survival of heart transplantation?

The MCS is an important alternative as a bridge to heart transplantations for children with critical heart failure, and many reviews have indicated their big potential to change the survival rates after the surgical procedure. The use of VAD as a bridge to heart transplantation has shown excellent short-term survival, with rates that are comparable with well-matched children not bridged with mechanical support [10]. However, this is achieved at the expense of a higher rate of stroke. Compared with VAD-bridged children, the long-term use of ECMO leads to significant lower rates of survival at 30 days, 6 months, and 1 year after the transplantation procedure and also to higher rates of post-heart transplantation renal failure [10]. The other postoperative complications are comparable between VAD, ECMO, and not-bridged with mechanical support children. Children bridged with ECMO use to have higher risk characteristics, including younger age, lower weight, more congenital heart disease, higher serum creatinine and bilirubin, a higher proportion of mechanical ventilation, and longer average ischemic time [10]. That's why ECMO is also considered a risk factor for the death of children on the waiting list for transplantation.

9. What are the challenges regarding the increase of MCS use?

The use of MCS in children demands some efforts to overcome obstacles such as the compatibility between children size and device capacity, associated pulmonary dysfunctions, ventricular interdependence, and low potential of utilization due to a low economical interest. Regarding these difficulties, it would be necessary financing for the development of new technologies for the devices, aiming to achieve the maximum compatibility with the pediatric patient, and investment in education and training for specialized services to improve their team technical capacity and motivation, the postoperative cares and the quality control.

Review About the Addressed Disease or Treatment

Mechanical circulatory support (MCS) devices are a consolidate option for patients who are on the list for a transplant or dramatically unstable and an important tool for children who underwent cardiogenic shock, especially in the context of scarcity of donors and in which there has been an important increase in hospitalizations for pediatric heart failure. Lately, new types of MCS devices are being and have been developed; for many decades, ECMO (extracorporeal membrane oxygenation) was the major option for pediatric patients as a bridge to transplant, until studies verified that it could be an important factor for decreasing survival on these patients when used in long term. Duration of ECMO longer than 14 days – along with cardiac diagnosis and renal dysfunction – has been listed as a predicting factor of non-survival [6]. Centrifugal pumps had slightly superior results compared with ECMO, being considered an adequate support for 4–8 weeks, but they're also associated with greater postoperative mortality [4].

As a long-term support tool and considered as a successful bridge to transplantation, pediatric VADs like the Berlin Heart EXCOR® can reliably support the circulation at any age, helping pediatric patients to survive until an adequate donor heart is available with good results [11]. However, use of VAD has been associated with a very increased incidence of stroke as a postoperative complication, which may be linked to thromboembolic events favored by the pump use or to anticoagulation-induced hemorrhages [10]. Nevertheless, there is a trending increase in the use of VAD as a bridge to transplant and in the use of ECMO as a bridge to VAD. The transition from ECMO to VAD is usually made in a window that ranges from 5 to 10 days, before ECMO-induced morbidities accumulate, so that VAD may be implanted electively [10]. An earlier transition may be demanded by some factors, such as cardiomyopathy leading to heart failure, asystole, worsening coagulopathy, and difficult ECMO run [10].

The challenges for the pediatric use of MCS remain a relevant issue, mainly to developing countries such as Brazil, where the investment in education and training required to manage these technologies is the key to achieve similar results as the centers of excellence abroad [5].

Bibliography

1. Kantor PF, Lougheed J, Dancea A, McGillion M, Barbosa N, Chan C, et al. Presentation, diagnosis, and medical management of heart failure in children: Canadian Cardiovascular Society guidelines. Can J Cardiol. 2013;29(12):1535–52.
2. Nandi D, Rossano JW. Epidemiology and cost of heart failure in children. Cardiol Young. 2015;25(8):1460–8.
3. Canter CE, Shaddy RE, Bernstein D, Hsu DT, Chrisant MR, Kirklin JK, et al. Indications for heart transplantation in pediatric heart disease: a scientific statement from the American Heart Association Council on Cardiovascular Disease in the Young; the Councils on Clinical Cardiology, Cardiovascular Nursing, and Cardiovascular Surgery and Anesthesia; and the Quality of Care and Outcomes Research Interdisciplinary Working Group. Circulation. 2007;115(5):658–76.
4. Caneo LF, Miana LA, Tanamati C, Penha JG, Shimoda MS, Azeka E. Use of short-term circulatory support as a bridge in pediatric heart transplantation. Arq Bras Cardiol [online]. 2015;104(1 [cited 2016-09-26]):78–84.
5. Caneo LF, Jatene MB. Pediatric mechanical circulatory support systems in Latin America. Artif Organs. 2016;40(10):925–8.
6. Almond CS, Singh TP, Gauvreau K, Piercey GE, Fynn-Thompson F, Rycus PT, Bartlett RH, Thiagarajan RR. Extracorporeal membrane oxygenation for bridge to heart transplantation among

children in the United States: analysis of data from the Organ Procurement and Transplant Network and Extracorporeal Life Support Organization Registry. Circulation. 2011;123(25):2975–84. https://doi.org/10.1161/.110.991505. Epub.

7. Rodriguez-Cruz E, Walters III H, Aggarwal S. Extracorporeal membrane oxygenation. Medscape. n.d. 2016. Available at: http://emedicine.medscape.com/article/1818617-overview?pa=4m5j7y3misjw4spk7vynl6ay0x+cgp6/vasrp+dbkqnmpgojiawq13dl1cs3aqazzoxaisyvxlpgq9sutv7w9gre+tdghihbdbpyiwrvfsa=#a3 (Accessed 26 Sept 2016).
8. Hetzer R, Stiller B. Ventricular assist devices for children. Nat Clin Pract Cardiovasc Med. 2006;3(7):377–86.
9. Jaquiss RDB, Imamura M. Berlin heart implantation for congenital heart defects. Oper Tech Thorac Cardiovasc Surg. Elsevier Inc; 1. 2016;15(2):162–71.
10. Kilic A, Nelson K, Scheel J, Ravekes W, Cameron DE, Vricella LA. Outcomes of heart transplantation in small children bridged with ventricular assist devices. Ann Thorac Surg. 2013;96:1420–7.
11. Hetzer R, Kaufmann F, Delmo Walter EM. Paediatric mechanical circulatory support with Berlin Heart EXCOR: development and outcome of a 23-year experience. Eur J Cardiothorac Surg. 2016;50(2):203–10. https://doi.org/10.1093/ejcts/ezw011.

Use of Venoarterial Extracorporeal Membrane Oxygenation (VA-ECMO) in an Adult Patient with Septic and Cardiogenic Shock

Henrique Louzan Machado, Leonardo Jadyr Silva Rodrigues Alves, and Helmgton José Brito de Souza

Clinical Presentation

A.C.F.F., female, 40 years old, on her 20th week of pregnancy with twins by in vitro fertilization, presented to the maternity ward with mild pelvic pain and vaginal bleeding. During the obstetric evaluation, protrusion of the amniotic sac of one of the fetuses was found, and the patient was admitted. During the second day of hospitalization, failure of the inhibition of preterm labor occurred, resulting in the rupture of the amniotic sac and septic abortion on the day after. The patient developed hypotension that required treatment with vasoactive amines. She was diagnosed with a uterine infection and then transferred to a tertiary hospital to undergo an emergency hysterectomy. During the procedure, the patient presented two episodes of cardiorespiratory arrest and was rapidly revived. The patient was referred, during postoperative period, to an intensive care unit with septic shock, with

H. L. Machado (✉) · L. J. S. Rodrigues Alves · H. J. B. de Souza
Unified School of Brasília (UNICEUB), Brasília, DF, Brazil

R. M. S. Almeida, F. B. Jatene (eds.), *Cardiovascular Surgery*,
https://doi.org/10.1007/978-3-319-57084-6_28

use of high doses of amines, presenting anuria and significant mixed acidosis. An echocardiogram was obtained, which revealed severe left ventricular dysfunction, with an ejection fraction of 18%. The circulatory assistance team was called in for case evaluation.

Diagnosis, Assessment, and Treatment

Patient is in her 20th week of pregnancy and admitted in a maternity with mild pelvic pain and vaginal bleeding. Ultrasonography evaluation demonstrated the protrusion of the amniotic sac of one of the fetuses. Polyhydramnios of both amniotic sacs was seen. At that time, the patient was in good general condition, eupneic, hydrated, acyanotic, anicteric, afebrile, and conscious and demonstrated natural skin tone and good mental status. Absolute rest was indicated, and indomethacin, utrogestan, and nifedipine were prescribed. On the second day of hospitalization, a failed attempt to inhibit preterm labor was performed, resulting in the rupture of the amniotic sac of one of the fetuses. Expectant management was maintained. After approximately 24 h, it was followed by tachycardia, tachypnea, hypotension, and leukocytosis, and she was diagnosed with septic abortion and uterine infection. She was then transferred to a tertiary hospital where an emergency hysterectomy was performed, due to severe septic endometritis. Vancomycin and meropenem were administered. During the procedure, the patient had two episodes of cardiorespiratory arrest, both rapidly reversed. After the completion of surgery, the patient was transferred to an intensive care unit with mechanical ventilation (MV; FiO_2 100% and 14 cmH2O), tachycardia (HR: 159 bpm), and shock (MAP 60 mmHg). A transthoracic echocardiography (TTE) revealed severe left ventricular dysfunction, with an estimated ejection fraction of 18%, requiring supramaximal doses of vasoactive drugs (noradrenaline 3.5 μg/kg/h, adrenaline, and vasopressin 0.05 U/min). The patient was anuric; thus, hemodialysis (HD) was indicated.

She also demonstrated hepatic insufficiency and disseminated intravascular coagulation (platelets 22,000/μL). Arterial blood gas analysis revealed mixed acidosis, with pH of 6,8, pO_2 52 mmHg, pCO_2 80 mmHg, HCO_3 27,9 mmol/L, and lactate 135 mg/dL.

Considering the patient's clinical history and evolution, a circulatory assistance device installation was indicated. In order to prevent imminent death and reverse the clinical condition with potential recovery of vital organs, ECMO in the venoarterial mode was installed as shown in Fig. 1.

Cannulation was performed through the right femoral artery (17F cannula) and the right femoral vein (23F cannula). After initiating the circulatory assistance, it was possible to reduce the VA drug infusion (adrenaline substituted by dobutamine 5 μg/kg/h, noradrenaline 0.7 μg/kg/h, and vasopressin 0.02 U/min). Platelet transfusion (10 IU) and 450 mL of red cell concentrate were required. The ECMO flow was initiated at 4300 mL/min.

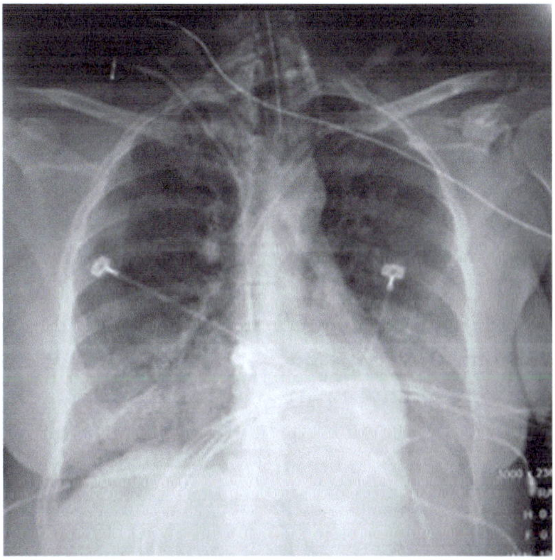

Figure 1 Chest X-ray after ECMO implant

During the initial hours of circulatory assistance, there was deterioration, with evidence of distal ischemia in the right lower limb (RLL) confirmed by bedside arterial Doppler examination. We opted to perform the reinstallation of the device in the contralateral LL. During the procedure, a significant volume of blood was lost – approximately 1000 mL – and transfusion was required.

On the second day of ECMO, hemodialysis was initiated (Prismaflex). The patient presented signs of thrombosis in her left lower limb (LLL); as a result, a catheter (8F) was installed for distal perfusion of the LLL. On physical examination, patient had decreased peripheral perfusion with bilateral absence of peripheral pulses, petechiae on the upper limb and LL, anasarca, distended abdomen with abolished hydroaerial sounds, and hypophonic heart sounds with no heart murmur and was acyanotic, pale, and afebrile. There was a hemodynamic improvement, with a reduction in the vasoactive amine infusion (noradrenaline, 0.3 μg/kg/min; vasopressin, 0.01 U/min; dobutamine, 10 μg/kg/min). Improvement in the blood gas parameters was also seen. On neurological evaluation, miotic and isochoric pupils and a Richmond Agitation-Sedation Scale score of 5 following sedation with midazolam and fentanyl were found. A transesophageal echocardiography (TEE) was performed, demonstrating severe left ventricular (LV) systolic dysfunction at the expense of diffuse hypocontractility, with an LV ejection fraction (LVEF) of 26%. A discrete improvement in the patterns of contractility in basal and mid segments of the back wall was verified when compared with the previous day's echocardiography. Laboratory exams evidenced an increase in transaminases, hypocalcemia at 0.9 mmol/L, creatinine at 2.4 mg/dL, thrombocytopenia at 39,000/μL, leukocytosis at 16,800/μL, indirect bilirubin at 1.01 mg/Dl, and direct bilirubin at 3.78 mg/dL. Arterial blood gas analysis revealed pH, 7.42; pO_2, 153 mmHg; pCO_2, 30 mmHg; HCO_3, 19.5 mmol/L, BE, 1; and lactate, 113 mg/dL.

On the third day of ECMO, the patient was evaluated using arterial Doppler, which identified a decrease of flow in the LL and right UL (RUL) and flow absence in the left UL (LUL). TEE identified an improvement of cardiac function with LVEF at 33%. In the ECMO circuit, fibrin and clots were present in the pre-membrane phase, but without intercurrence during the period.

On the fifth day of ECMO, laboratory exams evidenced hypomagnesemia and a decrease in C-reactive protein, CPK, and transaminases. On TEE, an LVEF of 42% and discrete pericardial effusion were seen. Heparin was at 16 U/kg/h, then decreased to 14 U/kg/h, and subsequently discontinued. The ECMO weaning process was then initiated with heparin discontinuation, flow reduction to 3.51 L/min, and frequency reduction to 3461 RPM.

On the sixth day of circulatory assistance, a TEE was performed, and an improvement in the cardiac function was identified, with LVEF at 70%. In the ECMO inspection, clots in the venous phase and fibrils in the arterial phase were identified. Arterial blood gas analysis exhibited a mixed acidosis with pH at 7.5, pO_2 at 83 mmHg, pCO_2 at 34 mmHg, HCO_3 at 25.7 mmol/L, and lactate at 54 mg/dL – as shown in Chart 1.

Considering the improvement in cardiac function, ECMO explantation was indicated. Noradrenaline was initially discontinued (MAP at 104 mmHg), but due to a decrease in blood pressure (MAP at 59 mmHg), it was resumed at a dose of 0.089 μg/kg/h. After the procedure, the patient developed atrial fibrillation with HR at 160 BPM; a loading dose of amiodarone (Atlansil) was administered and dobutamine reduced to 6 μg/kg/h.

Four days after ECMO withdrawal, bilateral amputation of the infrapatellar region of the lower limbs, left upper forearm (as shown in Fig. 2), and right upper limb digital pulps was performed.

One week after explantation of the circulatory assistance device, the patient evolve with a new sepsis episode resulting in death. The evolution of blood gas and hemodynamic parameters are shown at the Table 1.

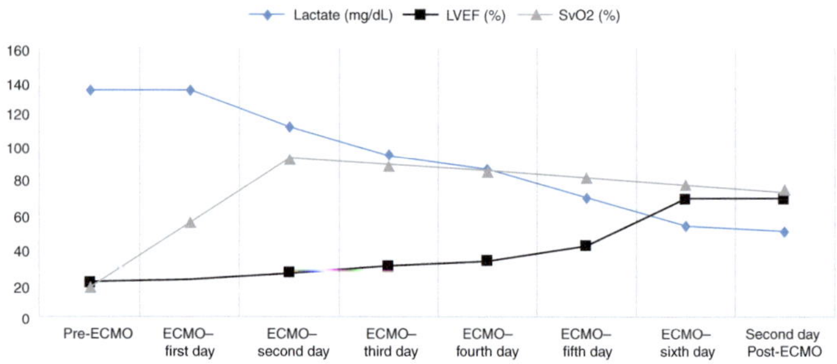

Chart 1 Evolution: Lactate, LVEF e SvO

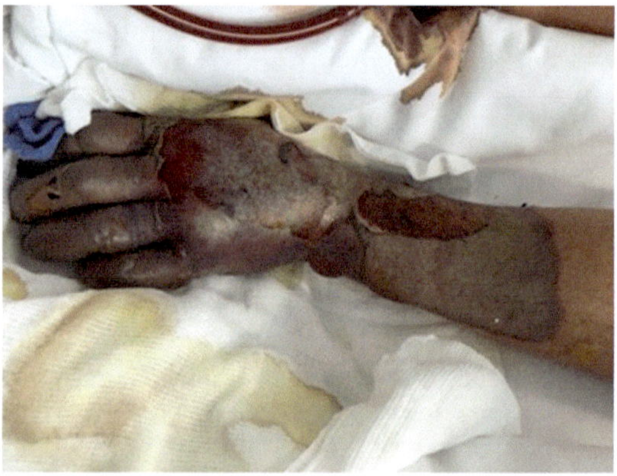

Figure 2 Left upper limb after the septic cyanosis

TABLE I Evolution of blood gas and hemodynamic parameters

	Pre-ECMO	ECMO – day 1	ECMO – day 2	ECMO – day 3	ECMO – day 4	ECMO – day 5	ECMO – day 6	Post-ECMO
pH	6.8	7.39	7.42	7.45	7.43	7.46	7.5	7.4
pO_2 (mmHg)	52	126	153	194	177	125	83	99
pCO_2 (mmHg)	80	44	30	40	37	28	34	35
HCO_3 (mmol/L)	27.9	25.4	19.5	25.9	25.3	19	25.7	22
Lactate (mg/dL)	135	135	113	96	88	71	54	50
LVEF (%)	20	22	26	30	33	42	70	70
SVO_2 (%)	18	56	94	91	87	82	78	75

Questions

1. What are the indications for weaning and explantation of the circulatory assistance device?

While monitoring ventricular function, signs of improvements in hemodynamics and ventricular performance and the presence of the pulse pressure must be observed.

For explant evaluation, the use of echocardiography and pulmonary artery catheter is recommended, and the following recovering indicators should be observed, with the flow of ECMO between 1,5 and 1,0 L/m: improvement of left ventricular function with an ejection fraction between 40% and 45%, appropriate hemodynamic standards, reduction of cardiac cavities, and a good opening of the aortic valve [7].

2. What are the thromboembolic complications in circulatory assistance?

The benefits of ECMO need to be weighed against its inherent risks. Embolic events are caused mainly by the inability to modulate coagulation-related parameters as required by mechanical circulatory assistance devices (MCADs).

Thromboembolic complications are more frequent during low flow and have difficult-to-measure incidence since the majority of events manifest in a hidden or subclinical form [4]. In a period shorter than 31 days, the major thromboembolic complications are clots formed in the circulatory assist device, especially in the oxygenator (11.5% of cases), bladder (5.7%), and hemofilter (4.2%). Disseminated intravascular coagulation (DIC) is also among the thromboembolic complications, with an incidence of 3.9% in the same period [9].

In general, anticoagulant MCAD therapy of short to medium durations is performed through intravenous heparinization, 12–24 h after implantation. Titration of the therapy must be performed until reaching a partial thromboplastin time (PTT) of 50–60 s per 24 h. After 24 h, the heparin dose must be increased and titrated until PTT reaches 60–80 s. Three to five days after implantation of ECMO, if there is no evidence of bleeding, the use of warfarin is recommended, maintaining the INR (international normalized ratio) between 2 and 3 [7].

3. What are the indications for circulatory assistance in patients with cardiogenic shock secondary to sepsis?

The indications for the installation of devices dedicated to circulatory assistance should depend on hemodynamic criteria for determining cardiac failure and the patient's clinical factors (age, clinical status, and prognostic factors: severe hepatic and/or renal dysfunction, coagulopathy, thrombocytopenia, pneumopathy, pulmonary hypertension, unstable arrhythmia, cerebrovascular disease, bacterial endocarditis, active infection, and incomplete surgical correction).

In the specific case of myocardial depression in sepsis, the mechanical circulatory support indication criteria are the same as those listed in the treatment of refractory cardiogenic shock, the extracorporeal membrane oxygenation (ECMO), as well as the Berlin Heart EXCOR® and CentriMag®, paracorporeal devices are disclosed. Recommendations for ECMO implantation are bridge to recovery (class I, level of evidence C) and bridge to transplant (class IIa, level of evidence C). In the case of paracorporeal circulatory pumps, recommendations are the same, except for class IIa for recovery bridge.

It should be noted that studies show that the success in the treatment of myocardial dysfunction in sepsis with circulatory support has proven effective only in those cases where there was no prior myocardial dysfunction to the infectious event.

4. What is the association between septic and cardiogenic shocks?

Septic shock can be defined as the presence of systemic inflammatory response syndrome (SIRS) with a known site of infection, combined with tissue hypoperfusion and persistent hypotension. Its connection with the impairment of cardiac function is related to an increase in the production of procoagulant substances and a decrease in anticoagulant factors, which may result in ischemia due to thrombus and valvular and vascular impairment. Furthermore, during sepsis, a large amount of nitric oxide is released, which is responsible for myocardial depression and cardiac injury due to the formation of peroxynitrite, a potential oxidant agent. Both contribute to cardiac dysfunction and failure.

5. What are the indications and the pharmacological treatment for inhibiting preterm labor?

The inhibition of preterm labor is indicated if there is cervical dilatation < 3 cm and if the gestational age is between 22 and 34 weeks. This procedure is contraindicated in cases of fetal death, severe fetal malformations, and diseases related to placental insufficiency.

For pharmacological inhibition, the use of oxytocin inhibitors, prostaglandin inhibitors, and calcium channel blockers is indicated, with the common objective of interrupting uterine contractions. Simultaneously, use of corticosteroids to reduce pulmonary complications in the newborn and prophylaxis against the vertical transmission of group B streptococcus should be administered.

6. What is the treatment for septic shock?

Initially, early therapy should be goal-driven with the main aim of correcting hemodynamic failures, including hypovolemia, myocardial depression, and increased endothelial permeability. The therapy should be aimed to obtain a central venous pressure (CVP) between 8 and 12 mmHg, mean arterial pressure (MAP) ≥ 65 mmHg, and central venous oxygen saturation ($ScvO_2$) ≥ 70%. Thus, the initial treatment should adjust preload, afterload, and cardiac contractility. Subsequently, the therapy should be based in administrate broad-spectrum intravenous antimicrobials for all likely pathogens, until the identification of the causative agent, when a more specific antibiotic should be chosen [3].

7. What is the pathophysiology of septic shock?

Septic shock may be triggered by a variety of injuries, particularly microbial infections, burns, trauma, and or pancreatitis. The common pathophysiology feature is a large production of inflammatory mediators from innate and adaptive immune cells that produce arterial vasodilation, vascular leakage, and venous blood pooling. These cardiovascular abnormalities result in tissue hypoperfusion, cellular hypoxia, and metabolic derangements that lead to organ dysfunction and, if severe and persistent, organ failure and death.

As the microbial infection begins, cells of the immune system, such as macrophages, neutrophils, dendritic cells, and endothelial cells, and complement system recognize several substances derived from microorganisms (PAMPs or pathogen-associated molecular patterns) and are activated. Once triggered, these cells initiate inflammatory responses that interact in an incompletely understood mechanism to produce septic shock and multiorgan dysfunction. The factors that have major roles in the pathogenesis of septic shock include *inflammatory and counter-inflammatory responses*, *endothelial activation and injury*, and *induction of a procoagulant state*.

The most likely initiator of inflammation in sepsis is signaling pathways that lie downstream of Toll-like receptors, which will recognize the PAMPs. Upon activation, innate immune cells produce tumor necrosis factor, interferon-y, and interleukin-1, interleukin-12, and interleukin-18. Reactive oxygen species and lipid mediators such as prostaglandins and platelet-activating factor (PAF) are also elaborated. These substances induce endothelial cells to produce more adhesion molecule expression and further stimulate cytokine and chemokine production. The complement system is also activated by microbial components, resulting in the production of anaphylatoxins (C3a, C5a), chemotactic fragments (C5a), and opsonins (C3b), all of which contribute to the pro-inflammatory state.

The hyperinflammatory state initiated by sepsis also activates counter-regulatory immunosuppressive mechanisms. As a result, septic patients may oscillate between hyperinflammatory and immunosuppressed states during their clinical course. Proposed mechanisms for the immune suppression include a shift from pro-inflammatory to anti-inflammatory cytokines, production of anti-inflammatory mediators (such as soluble TNF receptor, IL-l receptor antagonist, and IL-10) lymphocyte apoptosis, the immunosuppressive effects of apoptotic cells, and the induction of cellular energy.

Furthermore, microbial components can activate coagulation directly through factor XII and indirectly through altered endothelial function. The pro-inflammatory state leads loosen endothelial cell tight junctions, making vessels leaky and resulting in the accumulation of protein-rich edema throughout the body, which have deleterious effects on both nutrient delivery and waste removal, leading to tissue hypoperfusion. This condition also stimulates the production of nitric oxide and other vasoactive inflammatory mediators (e.g., C3a, C5a, and platelet-activating factor), which may contribute to vascular smooth muscle relaxation and systemic hypotension.

Pro-inflammatory cytokines increase tissue factor production by monocytes and endothelial cells and decrease the production of endothelial anticoagulant factors. The vascular leak and tissue edema decrease blood flow at the level of small vessels, producing stasis and diminishing the washout of activated coagulation factors. Acting in concert, these effects lead to systemic activation of thrombin and the deposition of fibrin-rich thrombi in small vessels, often throughout the body, further compromising tissue perfusion and leading to disseminated intravascular coagulation (DIC). In patients with DIC, the consumption of coagulation factors and platelets is so great that deficiencies of these factors appear, leading to bleeding and hemorrhage [10].

8. How to diagnose a septic shock?

By definition, septic shock refers to sepsis associated with circulatory and cellular/metabolic abnormalities capable of substantially increase mortality. In a clinical view, it is seen as sepsis related to the need for vasoactive drugs to raise mean arterial pressure above 65 mmHg and lactate > 18 mg/dL or 2 mmol/L after adequate volemic resuscitation.

Sepsis, in turn, is initially suspected through the use of qSOFA (quick sequential organ failure assessment score) during clinical screening, which has systolic BP less than 100 mmHg, respiratory rate > 22/min, and mental state (Glasgow coma scale <15) as assessment criteria. In order to confirm the diagnostic hypothesis, SOFA (sequential organ failure assessment) score is used, stating the presence of sepsis if there is suspicion or certainty of infection and an acute increase of 2 points or more in the SOFA [2]. See Table 2.

TABLE 2 Sequential Organ Failure Assessment (SOFA) score

	Score				
	0	1	2	3	4
PaO_2/FiO_2, mmHg (kPa)	≥400 (53.3)	<400 (53.3)	<300 (40)	<200 (26.7) with respiratory support	<100 (13.3) with respiratory support
Platelets, $\times 10^3/\mu L$	≥150	≥150	<100	<50	<20
Bilirubin, mg/dL (μmol/L)	<1.2 (20)	1.2–1.9 (20–32)	2.0–5.9 (33–101)	6.0–11.9 (102–204)	>12.0 (204)
Cardiovascular	MAP ≥70 mmHg	MAP <70 mmHg	Dopamine <5 or dobutamine (any dose)	Dopamine 5.1–15 or epinephrine ≤0.1 or norepinephrine ≤0.1	Dopamine >15 or epinephrine >0.1 or norepinephrine >0.1
Glasgow score	15	13–14	10–12	6–9	<6
Creatinine, mg/dL (μmol/L)	<1.2 (110)	1.2–1.9 (110–170)	2.0–3.4 (171–299)	3.5–4.9 (300–440)	>5.0 (440)
Urine output, mL/d				<500	<200

Review About the Addressed Disease or Treatment

The extracorporeal membrane oxygenation (ECMO) is a temporary invasive mechanical support therapy designed to promote a cardiopulmonary support for patients with cardiogenic shock refractory and/or acute breathing failure, unresponsive to oxygenation and recruitment maneuvers. This therapy is used in patients with potential functional recovery (class I, evidence level C), as a bridge to decision (class I, evidence level C), as a bridge to transplant (class IIa, evidence level C), or as a bridge for long-term mechanical circulatory assistance device – artificial heart for target therapy (class I, evidence level C).

There are two possible modalities for the use of this therapy: venoarterial (VA) and veno-venous (VV). The implant might be done in the central vessel (by thoracotomy) or peripheral, with cannulation by puncture or surgical dissection. In the VA-ECMO, the venous blood is drained by cannulation of a large caliber vein (jugular, femoral or directly from the right atrium) and conducted by a centrifugal pump through an oxygenation membrane, being returned, oxygenated, by a cannula inserted into the artery of large caliber, which may be an aortic artery, when access to the thoracotomy, or the peripheral, most commonly by one of the femoral arteries. In the VV-ECMO mode, both drainage and reinfusion are made exclusively from the venous system (femoral-femoral or femoral-jugular).

Due to complications related to the use of ECMO, such as hemolysis, thrombosis, bleeding, vascular accidents, infection, resistance of the oxygenation membrane, and impossibility of decompression of cardiac chambers, there is a limitation of its use time: a recommended 30-day maintenance. In cases of heart failure, uni- or biventricular, the persistence of the dysfunction may lead to replacement of the circulatory support device by prolonged use equipment.

Bibliography

1. Abrams D, Combes A, Brodie D. Extracorporeal membrane oxygenation in cardiopulmonary disease in adults. J Am Coll Cardiol. 2014;63(25 Pt A):2769–78.
2. Singer M, Deutschman CS, Seymour CW, et al. The third international consensus definitions for sepsis and septic shock (sepsis-3). J Am Med Assoc. 2016;315(8):801–10.
3. Howell MD, Davis AM. Management of sepsis and septic shock. JAMA. 2017. Available from: http://jamanetwork.com/journals/jama/fullarticle/2598892. Access on: Janciro, 2017.
4. Annich G, Lynch W, MacLaren G, Wilson J, Barlett R. Ecmo: extracorporeal cardiopulmonary support in critical care. 44th ed. Ann Arbor: ELSO Office; 2012.
5. Carvalho P, Trotta E. Avanços no diagnóstico e tratamento da sepse. J Pediatr. 2003;79(2):195–204.
6. Bittar R, Carvalho M, Zugaib M. Condutas para o trabalho de parto prematuro. Rev Bras Ginecol Obstet. 2005;27(9):561–6.
7. Ayub-Ferreira SM, et al. Diretriz de assistência circulatória mecânica da sociedade brasileira de cardiologia. Arq Bras Cardiolog. 2016;107(2 Supl. 2):1–33.
8. Felice CD, Susin CF, Costabeber AM. Shock: emergency diagnosis and treatment. Rev AMRIGS. 2011;55(2):179–96.
9. Extracorporeal Life Support Organization (ELSO). International summary of July – 2015. ECLS Registry Report. 23; 2015.
10. Robbins SL, Cotran RS. Pathologic basis of disease. 9th ed. Elsevier; 2015. p. 131–3.

Circulatory Assistance in a Patient with Respiratory Failure

Rafael Ramos Amaral, Thiago do Amaral Cavalcante, Leonardo Jadyr Silva Rodrigues Alves, and Helmgton José Brito de Souza

Clinical Presentation

The patient was admitted to the emergency room with respiratory failure after a suicide attempt with a blunt weapon. He was placed on mechanical ventilation and being diagnosed, after emergency intubation, with a bilateral pneumothorax. Following a bilateral thoracic drainage, he was transferred to the intensive care unit, developing after 3 days a respiratory infection and acute respiratory distress syndrome (ARDS), failing to respond after prone positioning and alveolar recruitment. Considering the worsening infection and multiple organ failure and in order to prevent imminent death, he was placed on veno-venous extracorporeal membrane oxygenation (VV-ECMO).

R. R. Amaral (✉) · T. do Amaral Cavalcante · L. J. S. R. Alves
H. J. B. de Souza
Unified School of Brasília (UNICEUB), Brasília, DF, Brazil

R. M. S. Almeida, F. B. Jatene (eds.), *Cardiovascular Surgery*,
https://doi.org/10.1007/978-3-319-57084-6_29

Diagnosis, Assessment, and Treatment

R.M.A., a previously healthy 33-year-old male drug user was admitted with respiratory failure following a suicide attempt. After emergency intubation, he was diagnosed with a bilateral pneumothorax (computerized tomography) and had a bilateral drainage. He developed a respiratory infection after 3 days (leukocytosis at 23,700/μL, rods at 6%). Piperacillin and tazobactam (Tazocin) were administered, and teicoplanin was also adopted afterward.

The arterial blood gas analysis revealed no improvement on the following days (pH 7.2; pO_2, 93 mmHg; pCO_2, 105 mmHg; $SatO_2$, 92%), despite mechanical ventilation at high parameters (FiO_2 100%, PEEP: 15; PaO_2/FiO_2: 0,93). The chest X-ray revealed opacification of the right hemithorax (Fig. 1). Alveolar recruitment maneuvers were realized but showed no clinical, blood gas, or X-ray improvements. Computerized tomography was realized again, in the fourth day after admission, revealing atelectasis of the right lower lobe and inflammatory/infectious process. The patient was placed on prone positioning but showed no improvement. On the fifth day, chest X-ray still revealed opacity on the right hemithorax, and bronchoscopic examination showed purulent

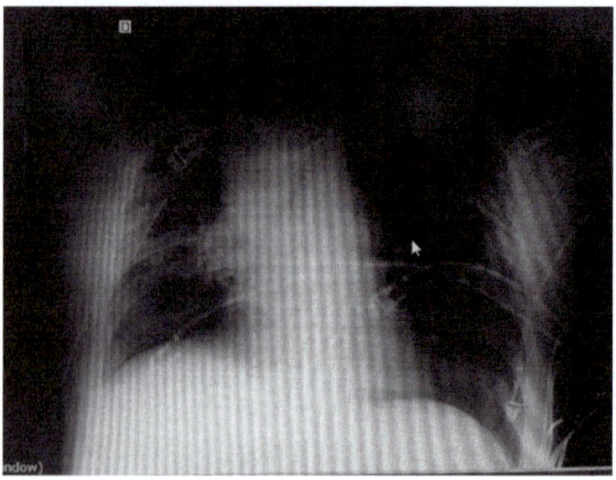

FIGURE 1 Chest X-ray before ECMO installation

secretion. The patient went on to develop hemodynamic instability, requiring administration of vasoactive drugs (noradrenaline 0.2 μg/kg/h). Prone positioning was attempted once again during 18 h, with no significant improvement and with persistent hypoxemia and hypercapnia (pH, 7.16; pO_2, 75 mmHg; PCO_2, 106 mmHg; HCO_3, 29 mmol/L; $SatO_2$, 90%; and lactate, 37 mg/dL). At this point, the Murray score, which evaluates the need for extracorporeal life support, was calculated at 3.25. Considering the high score, the patient's worsening respiratory condition, unresponsiveness to alveolar recruitment, and the increasing risk of death, extracorporeal membrane oxygenation (ECMO) in the veno-venous mode was indicated [1].

Installation was performed in the ICU. A 25 Fr (MAQUET) venous cannula was inserted with Seldinger technique puncture of the right femoral vein, and a 19 Fr (MAQUET) arterial cannula was inserted into the right jugular vein, with the same technique. The patient was then transferred to HOBRA-DF (Hospital Brasília, Distrito Federal, Brazil), where a trained multidisciplinary team was prepared to perform maintenance of the ECMO machine. On the first hours after admission, the first blood gas exam on circulatory assistance exhibited considerable improvement, with pH, 7.29; PCO_2, 72 mmHg; PO_2, 171 mmHg; HCO_3, 30.2 mmol/L; $SatO_2$, 99%; and lactate, 11 mg/dL. Sedation was changed to midazolam and fentanyl and initiated protective ventilation strategy with FiO_2: 100% and PEEP: 15. Hemodialysis was started in order to reduce the hydric balance and in an attempt of renal function recovery. Antibiotic therapy was changed to meropenem, vancomycin, and polymyxin B. Twelve hours after circulatory assistance with ECMO, the blood gas exhibited important decreasing acidosis (pH, 7.46; HCO_3, 27.2 mmol/L). Continuous heparin infusion was initiated, controlled by aPTT, as recommended by the service protocol.

Chest CT was realized on the second day of ECMO revealing hepatization of right lower lobe (Fig. 2). A chest X-ray was also performed in this day (Fig. 3). Hemodynamic

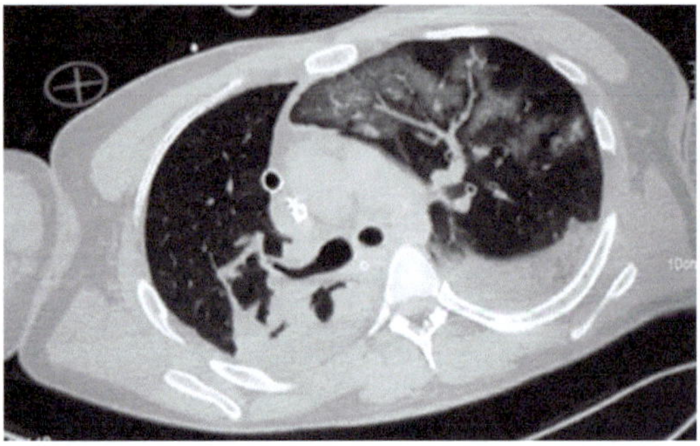

FIGURE 2 Thorax CT (second day of ECMO)

stability allowed weaning and suspension of noradrenaline. From the fourth day of circulatory assistance, yet without vasoactive drugs, he showed recovery signs of respiratory functions, with pCO_2, 35 mmHg; pO_2, 71 mmHg; and HCO_3, 25 mmol/L. Ventilation parameters, therefore, were reduced to FiO_2: 30% and PEEP: 10. On the seventh day of assistance, lung conditions were still improving, and a tracheostomy (n° 8 cannula) was performed, in order to facilitate ventilation weaning after ECMO explant. Following confirmation of respiratory function recovery (blood gas analysis with pH at 7.39; PO_2, 97 mmHg; PCO_2, 44 mmHg; $SatO_2$, 97%; and PO_2/FiO_2, 323), explant of the ECMO was performed in the ICU on the eighth day after its installation. He still remained on dialysis for 3 days until full renal recovery, and first blood gas after ECMO removal revealed further improvement of respiratory function, with pH, 7.39; pO_2, 144 mmHg; pCO_2, 42 mmHg; $SatO_2$, 99%; and HCO_3, 25.3 mmol/L. He was removed from the mechanical ventilator 8 days after the ECMO was explanted (post-ECMO arterial blood gas may be seen in Table 1). He was discharged from the ICU to a general ward 23 days after admission in the emergency room and discharged for rehabilitation after 60 days from his admission and 33 days after the ECMO explant. He left the hospital with a recommendation to keep on psychiatric care.

Table 1 Evolution of blood gas and respiratory parameters

	pH	pCO_2 (mmHg)	pO_2 (mmHg)	HCO_3 (mmol/L)	FiO_2 (%)	Sat O_2 (%)	PEEP	Lactate (mg/dL)
PRE-ECMO	7,26	105	93	32	100	92	15	16
ECMO – first day	7,41	38	148	32	100	99	10	11
ECMO – second day	7,4	38	148	31	21	92	12	8
ECMO – third day	7,43	39	133	26	30	100	14	5
ECMO – fourth day	7,43	35	97	25	60	98	12	5
ECMO – fifth day	7,41	24	269	15,2	100	92	10	5
ECMO – sixth day	7,44	41	74	27,5	70	95	10	6
ECMO – seventh day	7,42	45	110	23	30	98	12	5
ECMO – eighth day	7,44	39	165	26,5	35	98	12	6
POST-ECMO	7,39	42	144	25,3	40	99	10	6

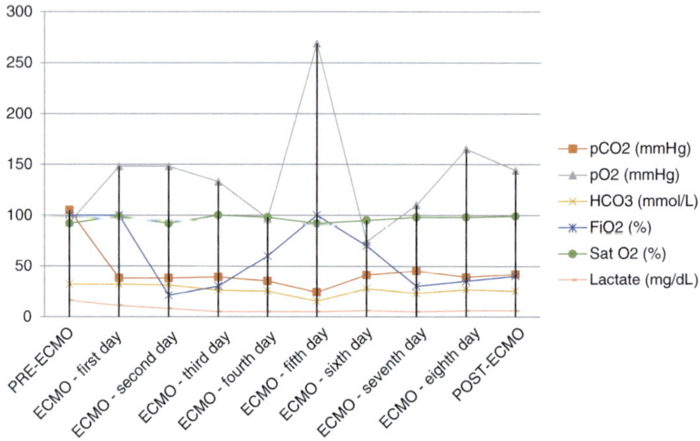

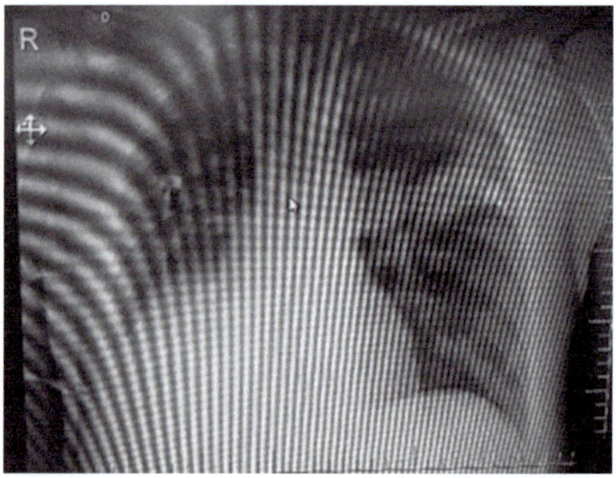

Figure 3 Chest X-ray (second day of ECMO)

Questions

1. What are the principles of extracorporeal circulation?

Circulation and ventilation with mechanical support, extracorporeal circulation, or cardiopulmonary bypass have been used in cardiac surgeries since 1953, when it was first adopted by Gibbon, facilitating cardiac surgical processes [2]. This technique temporarily replaces cardiac and pulmonary functions during surgery by means of mechanical devices, maintaining the circulation of blood and oxygen throughout the body. A pump and an oxygenator, its two functional units, work so that the poorly oxygenated blood is removed from the patient's body, oxygenated and returned via cannulae. This way, blood cells are able to maintain cellular respiration outside the body during surgery [3]. Currently, there are few risks associated with the use of this feature, as long as it is used properly [2].

2. How does ECMO differ from traditional cardiopulmonary bypass?

Extracorporeal life support, also known as ECMO (extracorporeal membrane oxygenation), is a variation of cardiopulmonary bypass. Whereas cardiopulmonary bypass facilitates open surgery for a few hours, ECMO allows the patients with respiratory or cardiac failure to be on circulatory assistance outside the operating room under observation. Acknowledging the differences, the ECMO circuit is similar to the cardiopulmonary bypass, although cannulation is often not the same. Veno-venous cannulation is used to replace respiratory functions only so that a double lumen cannula is placed into a major vein (usually the vena cava) and the deoxygenated blood flow into the pump-oxygenator setup and oxygenated blood is returned to the right atrium. Venous-arterial cannulation bypasses both the heart and lungs with insertion in a major artery (usually the femoral) and one of the major veins, often used in cardiac failure conditions, with or without respiratory failure [4].

3. What is the Murray score? How is it used in the indication of ECMO?

The Murray scoring system evaluates the presence and extent of pulmonary damage and includes four criteria which are related to ARDS development:

- Hypoxemia
- PEEP
- Lung compliance
- Chest radiograph

Each criterion receives a score from 0 to 4 according to the severity of the condition. The final score is obtained by dividing the collective score by the number of components that were used. A score of zero indicates no lung injury, a score of 1–2.5 indicates mild to moderate lung injury, and a final score of more than 2.5 indicates the presence of ARDS [5].

4. In what circumstances is veno-venous circulatory assistance indicated?

According to ELSO [6] (Extracorporeal Life Support Organization) General Guidelines:

(a) In hypoxic respiratory failure due to any cause (primary or secondary), ECLS should be considered when the risk of mortality is 50% or greater and is indicated when the risk of mortality is 80% or greater. (a) Fifty percent mortality risk is associated with a $PaO_2/FiO_2 < 150$ on $FiO_2 > 90\%$ and/or Murray score 2–3. (b). Eighty percent mortality risk is associated with a $PaO_2/FiO_2 < 100$ on $FiO_2 > 90\%$ and/or Murray score 3–4 despite optimal care for 6 h or more.
(b) CO_2 retention on mechanical ventilation despite high Pplat (>30 cmH2O)
(c) Severe air leak syndromes
(d) Need for intubation in a patient on lung transplant list
(e) Immediate cardiac or respiratory collapse (PE, blocked airway, unresponsive to optimal care)

5. What are patient-related management issues during veno-venous ECMO?

According to ELSO [6] General Guidelines:

- Medication and infusions should be used to control hemodynamics.
- Ventilation should be preferably on low settings, so that the lungs can rest (also valid to venoarterial assistance), with a low rate and long inspiratory time, low FiO_2, and PEEP at any level. Lung recruitment maneuvers should not be attempted if the patient has respiratory failure during acute inflammatory stage.
- Sedation is always recommended during cannulation and management in the first 12 to 24 h. The main reason for sedation in veno-venous ECMO is to tolerate endotracheal intubation.

- Management should aim for a normal hematocrit, body weight (regulated fluid balance), and blood volume.
- Diuresis should happen spontaneously or by medication until the patient is close to dry weight and has no edema. Renal failure may occur and should be treated with continuous hemofiltration.
- Cannula sites should be constantly cleaned with antiseptic solution to prevent infections.
- Patient positioning should be mobile and as normal as possible.

6. How should the weaning for the veno-venous ECMO be realized?

According to the Extracorporeal Life Support Organization, when management is carried out using the lowest flow to provide adequate support at low ventilator settings and pressor doses, the weaning should be automatic, and the organ function improves as the assistance is decreased [6].

7. What is the pathophysiology of acute distress respiratory syndrome?

ARDS is a disease in which the lungs suffer from severe inflammation with hypoxemia and respiratory failure. This interferes with lung compliance and results in bilateral and diffuse damage. It may be infective or noninfective. In its initial phase, there is alveolar flooding, causing a noncardiogenic edema. Increased capillary permeability is the strongest evidence of ARDS. Damage to the capillary endothelium and alveolar epithelium, together with the removal of fluid from the alveolar space, causes an accumulation of protein fluid within the alveolus, thus triggering alveolar damage. Neutrophils are attracted to the lungs due to the release of proinflammatory cytokines (TNF, IL-1, IL-6) and release mediators as reactive oxygen species and proteases. The release of these free radicals has an endogenous antioxidant effect causing damage to alveolar cells. The lesion of the alveolar epithelium can be classified into two different types. Type 1 leads to pulmonary edema and consequent rupture of the epithelial barrier exposing the basement membrane, facilitating a bacterial infection or sepsis. Type 2 leads to decreased surfactant synthesis and metabolism resulting in increased alveolar surface tension leading to collapse of the structure. Pulmonary hypertension is also widely recognized as a feature in ARDS. The etiology of this disease includes destruction of the parenchyma and collapse of the airways, pulmonary hypoxemia due to vasoconstriction, and presence of other pulmonary vasoconstrictors and vascular compression [7].

8. What is the main treatment for this condition?

Treatment usually involves mechanical ventilation in an intensive unit care, while also supporting other associated comorbidities (infections, stress ulcer, thrombosis). Ventilation therapy includes positive pressure to ensure adequate oxygenation, although the optimal levels of positive end-expiratory pressure are controversial. Other than ventilation, techniques used in severely ill patients are ECMO, which has been adopted in many specialized centers as a rescue therapy for refractory hypoxemia, and prone positioning, which can improve oxygenation. ECMO helps oxygenate the patient's blood out of their body through a membrane that oxygenates the blood and functions as an artificial lung, allowing an adequate control of gas exchange without vigorous mechanical ventilation. Prone positioning strategy can cause a significant increase in oxygenation in patients with respiratory hypoxemia. The mechanisms that enhance this improvement are recruitment of dependent lung units, redistribution of blood flow to the more unaffected lung regions, reduction of ventilation perfusion mismatch, minimization of compression of the lung from anterior mediastinal structures, and facilitation of respiratory secretion clearance [8].

Review About the Addressed Disease or Treatment

Some patients referred to ECMO have ARDS, in addition to fulfilling the prerequisites for ECMO implantation, such as PaO_2/FIO_2 ratio of 70–80 mmHg, Murray score > 3, and pH <7.2. Even though this condition is generally caused by pneumonia, its development by blunt thoracic trauma does not contraindicate the use of extracorporeal life support. In fact, although respiratory failure caused by severe thoracic trauma is still a challenge to intensive care specialists, the veno-venous ECMO reveals itself as a safe and life-saving treatment option for this condition. The onset of ARDS due to exposure caused by trauma triggers an acute response by tissue injury and organ involvement; therefore, the reported case is shown as an example of a rapid implementation of ECMO and successful treatment. The publications of the last decade showed that even with some complications associated with this scenario, such as increased risk of prior massive blood loss, coagulopathy, coexisting solid organ, or traumatic brain injury, the use of ECMO as a tool in early diagnoses has shown an important decrease in long-term morbidity. As for these studies, the use of ECMO (with or without systemic anticoagulation) for refractory severe ARDS generally survived with minimal complications. Ultimately, it is also cost-effective (especially if realized early) and has survival rates which vary from 74% to 79% [9, 10].

Bibliography

1. Peek GJ, et al. Efficacy and economic assessment of conventional ventilatory support versus extracorporeal membrane oxygenation for severe adult respiratory failure (CESAR): a multicentre randomised controlled trial. Lancet (London, England). 2009;374(9698):1351–63.
2. Harlan BJ, Starr A, Harwin FM. Manual Ilustrado de Cirurgia Cardíaca. 1a edn. Revinter; 2000.
3. Stoney WS. Evolution of cardiopulmonary bypass. Circulation. 2009;119(21):2844–53. https://doi.org/10.1161/circulationaha.108.830174.
4. Gaffney AM, Wildhirt SM, Griffin MJ, Annich GM, Radomski MW. Extracorporeal life support. BMJ. 2010;341(nov02 1):c5317. https://doi.org/10.1136/bmj.c5317.
5. Murray JF, Matthay MA, Luce JM, Flick MR. An expanded definition of the adult respiratory distress syndrome. Am Rev Respir Dis. 1988;138(3):720–3. https://doi.org/10.1164/ajrccm/138.3.720.

6. Extracorporeal Life Support Organization (ELSO). General guidelines for all ecls cases (Version 1.3). Extracorporeal Life Support Organization; 2013. http://www.elso.org/resources/guidelines?download=17:elso-guidelines-generalv11.
7. Pierrakos C, et al. Acute respiratory distress syndrome: pathophysiology and therapeutic options. J Clin Med Res. 2012;4(1):7–16.
8. Dushianthan A, Grocott MPW, Postle AD, Cusack R. Acute respiratory distress syndrome and acute lung injury. Postgrad Med J. 2011;87(1031):612–22. https://doi.org/10.1136/pgmj.2011.118398.
9. Bosarge PL, Raff LA, McGwin G, Carroll SL, Bellot SC, Diaz-Guzman E, Kerby JD. Early initiation of extracorporeal membrane oxygenation improves survival in adult trauma patients with severe acute respiratory distress syndrome. J Trauma Acute Care Surg. 2016;1. https://doi.org/10.1097/ta.0000000000001068.
10. Jacobs JV, Hooft NM, Robinson BR, Todd E, Bremner RM, Petersen SR, Smith MA. The use of extracorporeal membrane oxygenation in blunt thoracic trauma. J Trauma Acute Care Surg. 2015;79(6):1049–54. https://doi.org/10.1097/ta.0000000000000790.

Part X
Pericardial Disease

Constrictive Pericarditis: A Late Complication of Tuberculosis

Carla Mayara Forte dos Santos, Bárbara Liss de Sousa Freire, Amanda Késsia da Silva Sales, Joaquim David Carneiro Neto, and Mamede Francisco Johnson de Aquino Filho

Clinical Presentation

A 37-year-old man, brown, born and raised in Brazil, reports severe dyspnea for 20 days associated with a ventilatory-dependent pain on the left hemithorax and cystic formation in scar area located in fifth left intercostal space (Fig. 1).

He underwent a pericardiectomy 1 year ago with antero-lateral left excision by important pericardial effusion held in the city of Rio de Janeiro, Brazil. He has been in treatment of tuberculosis for 5 months.

On the patient's physical examination he was afebrile, epneic, pale, hydrated, conscious and responsive, hemodynamically stable, with swollen lymph nodes in the neck an supraclavicular, preserved ambulation and decreased auditory acuity.

Blood pressure: 100/65 mmHg

Heart rate: 80 beats per minute

Respiration rate: 12 breaths per minute

Temperature: 36 °C

C. M. F. dos Santos (✉) · B. L. de Sousa Freire · A. K. da Silva Sales
J. D. C. Neto · M. F. J. de Aquino Filho
Federal University of Ceará (UFC), Sobral, CE, Brazil

R. M. S. Almeida, F. B. Jatene (eds.), *Cardiovascular Surgery*,
https://doi.org/10.1007/978-3-319-57084-6_30

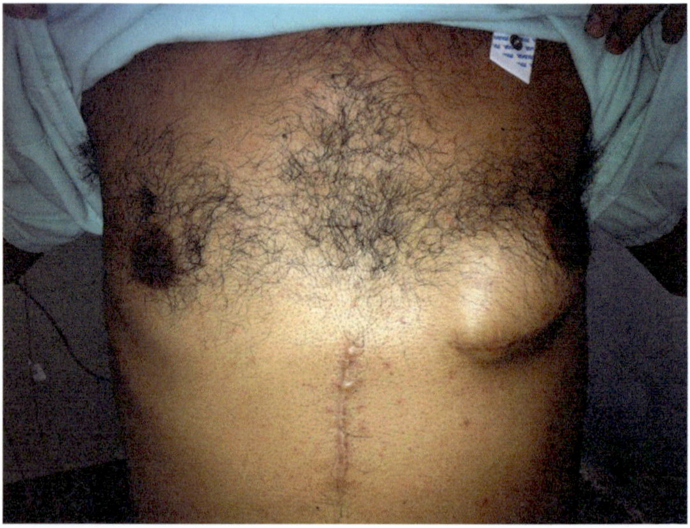

Figure 1 Cystic formation in scar area located in the fifth left intercostal space

Cardiovascular system: regular heart rhythm with normophonetic sounds, without murmurs

Respiratory system: vesicular breath sounds without adventitious sounds and with tachypnea

Abdomen: flaccid, with no palpable visceromegaly; bowel sounds negative

Extremities: perfused, heated, and without edema

Genitourinary system: no changes

Gastrointestinal tract: no changes

Nervous system: no changes

Diagnosis, Assessment, and Treatment

The patient was referred to the intensive care unit (ICU) for hospitalization due to the risk of complication and to perform general examinations because of the clinical presentation of intense dyspnea. In the intensive care unit, intensive treatment for congestive heart failure (CHF) was initiated, associated with collection of vital signs and physical examination on a daily basis.

From the clinical picture, the following laboratory tests were initially requested. Hemogram showed hematocrit = 40.3%, hemoglobin = 12.2 g/dL, leucogram = 5100 leukocytes/mm^3, basophils = 0, eosinophils = 1, metamyelocytes = 0, bands = 0, segmented = 87, platelets = 212,000 Plt/mm^3, creatinine = 0.7 mg/dL, urea = 21 mg/dL, sodium = 140 mEq/L, and potassium = 4.2 mEq/L. From the above data, and considering patient's previous tuberculosis disease, it was hypothesized that it would be a picture of pericardial tuberculosis. In this situation, the pericardium can be affected by Koch's bacillus through hematogenous dissemination during the course of endogenous reactivation of pulmonary focus or by direct extension of the disease in the lung, pleura, and tracheobronchial lymph nodes into the pericardial cavity. Due to this situation, the adenosine deaminase laboratory test was requested, and the patient's exam was 103.88 U/L. The adenosine deaminase measurement in the pleural fluid is a sensitive and specific method for diagnosis of pleural tuberculosis, and its use may preclude the need for pleural biopsy in the initial work-up of pleural effusion patients. An adenosine deaminase cutoff value of 40 U/L is recommended.

Electrocardiogram revealed sinus rhythm, low voltage, and right bundle branch block (Fig. 2).

An echocardiography was requested for structural evaluation, presenting: pericardial effusion predominantly related to the inferolateral heart wall, anechoic and cystic image, extracardiac and subcutaneous, of the thorax that communicates with pericardial effusion observed with color Doppler (Fig. 3). A dilated inferior vena cava (26 mm) was also observed with respiratory oscillation below 50% compatible with pericardial effusion that generates hemodynamic repercussion.

After evaluation of all data collected from the patient, a surgical procedure was performed, being described as anterolateral left incision (in previous scars and cystic mass) with

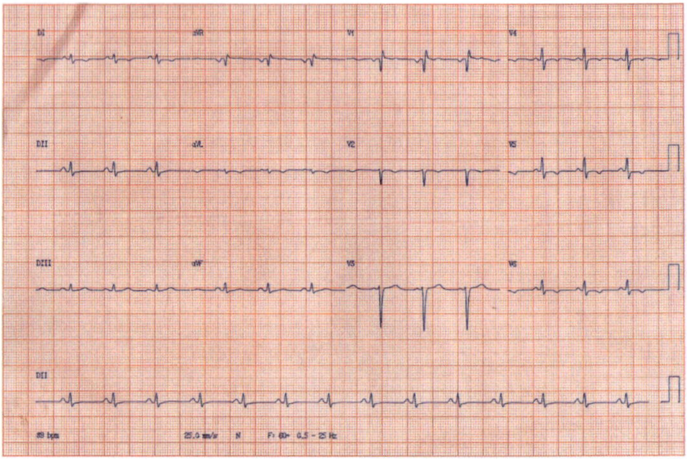

FIGURE 2 Electrocardiogram: sinus rhythm e right bundle branch block

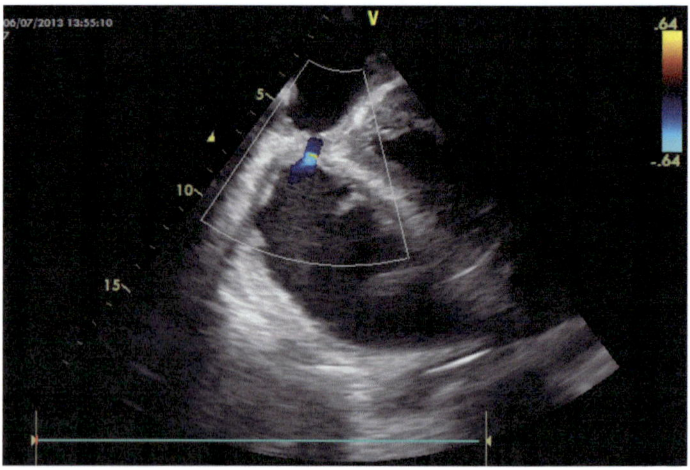

FIGURE 3 Anechoic and cystic image (extracardiac and subcutaneous cystic mass of the thorax) that communicates with pericardial effusion being observed on Doppler echocardiography

drainage of serohematic secretion (Fig. 4). In the intraoperative it was possible to observe a "herniation" of the pericardial effusion into the subcutaneous tissue, forming a cyst with pericardial fluid, caused by the partial absence of the pericardium (previous partial pericardiectomy). At the conclusion of the procedure, partial fluid drainage was performed due to extensive fibrosis and tissue adhesion to avoid access to the posterior pericardium.

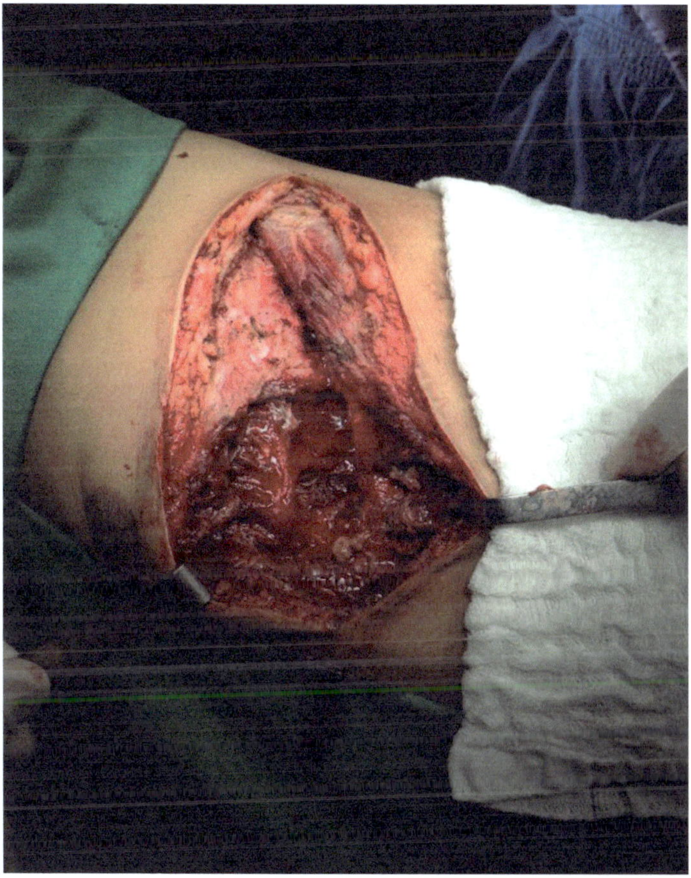

FIGURE 4 Incision anterolateral left

In the postoperative period, the patient regained consciousness, was oriented, active, eupneic, pale and hydrated. Patient was maintained in the hospital bed to use the mediastinal drainage bag in which 400 mL was drained within the first 24 h. Physical examination with mild pericardial friction and subcutaneous emphysema.

Computed tomography of the chest was performed to evaluate the postoperative evolution of the patient, being evidenced: emphysema at the site of drainage of the left hemithorax associated with abscess in the left ventricular projection with less extension, pericardial effusion, measuring 12.2 × 9.2 cm, atelectasis of the lower lobe of the left lung, posterior pleural thickening and small bilateral left pleural effusion.

The patient was subsequently maintained in an infirmary bed with oral diet, symptomatic medications for fever and pain, pyrazinamide and isoniazid once daily.

Questions

1. What are the main causes of acute pericarditis, and how does the clinical evolution of the disease occur?

Although many causes are possible, the most common is viral infection and idiopathic causes. The clinical syndrome is often relatively short (days to weeks) in duration and uncomplicated, but it is prudent to be aware of the progression to tamponade.

2. What are the possible differential diagnoses?

The differential diagnoses for pericarditis are pulmonary embolism, right ventricular infarction, chronic obstructive pulmonary disease, and restrictive cardiomyopathy.

3. What are the pathophysiological mechanisms involved in the pathogenesis of pericarditis?

When an inflammation or injury occurs, the pericardium reacts forming an exudate (pericardial effusion) in variable volume. If the liquid quickly accumulates or its volume is large, the ventricles may be compressed. In practice, 1–2 L slowly accumulated in pericardial sac is well tolerated. During the healing process, the pericardium gets thick and sometimes calcifies, and then the constriction may arise. With the constriction, venous pressure rises, including an inspiratory increase (Kussmaul sign). The pericardial thickening process may extend to the myocardium, causing sometimes a reduction in myocardial contractility, although the main problem of constrictive pericarditis is the hipodiastolia (restriction of ventricular filling). With restriction of ventricular filling, right and left ventricular diastolic pressure increases, leading to large-sized atrial pressures. The acceleration of venous return from the vena cava to the right atrium, which normally occurs in inspiration, will be prevented in constrictive pericarditis. Thus the average venous pressure will not decrease in inspiration and occasionally will increase (Kussmaul sign).

4. What are the main diagnostic methods for the case?

Echocardiography is the most used imaging technique. It is sensitive, specific, simple, and noninvasive, may be performed at the bedside, and can identify cardiac tamponade. The presence of pericardial fluid is recorded as a relatively echo-free space between the posterior pericardium and left ventricular epicardium in patients with small effusions and as a space between the anterior right ventricle and the parietal pericardium just beneath the anterior chest wall in patients with large effusions. The heart may swing freely within the pericardial sac. When severe, the extent of this motion alternates and may be associated with electrical alternans. Echocardiography allows localization and identification of the quantity of pericardial fluid. The diagnosis of pericardial fluid or thickening may be confirmed by computed tomography (CT) or magnetic resonance imaging (MRI). These techniques may be superior to echocardiography in detecting loculated pericardial effusions, pericardial thickening, and the identification of pericardial masses. Electrocardiographic changes are common. During the early days, diffuse ST-segment elevations occur (peripheral and precordial derivations) in the absence of reciprocal ST-segment depressions.

PR-segment depression is also common and reflects the atrial involvement. After several days, ST segments normalize and T waves reverse. In a large pericardial effusion, tachycardia, loss of R-wave voltage, and electrical switching may be seen. Blood tests reflect an inflammatory state, with blood sedimentation speed, reactive C-protein levels, and generally high leukocyte count.

5. What is the best indication of treatment?

In the absence of significant pericardial effusion, the treatment is directed primarily to relieve the patient's symptoms. Nonsteroidal anti-inflammatory drugs are used or glucocorticoids when resistance occurs. When the pericardial effusion is clinically suggested, treatment must be started immediately. If echocardiography shows at least 1 cm of liquid in front of the medium part of the right ventricle free wall, it can usually perform a percutaneous pericardiocentesis safely. The maximum of liquid must be removed with the monitoring of filling pressures. The liquid must be submitted for evaluation. The hemodynamically significant effusions of less than 1 cm must be surgically approached through a pleuro-pericardial window.

6. What are the main clinical manifestations of pericarditis?

Acute pericarditis usually manifests with continues tightness chest pain that increases with deep inspiration. The relief occurs when the patient assumes a genupectoral position (a prone posture resting on the knees and upper part of the chest). The pain results from the friction between the pericardial leaflets and improves when there is accumulation of fluid (pericardial effusion), and these leaflets stay away. The pain may be preceded by a low-grade fever, and the symptoms are sudden and severe since the beginning.

7. How to make the evaluation in case of chronicity of pericarditis?

The assessment should exclude the possibility of tuberculosis by performing a skin test, chest radiography, and gastric aspirate analysis. Pericardial biopsy is most commonly used for the diagnosis of tuberculosis pericarditis than microscope slide or culture of pericardial fluid. Aggressive drug treatment is indicated.

8. What are the different etiologies of pericarditis?

I. Infectious pericarditis

   A. Viral (coxsackievirus A and B, adenovirus, hepatitis, HIV, etc.)
   B. Pyogenic (pneumococcus, *Streptococcus*, *Staphylococcus*, *Neisseria*, etc.)
   C. Tuberculous
   D. Fungal (histoplasmosis, coccidioidomycosis, *Candida*, blastomycosis)
   E. Other infections (syphilitic, protozoal, parasitic)

II. Noninfectious pericarditis

   A. Acute myocardial infarction
   B. Uremia
   C. Neoplasia
   D. Myxedema
   E. Cholesterol
   F. Chylopericardium
   G. Trauma
   H. Aortic dissection (with leakage into pericardial sac)
   I. Postirradiation
   J. Familial Mediterranean fever
   K. Familial pericarditis
   L. Acute idiopathic
   M. Whipple's disease
   N. Sarcoidosis

III. Pericarditis presumably related to hypersensitivity or autoimmunity

   A. Rheumatic fever

B. Collagen vascular disease (systemic lupus erythematosus, rheumatoid arthritis, ankylosing spondylitis, scleroderma, acute rheumatic fever, granulomatosis with polyangiitis [Wegener's])
C. Drug-induced (e.g., procainamide, hydralazine, phenytoin, isoniazid, minoxidil, anticoagulants, methysergide)
D. Postcardiac injury

Review About the Addressed Disease or Treatment

The involvement of the pericardium by *Mycobacterium tuberculosis* is rare and observed in only 1–4% of cases of pericarditis and less than 1% of people with tuberculosis. It occurs most frequently in developing countries.

The tuberculous pericarditis occurs secondary to hematogenous spread during the course of endogenous reactivation of pulmonary focus or direct extension disease in the lung, pleura, lymph nodes, and tracheobronchial to the pericardial cavity, with most cases arising from injury by contiguity from tuberculosis of the mediastinal lymph nodes.

The clinical presentation of patients with tuberculous pericarditis is variable and unspecific, which makes diagnosis difficult, attending with cough, early dyspnea, chest pain, night sweats, orthopnea, weight loss, and lower extremities edema. The most frequent signs are cardiomegaly, pericardial friction, and tachycardia. In cases of constrictive pericarditis, arise jugular venous distension and paradoxical pulse.

Among the diagnostic methods, chest X-ray shows increased cardiac area in the early stages, which can take the typical image of "Water Jar." The long-term calcification arises as a result of the healing process. The chest CT allows delimiting the extent of involvement of pericardium and the mediastinal lymph node enlargement. The echocardiogram is the most effective test for diagnosis of the disease. It allows to evaluate the volume of liquid and early detection of cardiac tamponade. Proof of diagnosis is performed by demonstration of tubercle bacilli in pericardial material, through pericardial culture or pericardial fluid biopsy.

Bibliography

1. Braunwald F, Kasper H, Longo J. Harrison Medicina Interna. Rio de Janeiro: Mcgraw-Hill; 2008.
2. Braunwald E. Heart disease – a textbook of cardiovascular disease. 9th ed. Saunders Company: Philadelphia; 2012.
3. Ausiello D, Goldman L. Cecil; Tratado de Medicina Interna. 23rd ed. Rio de Janeiro: Elsevier; 2009.

Hodgkin's Disease and Pericardial Effusion

Bárbara Liss de Sousa Freire, Emanuel Sampaio Araújo, Rodrigo Mont'Alverne Guimarães, Joaquim David Carneiro Neto, and José Antônio de Lima Neto

Clinical Presentation

A 22-year-old man, white, single, student, born and raised in the Northern (CE) region, was referred to a tertiary care hospital presenting dyspnea complaints, chest pain on pressure, dysphagia, sporadic palpitations, and dry cough with fever episodes not measured. All symptoms started gradually within 2 weeks. The patient reported severe pain radiating to the back, correlated to dyspnea with minimal exertion. He referred improvement of symptoms in the genupectoral position. The admission electrocardiogram showed low-voltage QRS complex (Fig. 1).

Previous diagnosis: type 2 diabetes mellitus and stage IIIB Hodgkin's lymphoma (presenting night sweats, fever, and significant weight loss for the past three and a half years; underwent 4 cycles of ABVD chemotherapy regimen: Adriamycin + Bleomycin + Vinblastine + Dacarbazine). Patient denies hypertension and familiar cardiovascular risk factors. The patient was hospitalized previously for reasons of immunosuppression, anemia, cardiac tamponade, and nosocomial pneumonia treated with antibiotics (14 days on cefepime and ciprofloxacin).

B. L. de Sousa Freire (✉) · E. S. Araújo
R. Mont' Alverne Guimarães · J. D. C. Neto · J. A. de Lima Neto
Federal University of Ceará (UFC), Sobral, CE, Brazil

R. M. S. Almeida, F. B. Jatene (eds.), *Cardiovascular Surgery*,
https://doi.org/10.1007/978-3-319-57084-6_31

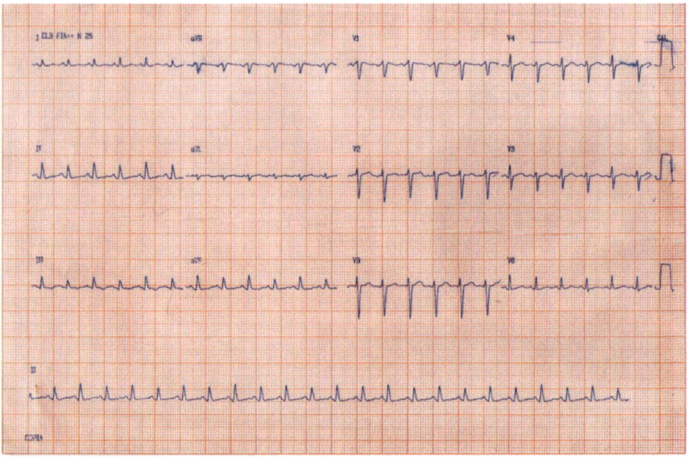

FIGURE 1 Electrocardiogram: sinus tachycardia, alterations of ventricular repolarization, and T wave flattened

Physical exam:

- General: poor general state, hypotrophic, anicteric, acyanotic, feverish, dyspneic, normal skin color, vigil and awake
- Vital signs: BP = 100/60 mmHg, HR = 74 bpm, RR = 19 bpm, axillary temperature = 38.1 °C
- Head and neck: no notable changes in the ears, eyes, nose, and oral cavity. Presence of tangible fixed and painless lymph nodes in the neck chains
- Neurologic: absence of focal signs
- Chest:

  (a) Cardiac auscultation: B1/B2 regular heart rhythm, muffled heart sounds, without murmurs
  (b) Respiratory auscultation: vesicular murmur universally present, with bibasal pulmonary crackles
  (c) Examination of peripheral vessels: increased jugular venous pulse and hypotension associated with paradoxical pulse

- Abdomen: Observation - no scars or striae; Auscultation - normal bowel sounds, no bruits; Palpation - no tenderness, masses or guarding
- Extremities: perfused ends with palpable peripheral pulses and no edema or cyanosis

Diagnosis, Assessment, and Treatment

Additional tests:

Laboratory tests

- Hemogram: hematocrit, 26% (36–50%); hemoglobin, 7.8 g/dL (12–17)
- Leukogram: 14,500 leukocytes/mm^3 (5–11 × 10^3)
- Glucose: 236 mg/dl (70–125)
- LDH = 196 U/L (240–480); total protein, 6 g/dL (6.1–7.9); albumin, 3 g/dL (3.5–4.8); globulin, 3 g/dL (1.2–2.2); A/G ratio = 1

Image exams

- Chest radiograph: right perihilar thickening, linear atelectasis of the lower third of the right lung, convex diaphragm and free costophrenic sinus, and enlarged cardiac silhouette – mainly the left ventricular arch, elongated aorta (Fig. 2). Transthoracic echocardiogram: significant pericardial effusion with diastolic restriction and LVEF = 62% (Fig. 3).
- Chest CT, mediastinal region: lymphadenomegaly in prevascular and pre-tracheal chains. Mediastinal vessels permeable and with normal dimensions. There is an extensive pericardial effusion. Pleuropulmonary region: atelectasis of the lower lobe of the right lung, moderate right pleural effusion, and small left pleural effusion. Fibrotic aspect of veiling in the medial segment of the middle lobe of the right lung (Fig. 4).

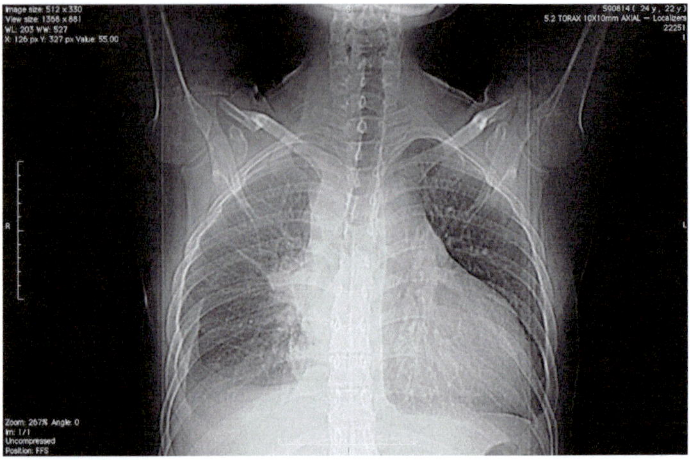

FIGURE 2 Chest radiograph showing elevation of cardiothoracic ratio

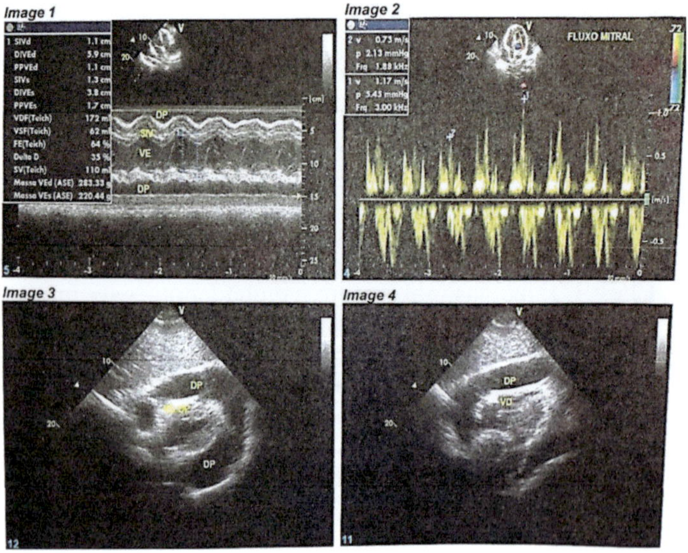

FIGURE 3 Doppler echocardiography showing pericardial effusion (DP) important

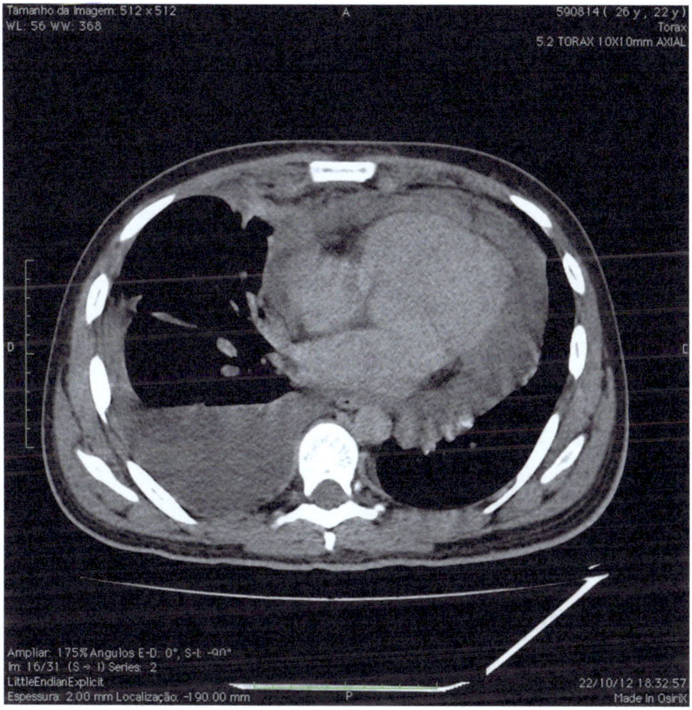

FIGURE 4 Chest tomography showing pericardial effusion and pleural effusion in the right hemithorax

Questions

1. What is the most likely diagnosis?

The patient in question has symptoms of pericardial effusion. Its effusion can be associated with various pathologics such as infectious, inflammatory, and neoplastic processes.

2. Is it possible to find a correlation between the lymphoma and the pathology in question?

In this particular situation, the etiology is neoplastic, being Hodgkin's lymphoma the underlying disease. It affects primarily young people, aged between 20 and 30 years old, and males. However, sometimes it has an aggressive and refractory profile, manifesting severe symptoms, including pericardial effusion, possibly leading to cardiac tamponade.

3. What evidence on the clinical history/symptoms give us subsidies to strengthen the main diagnostic hypothesis?

Among the clinical history data that lead us to suspect of pericardial effusion, we can mention that genupectoral position relieved dyspnea and chest pain on pressure, dysphagia, and dry cough. On physical examination, mainly in larger pericardial effusions, muffled heart sounds, elevated jugular venous pulse, and arterial hypotension are common, featuring the Beck's triad. Kussmaul sign or paradoxical pulse (with reduction of systolic blood pressure during inspiration, higher than 10 mmHg) can also be present.

4. Knowing that when analyzing a clinical case, we should try to fit it into a single diagnosis, how do we explain the symptoms of dysphagia, dry cough, and dyspnea?

These symptoms are characteristic of the compression syndrome of structures such as bronchi, esophagus and pulmonary parenchyma. In addition to these symptoms, we can see in some other cases hiccup and hoarseness resulting from compression of the phrenic nerve and laryngeal recurrent. The weight of the pericardial fluid on the abdomen can take the feeling of nausea and abdominal discomfort.

5. In case of chest pain, what factors contribute to distinguish ischemic from pericardial syndrome? Are ECG changes important to identify them?

The causes of chest pain with similar symptoms lead us to suspect cardiac ischemia or pericardial effusion. To avoid misunderstanding regarding these etiologies, we can use the electrocardiogram, which in case of pericardial effusion, QRS complex presents with low voltage (<15 mm in frontal derivations) and T wave flattened. While in acute myocardial infarction, we should seek changes indicative of injury and myocardial necrosis such as ST-segment elevation, pathological Q-wave onset, and T-wave inversion.

6. Are the imaging tests needed for diagnosis? If so which one(s)?

Currently diagnosis is guided by imaging tests such as cardiac CT and MRI. Usually it is not needed, but when in a bad echo window or dissociation between clinical and echo findings, these methods are used to detail pericardial effusion and suggest specific etiologies. Measuring the effusion is also more accurate with these two tests. Pericardial effusion with more than 3 weeks of evolution, which does not respond to NSAIDs, colchicine or corticosteroids, is established as an indication for pericardiocentesis. The diagnostic pericardiocentesis should always be made guided by echocardiography to avoid possible complications. The conduit applied to our patient was the pleuropericardial window, aimed to provide symptom and heart pumping relief.

When in a chest X-ray, the presence of 250 ml or more of fluid in the pericardial cavity is enough to increase the cardiac silhouette. A clue to differentiate pericardial effusion from dilated cardiomyopathy is the globular cardiac silhouette (Enlarged globular shaped heart).

Can be expected to the echocardiography, moderate to severe diastolic restriction and also sometimes significant LVEF reduction.

7. What are the main differential diagnoses?

- Constrictive pericarditis
- Dilated cardiomyopathy
- Myocardial infarction
- Mediastinal metastasis
- Viral infections (*Cytomegalovirus*, Coxsackievirus, Echovirus, HIV)
- Pericardial tuberculosis
- Uremia by severe renal impairment
- Pericardial injury surgery
- Autoimmune diseases: lupus erythematosus and rheumatoid arthritis
- Hypothyroidism

8. What is the most appropriate conduct in frames with more than 3 weeks of evolution unresponsive to drug therapy?

The indications of pericardiocentesis are effusions with more than 3 weeks of evolution and no response to therapy with NSAIDs, corticoids, or colchicine.

Diagnosis should be made always guided by echocardiogram, in order to avoid possible complications. The conduct applied to the following patient was the pleuropericardial window with the goal of providing relief of symptomatology and heart function.

Surgical procedure should be considered in cases with significant hemodynamic repercussions.

Bibliography

1. Braunwald E. Braunwald's heart disease – a textbook of cardiovascular medicine. Philadelphia: Elsevier; 2011.
2. Lopes AC. Tratado de Clínica Médica. São Paulo: Roca; 2009.
3. Longo DL. Medicina interna de Harrison. Porto Alegre: AMGH; 2013.
4. Spodick DH. Acute cardiac tamponade. N Engl J Med. 2003;349:684–90.

Pericardiocentesis: A Lifesaving Procedure

Gabriel Lorente Mitsumoto, Henry Eiji Toma, Daniel Bartholo de Hyppolito, and Valquiria Pelisser Campagnucci

Clinical Presentation

WSF, 61-year-old male, retired and born in São Paulo. Patient was admitted in the emergency department, referring tachypnea and shortness of breath which started 15 days ago, associated with lower limb edema and worsening of his respiratory symptoms. He referred to be diagnosed with adenocarcinoma of the right lung a couple of weeks ago.

The patient is a former smoker, 30 pack-year, and quit smoking 1 month ago.

The physical examination at admission was as follows. Patient was awake and alert; afebrile, with no signs of cyanosis; dehydrated; and pale.

Vitals:

- Heart rate: 120 bpm
- Respiratory rate: 22 bpm
- Blood pressure: 100/60 mmHg
- O_2 saturation: 91%

G. L. Mitsumoto (✉) · H. E. Toma · D. B. de Hyppolito
V. P. Campagnucci
Santa Casa de São Paulo School of Medical Sciences (FCMSCSP), São Paulo, SP, Brazil

R. M. S. Almeida, F. B. Jatene (eds.), *Cardiovascular Surgery*,
https://doi.org/10.1007/978-3-319-57084-6_32

Cardiovascular: Heart sounds with S1 and S2 with normal intensity, tachycardia, regular rhythm, and no murmurs. There was no hepatojugular reflux.

Respiratory: Breath sounds were present and symmetrical but diminished in right lower hemithorax with rhonchi diffusely spread across all parenchyma.

Abdominal: Normal bowel sounds, soft, resonant to percussion, without pain or palpable masses.

Extremities: cold and with right arm and bilateral lower limbs edema. Palpable arterial pulses.

Diagnosis, Assessment, and Treatment

The first hypotheses were of acute respiratory failure due to pneumonia or congestive heart failure.

Initial measures: morphine, furosemide, hydrocortisone, oxygen mask, and assessment of general laboratory tests and cultures; an x-ray was also requested.

Laboratory exams at admission are listed in Table 1:

Table 1 Laboratory exams

Exams	Values
Hemoglobin	11.9 g/dL
Platelets	305,000 U/uL
Creatinine	1.4 mg/dL
Leukocyte	14.480 U/uL
Neutrophils	83%
Metamyelocytes	1%
Band cells	4%
Segmented	78%
Lymphocytes	10%
Monocytes	7%
Urea	62 mg/100 mL
K^+	4.6 mEq/L
Na^+	145 mEq/L

X-ray presented at admittance:

The x-ray (Fig. 1) showed a parenchymatous opacification close to right hilum and a large pleural effusion; also the cardiothoracic ratio is in its upper limit.

Due to his previous hospitalization and the findings in his chest x-ray, the possibility of a hospital-acquired pneumonia was considered, and the patient was started on piperacillin-tazobactam. Also, as a treatment of the right effusion, it was requested drainage of the pleural effusion. Moreover, due to the enlarged cardiac area and to exclude other diagnosis as well as to evaluate the heart, a transthoracic echocardiogram was requested.

The exam showed no indirect signs of pulmonary embolism but revealed the presence of pericardial effusion. He was

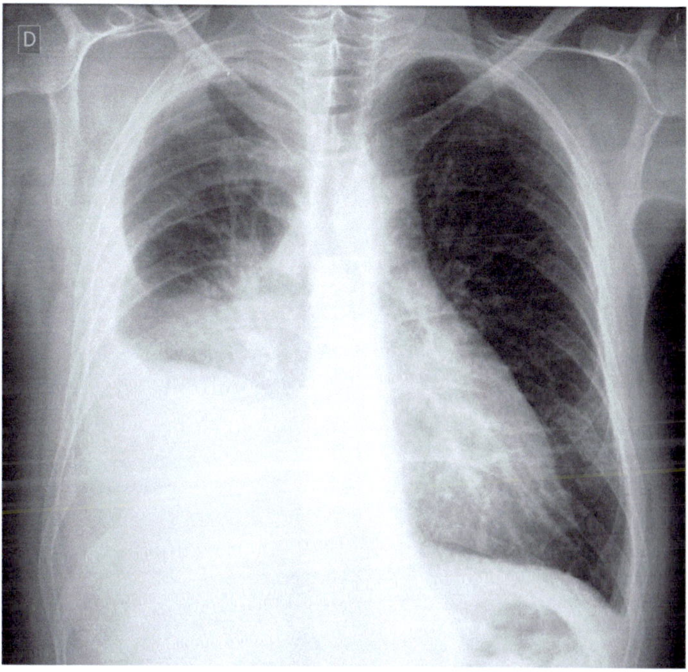

FIGURE 1 Chest x-ray at admission in the emergency department

then evaluated by the cardiac surgery service which determined the need of a pericardiocentesis. Before the procedure, another x-ray was requested (Fig. 2).

A pericardiocentesis (Marfan puncture) was performed using a double-lumen catheter, as described below.

1. Patient was positioned in horizontal dorsal decubitus with a headboard in 30-degree inclination, with continuous cardiac monitoring and an oxygen mask.
2. Asepsis and antisepsis followed by positioning of the surgical fields.
3. Identified puncture point lateral to xiphoid process, followed by local anesthesia with a 2% lidocaine solution.

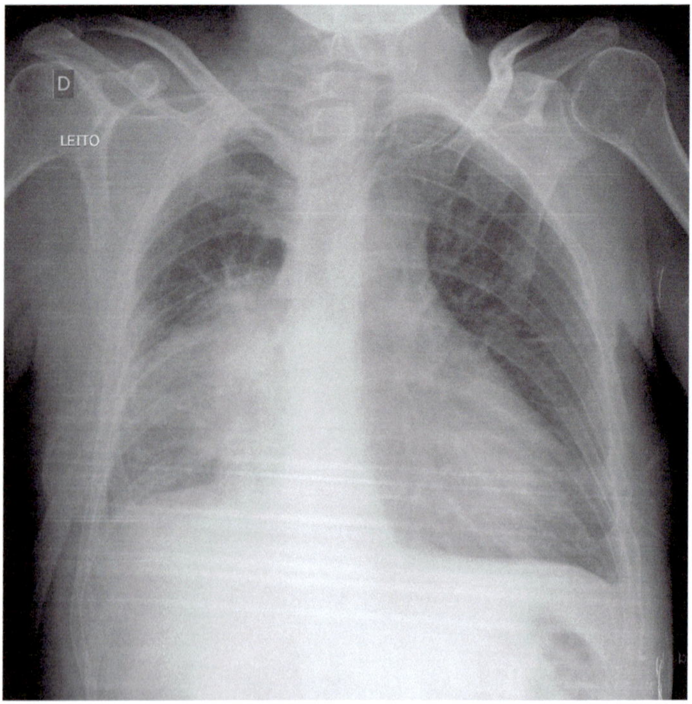

Figure 2 Chest x-ray just before pericardiocentesis

4. The pericardium puncture was performed using the modified Seldinger technique with a central venous catheter needle, and 250 ml of citrine liquid was aspirated.
5. A double-lumen catheter filled with saline solution was left for pericardial drainage, and a sample of pericardial liquid was sent to analysis.
6. Occlusion.

The patient remained hemodynamically stable for the next few days, and a follow-up x-ray assessed the position of the drain (Fig. 3).

Considering the recurrent pleural effusion which required several drainages, it was opted to perform a pleurodesis using sterile talcum.

The biochemical, cytological, and culture analysis of pericardial effusion are listed in Table 2:

Tazocin was suspended due to culture exam results being negative.

The final aspect is shown in the Fig. 4.

Due to the analysis results, the patient was transferred to oncology sector for proper neoplastic treatment, and the pericardial catheter was removed after 7 days.

Questions

1. What are the most frequent causes of pericarditis in developed and in developing countries, respectively?

Pericarditis has different causes in developed and in developing countries: viral/idiopathic and tuberculosis, respectively.

2. What are the components of Beck's triad?

Beck's triad components are jugular venous distention due to elevated systemic venous pressure, muffled heart sounds, and hypotension.

3. What are the main suggestive signs and symptoms of pericarditis?

The main suggestive signs and symptoms of pericarditis are pericardial friction rub, precordial pain, and fever.

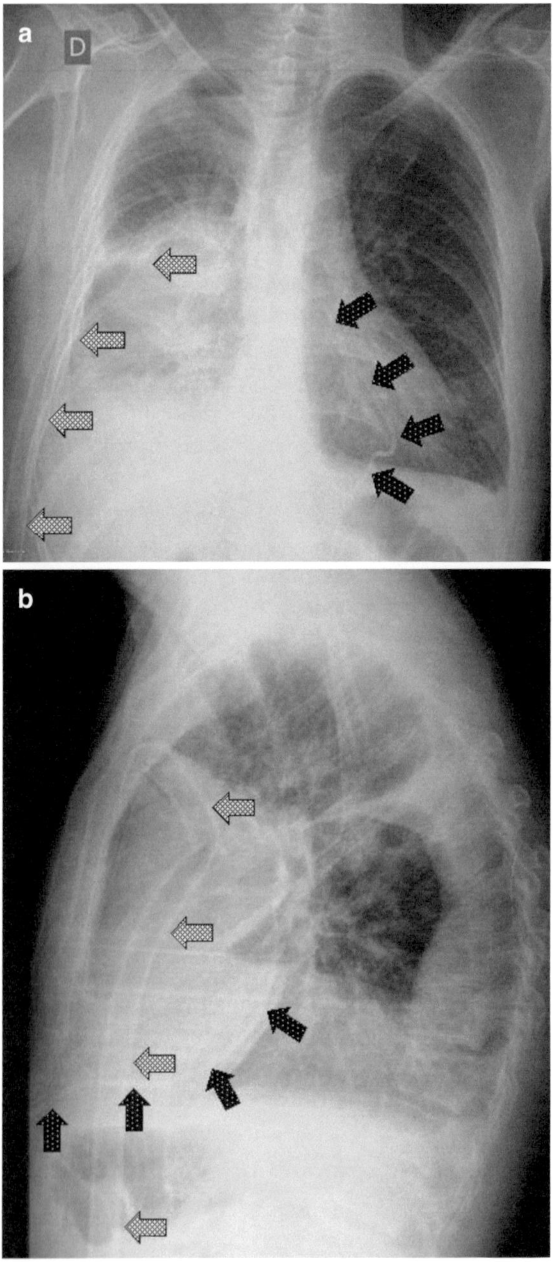
a
D
b

4. What are the signs of pericarditis in ECG?

ECG presents with diffuse ST segment elevation (Fig. 8).

5. What are the signs of cardiac tamponade in ECG?

The signs of cardiac tamponade in ECG are low QRS voltage (Fig. 5) and electrical alternance (Fig. 6).

6. What is the main indication for pericardiocentesis?

The main indication for pericardiocentesis is cardiac tamponade.

TABLE 2 Laboratory exams

Exams	**Values**
pH	7.7
Glucose	140 mg/dL
Total protein	2.7 g/dL
Albumin	1.5 g/dL
Volume	4 mL
Gross appearance	Sanguineous
Fibrin clot	Present
Nucleated cells	230 U/mm^3
Leucocytes	40%
Lymphocytes	56%
Neutrophils	44%
Eosinophils	0
Mesothelial	40%
Histiocytic	20%
Red blood cells	2900 U/mm^3
Neoplastic cell research	Negative
No growth of bacteria after 48 h of seeding	

FIGURE 3 (**a**, **b**) Chest x-ray after pericardiocentesis showing the double-lumen catheter (indicated by the ⬅ arrow) and the chest tube (indicated by the ⇦ arrow)

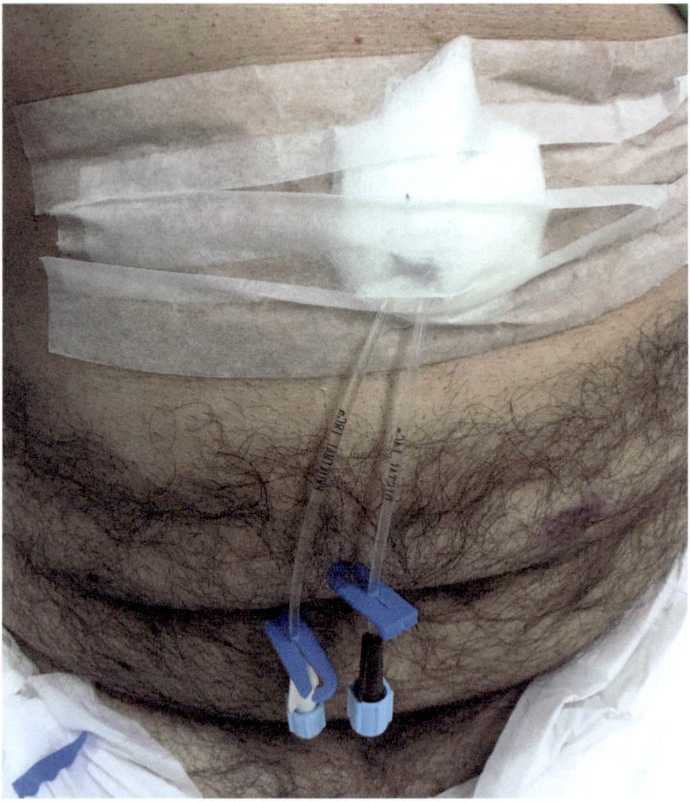

FIGURE 4 Double-lumen catheter appearance

7. What is the treatment for viral pericarditis?

Viral pericarditis treatment is the administration of nonsteroidal anti-inflammatory drugs and colchicine.

8. What is the treatment for non-viral pericarditis?

Non-viral pericarditis treatment is based on treating the underlying disease.

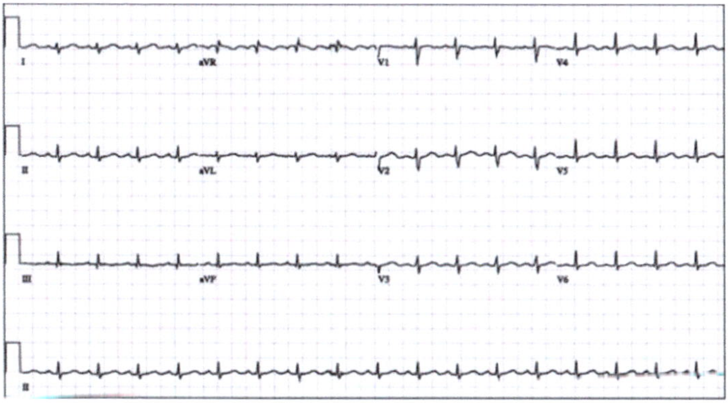

FIGURE 5 ECG showing low QRS voltage

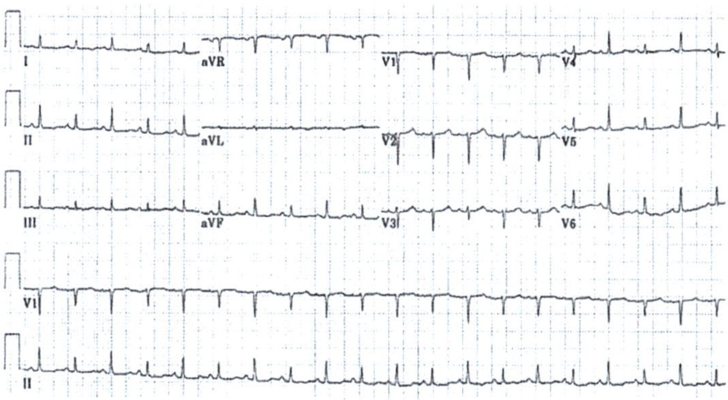

FIGURE 6 ECG showing electrical alternance

Review About the Addressed Disease or Treatment

The normal pericardial sac contains 10–50 ml of pericardial fluid as a plasma ultrafiltrate that acts as a lubricant between the pericardial layers. Any pathological process usually causes inflammation with the possibility of increased production of pericardial fluid, as pericarditis (exudate). An alternative mechanism of accumulation of pericardial fluid may be decreased reabsorption due to a general increase in systemic venous pressure as a result of congestive heart failure or pulmonary hypertension (transudate). Pericardial effusion may be classified according to its onset (acute or subacute vs. chronic when lasting >3 months), distribution (circumferential or loculated), hemodynamic impact (none, cardiac tamponade, effusive-constrictive), composition (exudate, transudate, blood, rarely air, or gas from bacterial infections), and, in particular, its size based on a simple semiquantitative echocardiographic assessment as mild (<10 mm), moderate (10–20 mm), or large (>20 mm).

A significant proportion of patients with pericardial effusion are asymptomatic, and pericardial effusion constitutes an incidental and unexpected finding on x-ray or echocardiogram performed for other reasons, as in this case.

The clinical presentation of pericardial effusion varies according to the speed of pericardial fluid accumulation. If pericardial fluid accumulates rapidly, such as after wounds or iatrogenic perforations, the evolution is dramatic, and even small amounts of blood may cause an increase in intrapericardial pressure within minutes and overt cardiac tamponade. On the other hand, a slow accumulation of pericardial fluid allows the collection of a large effusion in days to weeks before a significant increase in pericardial pressure causes symptoms and signs, that is, due to the restricted, but yet distensible, pericardial sac, in which large amounts of fluid can accumulate gradually without hemodynamic effects. The intrapericardial pressure then increases until it equals the right ventricular diastolic pressure and then the left ventricular diastolic pressure, which leads to impaired cardiac filling and decreased cardiac output.

The classic presentation of patients with pericardial tamponade includes Beck's triad of jugular venous distention due to elevated systemic venous pressure, muffled heart sounds, and hypotension. Most patients will have at least one of these signs. However, studies points Beck's triad symptoms to be found significant only in 54%, 28%, and 22% of the cases, respectively. Despite that, tachypnea is a common clinical finding in patients with cardiac tamponade, and dyspnea is the most frequently reported symptom on presentation, with a sensitivity of about 87–88% for cardiac tamponade.

Classic symptoms include shortness of breath on exertion progressing to orthopnea, chest pain, and/or fullness. Additional occasional symptoms due to local compression may include nausea (diaphragm), dysphagia (esophagus), hoarseness (recurrent laryngeal nerve), and hiccups (phrenic nerve). Non-specific symptoms include cough, weakness, fatigue, anorexia, and palpitations, reflecting the compressive effect of the pericardial fluid on contiguous anatomic structures or reduced blood pressure and secondary sinus tachycardia. Also, the signs of cardiac tamponade in ECG are low QRS voltage (Fig. 5) and electrical alternance (Fig. 6), illustrated in the figures below.

When pericardial effusion is detected, the first step is to assess its size, hemodynamic impact (specially the presence of cardiac tamponade), and possibility of associated diseases (either cardiovascular or systemic diseases). Therapy of pericardial effusion should include treatment of the etiology as often as possible; however, this patient's lung cancer treatment would not allow recovery as fast as it would be necessary to control or even reduce the effusion.

Pericardiocentesis is indicated for cardiac tamponade or for symptomatic moderate to large pericardial effusions not responsive to medical therapy, and for suspicion of unknown bacterial or neoplastic etiology (class Ic). Pericardiocentesis alone may be necessary for the resolution of large effusions, but recurrence is common, and pericardiectomy or less invasive options (i.e., pericardial window) should be considered whenever fluid re-accumulates and becomes loculated or biopsy material is required.

Considering that the patient has lung cancer and medical therapy was not successful, the algorithm (Fig. 7) below was followed (large arrows), and a pericardiocentesis was performed.

The prognosis of pericardial effusion is essentially related to the etiology. The size of the effusion correlates with the

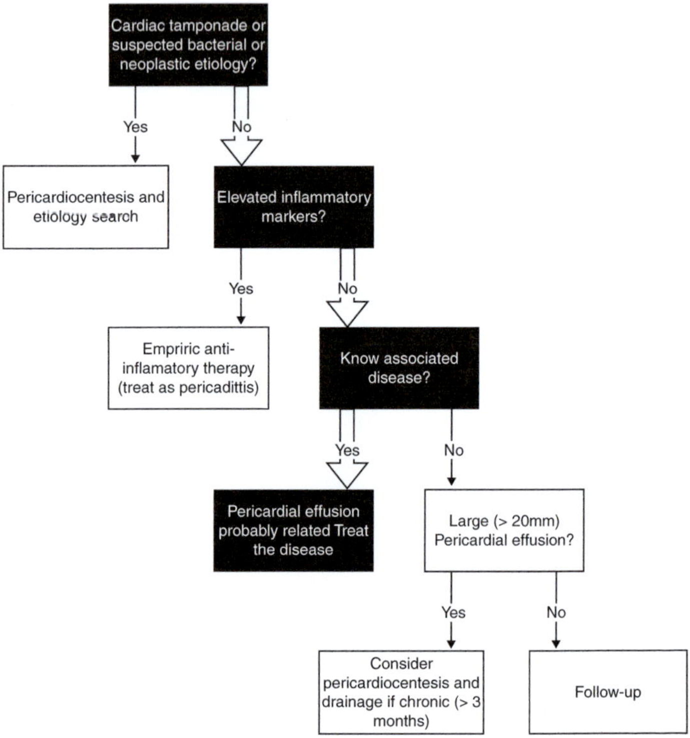

FIGURE 7 Simplified algorithm for pericardial effusion triage and management

prognosis, as moderate to large effusions are more common for specific etiologies such as bacterial and neoplastic conditions. In patients with pericardial tamponade, emergency pericardiocentesis to aspirate pericardial fluid can restore normal cardiac function and peripheral perfusion. It can be a lifesaving procedure.

The x-ray film after completing the procedure serves to assess not only drain position but also complications such as a pleural effusion or pneumothorax. Continuous monitoring of the patient for signs of hemodynamic instability and for physical findings which suggests fluid is still accumulating is mandatory. Definitive care may include placement of a soft catheter in the pericardial space or surgical placement of a pericardial window to allow for continuous drainage. In this case, a double-lumen catheter was the drainage choice.

Once again, one of the main causes of cardiac tamponade is pericarditis, which has different causes in developed and in developing countries: viral/idiopathic and tuberculosis, respectively. Pericarditis is divided in viral etiology and non-viral etiology, with different treatments. Viral pericarditis treatment is the administration of nonsteroidal anti-inflammatory drugs and colchicine and for non-viral pericarditis is the treatment of the underlying disease. Studies showed that colchicine diminishes viral proliferation and corticoids augment it. The main suggestive signs and symptoms of both types of pericarditis are pericardial friction rub, precordial pain, and fever, and ECG presents with diffuse ST segment elevation (Fig. 8).

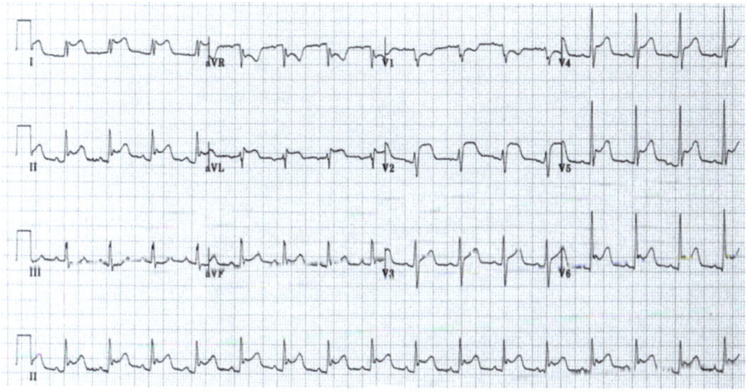

FIGURE 8 ECG showing diffuse ST segment elevation

Bibliography

1. Adler Y, Charron P, Imazio M, Badano L, Barón-Esquivias G, Bogaert J, Brucato A, Gueret P, Klingel K, Lionis C, Maisch B, Mayosi B, Pavie A, Ristić A, Sabaté Tenas M, Seferovic P, Swedberg K, Tomkowski W. 2015 ESC guidelines for the diagnosis and management of pericardial diseases. Eur Heart J. 2015;36(42):2921–64.
2. Fitch M, Nicks B, Pariyadath M, McGinnis H, Manthey D. Emergency pericardiocentesis. N Engl J Med. 2012;366(12):e17.
3. Jacob S, Sebastian J, Cherian P, Abraham A, John S. Pericardial effusion impending tamponade: a look beyond Beck's triad. Am J Emerg Med. 2009;27(2):216–9.
4. Kouchoukos N, Kirklin J. Kirklin/Barratt-Boyes cardiac surgery. Philadelphia: Elsevier/Saunders; 2013.

Part XI
Pulmonary Embolism

Chronic Thromboembolic Pulmonary Hypertension (CTEPH): A Surgically Curable Cause of Pulmonary Hypertension

Leandro Pedro Goloni Bertollo, Guilherme Henrique Ribeiro de Carvalho, Vanessa Lopes Vieira, Fabio Biscegli Jatene, and Orival de Freitas Filho

Clinical Presentation

A 45-year-old former smoker (10 years/1 pack/day) female patient presented a report of chest discomfort, tiredness, and progressive dyspnea on moderate efforts 4 years ago. She was assessed by a cardiologist at her hometown, who requested a transthoracic echocardiography, but the patient did not return. Two years later, she had worsened, presenting dyspnea even at rest and requiring home supplemental oxygen. She was then evaluated by a general practitioner, who requested a new echocardiography and a chest CT angiography.

After another year, she was evaluated by a local thoracic surgery team that suspected of a mediastinal malignant neoplasm or a fibrosing mediastinitis. The PET-CT performed

L. P. G. Bertollo (✉) · G. H. R. de Carvalho · V. L. Vieira
F. B. Jatene · O. de Freitas Filho
Faculty of Medicine of University of São Paulo (FMUSP), São Paulo, SP, Brazil

R. M. S. Almeida, F. B. Jatene (eds.), *Cardiovascular Surgery*,
https://doi.org/10.1007/978-3-319-57084-6_33

did not capture any thrombus. She underwent a cervical mediastinoscopy in which there was no sign of malignant cells or tissue fibrosis. A lung scintigraphy was performed and showed multiple areas of radiopharmaceutical concentration reduction, indicating high probability of chronic thromboembolic pulmonary hypertension (CTEPH). The patient was then referred to the CTEPH team at INCOR-HCFMUSP for investigation and evaluation of surgical treatment, in use of Clexane 120 mg/day and warfarin 2.5 mg/day. The physical examination at our institution showed O_2 Sat of 95% at rest and of 75% at effort without the 02 catheter. She also had P2 hyperphonesis at cardiac auscultation. All other aspects of the physical examination showed no alterations.

Diagnosis, Assessment, and Treatment

For the etiologic investigation, a transthoracic echocardiography was firstly requested as a screening exam for CTEPH, showing significantly increased right chambers, preserved left ventricular systolic function, and preserved myocardial thickness. Doppler findings were compatible with left ventricular relaxation alteration, right ventricular moderate hypokinesia, paradoxical movement of the interventricular septum, and moderate tricuspid valve regurgitation. Pulmonary artery systolic pressure (PASP) was 93 mmHg.

Another screening exam for CTEPH was then requested: the ventilation/perfusion lung scintigraphy. The perfusion study showed a heterogeneous pattern of radiopharmaceutical distribution, with hypoperfusion in right upper lobe projection, lateral segment of the right middle lobe, and segments of the right lower lobe; basal segments of the left lower lobe were hypoperfused as well. The inhalation study showed a radiopharmaceutical distribution pattern which was discordant of the perfusion pattern, with aeration preserved in both lungs.

Since there was a high probability of CTEPH, a chest CT and a pulmonary arteriography were requested to confirm the diagnosis and to access the operability of the thrombus.

The chest tomography showed chronic thromboembolic pulmonary signs, characterized by eccentric thrombus in the distal portion of the right pulmonary artery, extending to the corresponding lobar branches. There was complete obliteration of the right upper lobe artery and reduction in size of the origins of the arteries of the middle and lower lobes on this side. Complete obstruction of the left lower lobe artery and its segmental branches was also observed, with thinning of the lingular segment artery. Increased caliber of the pulmonary artery trunk (3.7 cm) and cardiomegaly at the expense of the increase of the right chambers were observed as well (Figs. 1 and 2).

The pulmonary arteriography demonstrated increased caliber of the pulmonary artery trunk, smooth walls, and patency of the main trunk of the right and left pulmonary arteries. Left pulmonary artery presented mild dilation of the main trunk and regular walls. Absence of opacification on the left lower lobe and on the right upper lobe was observed. Right pulmonary artery presented an increased diameter, habitual disposition, and slight parietal irregularities. It is observed return of the pulmonary veins with posterior aortic hallmarking. The pulmonary artery had a systolic blood pressure (BP) of 84 mmHg (reference ranges, 15–30 mmHg), a mean BP of 63 mmHg (10–20 mmHg), and a diastolic BP of 39 mmHg (8–15 mmHg). The right atrium presented a mean pressure of 19 mmHg (2–6 mmHg). These measurements were compatible with CTEPH (Fig. 3).

To support the etiologic investigation and as patients with CTEPH have hypercoagulability predisposition, thrombophilia was searched in the patient: Leiden factor V and prothrombin-negative mutant; antithrombin 3 (AT3), lupus anticoagulant, and anticardiolipin normal.

Finally, a right cardiac catheterization was made to access hemodynamic factors which were important for the evaluation of surgical indication. The results were right atrium = 9 mmHg (reference ranges, −1–7 mmHg); right ventricular systolic BP = 86 mmHg (15–30 mmHg); right ventricular systolic BP = 6 mmHg on the first moment and

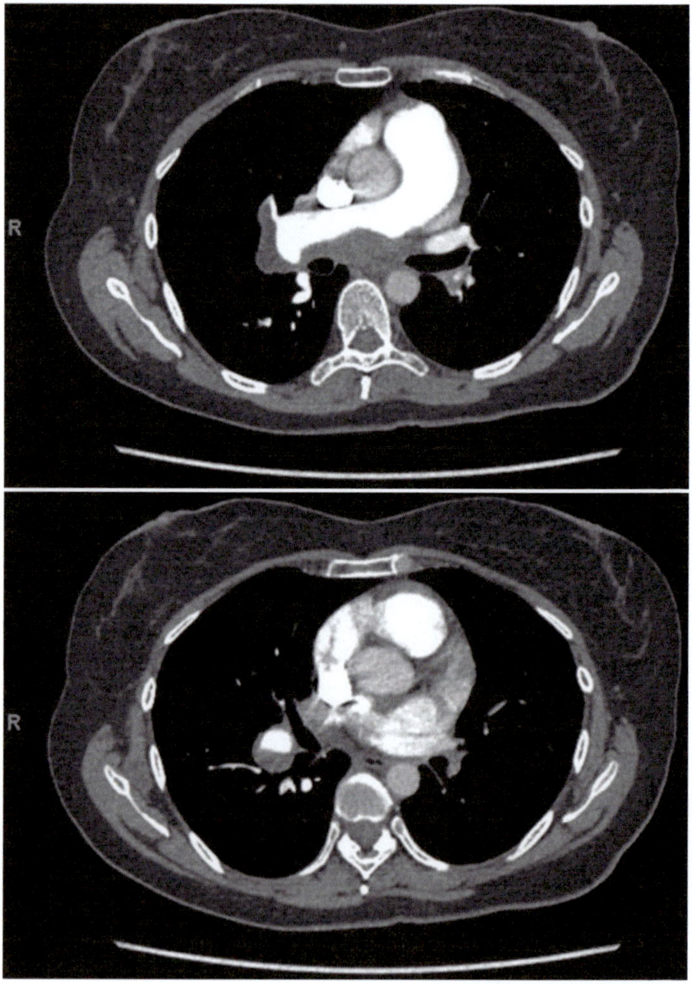

FIGURE 1 Above: computed tomography angiography (mediastinal window) showing proximal thrombus in the right pulmonary artery. Below: proximal thrombus in the lumen of the right interlobar artery

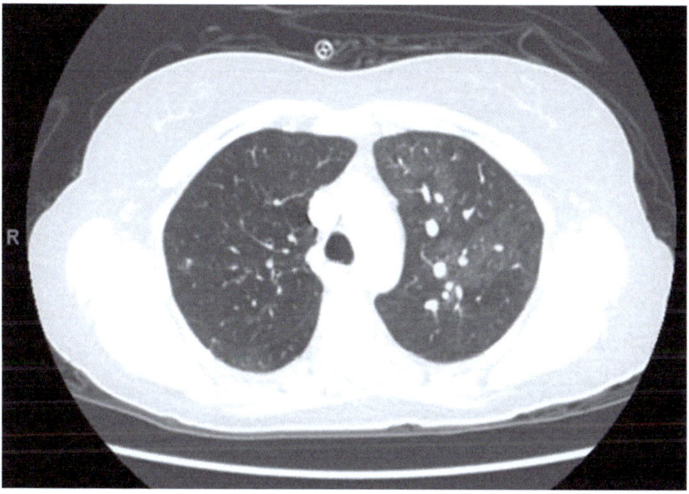

FIGURE 2 Computed tomography angiography (pulmonary window) showing mosaic perfusion pattern more evident in the left lung, with areas of hypo- and hyperperfusion

10 mmHg later (0–8 mmHg); pulmonary trunk systolic BP = 86 mmHg (15–30 mmHg); pulmonary trunk diastolic BP = 35 mmHg (8–15 mmHg); pulmonary trunk mean BP = 58 mmHg (10–20 mmHg); pulmonary capillary mean BP = 14 mmHg (8–12 mmHg), cardiac output = 3.5 L/min (Fick); and pulmonary vascular resistance (PVR) = 12.5 Wood units (0.25–1.6 Wood units).

Other standard preoperative exams were performed (such as hepatic and renal functions), without any abnormalities.

The patient was then indicated for pulmonary thromboendarterectomy, due to favorable hemodynamic parameters (especially the PVR) and operable location of the thrombus.

About 1 year later, she was referred to INCOR-FMUSP, and 4 years from the beginning of the symptoms, she

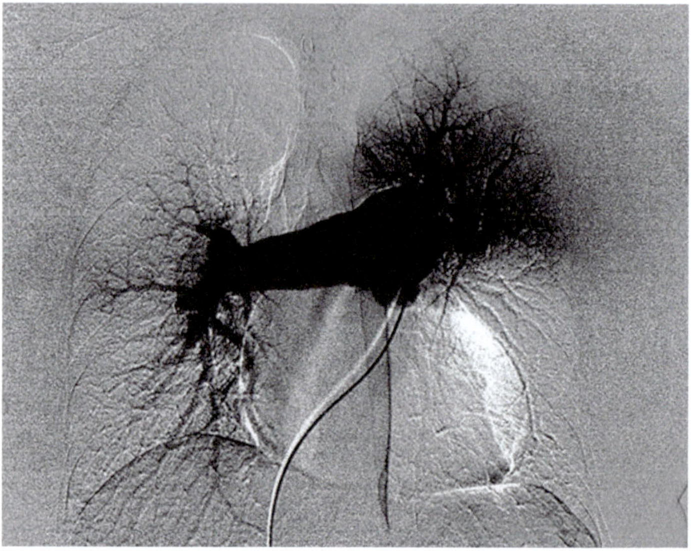

FIGURE 3 Pulmonary arteriography showing proximal obstruction in the right and left branches of the pulmonary artery. It also evidences that the only perfused area is the left superior lobe

underwent the pulmonary thromboendarterectomy, in June 2015. The surgery was performed by general anesthesia and longitudinal sternotomy with deep hypothermia (16 °C) and two periods of circulatory arrest (18 and 22 min). Thrombi type I was found on the right and left sides and operation was successful. The patient was extubated on the first postoperative day. Pulmonary artery systolic pressure decreased from 86 mmHg (preoperative) to 43 mmHg (immediate postoperative). In the first postoperative day it was 46 mmHg and 35 mmHg in the second postoperative day. The Swan-Ganz catheter was removed on the third postoperative day. The patient remained in ICU until the 7th postoperative day and was discharged on the 16th day after surgery.

One month postoperative echocardiography (July/2015) showed a slightly increased right ventricle and minimal tricuspid valve insufficiency (Fig. 4).

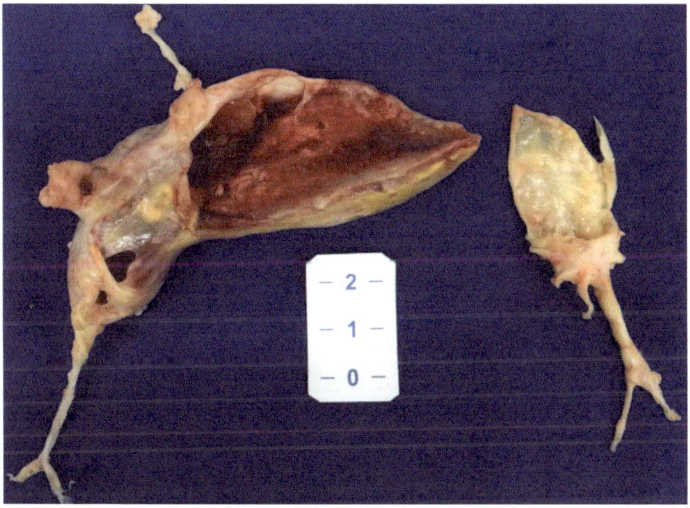

FIGURE 4 Surgical specimen: thrombus on the right and left sides. The right lung thrombus occluded the right pulmonary artery

Questions

1. What is the definition of CTEPH?

Chronic thromboembolism pulmonary hypertension (CTEPH) is a chronic obstruction of the pulmonary arteries. It is defined as pulmonary hypertension observed after a minimum period of 3 months after at least one episode of pulmonary embolism, excluding other causes of pulmonary hypertension [1]. Inadequate anticoagulation, massive thrombus, residual thrombus, and recurrent embolic event contribute to the development of CTEPH. Prospective epidemiological data show an incidence of symptomatic CTEPH of 1% in the sixth month, 3.1% in the first year, and 3.8% at the end of the second year after acute episode pulmonary thromboembolism [2].

2. How is the clinical presentation of CTEPH?

The most common symptoms are chest pain, dyspnea, syncope, angina, and hemoptysis. However, few patients receive the diagnosis in long-term follow-up after the pulmonary embolism, due to nonspecific symptoms and variable presentation. In addition, there may be absence of previous symptoms of acute pulmonary thromboembolism in 63% of patients with CTEPH [2].

3. Which is the differential diagnosis?

Other causes of obstruction of the pulmonary artery should be considered: angiosarcoma of the pulmonary artery, pulmonary arteritis, mediastinal fibrosis, hydatid cyst embolism, and tumor embolism – from both benign tumors (uterine leiomyoma) and malignant (primary renal cancer, thyroid, testicular, or uterine) [3].

4. Which exams help the diagnosis?

If you suspect the diagnosis, investigation should be guided with transthoracic echocardiography, chest CT angiography, and ventilation-perfusion pulmonary scintigraphy. The definitive diagnosis as well as the vascular staging will be set with pulmonary arteriography.

5. Which is the importance of the pulmonary scintigraphy?

The ventilation-perfusion (V/Q) pulmonary scintigraphy is an important initial exam for screening in patients with suspected CTEPH. It has a high sensitivity to detect embolic disease as a potentially curable cause of pulmonary hypertension, showing a higher sensitivity than multidetector CT pulmonary angiography [4]. The transthoracic echocardiography is also an important screening exam, being recently suggested as the initial exam to investigate CTEPH, since it is more easily available and provides parameters that can suggest the diagnosis, such as the estimated right ventricular systolic pressure (RVSP), dilation of the right ventricle with impaired contractility, impingement on the left ventricle, D-shaped left ventricle, and the tricuspid annular plane systolic excursion (TAPSE) [5].

6. Is the surgery a good option for treatment?

Medical therapy with anticoagulant drugs, thrombolytic agents, or vasodilator drugs has not been shown to affect the prognosis. Surgical therapy is curative and with few exceptions is regarded as permanent [6].

7. Which are the indications for the surgery?

The main indications for the thromboendarterectomy are New York Heart Association functional class III and IV, pulmonary arterial resistance >300 dynes.s.cm-5 (or 3.75 W), predominance of central obstructive lesions (large arterial branches or lobar), and prediction of reduction in pulmonary artery pressure (PAP) of at least 50% after thromboendarterectomy [3]. The largest risk factor for operation remains the degree of operability as assessed by PVR. A high PVR without gross changes on angiogram signifies secondary vasculopathy – an inoperable change and a degree of postoperative pulmonary hypertension that will likely hinder recovery. The mortality rate was 30.6% when the residual PVR was higher than 500 dynes.s.cm(−5) but only 0.9% when it was below this level [6]. More recently, it has been shown that the preoperative PA (pulmonary artery diameter)/BSA (body surface area) ratio was an independent predictor for hemodynamic outcome after thromboendarterectomy [7].

8. Which are the preoperative exams?

The pre-op routine includes the evaluation of vasculopathies (previous stroke, vascular malformations, arteriopathies), hepatic function (serum hepatic enzymes, bilirubin, and coagulation factors), renal function (serum creatinine, urea, and electrolytes), and catheterization – especially to establish the pulmonary vascular resistance (PVR), an important parameter to analyze the surgery indication.

9. Which are the steps of the surgery?

The surgical procedure involves median sternotomy with extracorporeal circulation and periods of circulatory arrest with hypothermia. Sternotomy provides access to the central vessels of both lungs, since there is need for bilateral desobstruction in most cases. It is important to emphasize the need to perform a thromboendarterectomy and not an embolectomy. The plane of dissection should be performed in the middle layer of the arteries, which is partially withdrawn, together with the inner layer and the organized thrombus [8].

10. Which are the possible complications of the surgery?

As a result of the thromboendarterectomy procedure, the patient may present complications in 46% of the cases. They are related to some technical peculiarities such as circulatory arrest, deep hypothermia, pulmonary reperfusion, and post-op ventricular dysfunction. Possible complications include pulmonary reperfusion syndrome (33.3%), one of the major causes of death (66.7%), coagulopathies (21.3%), and renal (16.3%) and neural (16%) dysfunctions [9].

Review About the Addressed Disease or Treatment

Although CTEPH is a rare complication of acute pulmonary embolism, its delay in diagnosis and lack of knowledge in the medical community leading to patients with chronic and worsening dyspnea make it important to talk about it. The etiology behind CTEPH is also largely unknown and full of speculations. Some mechanisms have been proposed, as increased hypercoagulability, reduced fibrinolytic capacity, and genetic polymorphisms in fibrin that make it resistant to fibrinolysis, but none of these hypotheses explain the development of CTEPH in the majority of the patients, being consistent with only a minor percentage of the cases [5]. Recently, researchers have explored alternative causes of CTEPH including impaired angiogenesis, inflammation, and possible similarities on a cellular level to cancerous transformation [5].

Regarding the diagnosis, it is very important to consider the hypothesis of CTEPH in patients with pulmonary hypertension (PH) or chronic worsening dyspnea, as CTEPH is the only cause of PH that is potentially curable. The differential diagnoses are conditions such as angiosarcoma of the pulmonary artery, pulmonary arteritis, mediastinal fibrosis, hydatid cyst embolism, and tumor embolism. For screening of CTEPH, the recommended exam remains the pulmonary scintigraphy (ventilation/perfusion (V/Q) scan). The echocardiogram has been gaining a role as a screening exam more recently [5]. The gold standard exam to confirm the diagnosis is pulmonary angiography, but high-quality computed tomography angiography and magnetic resonance angiography are also increasing in use for this purpose at experienced centers [5].

The treatment of choice for CTEPH is the pulmonary thromboendarterectomy (PTE). Long-term survival is excellent with 5-year survival rates of 88–90% [5], and an in-hospital mortality of less than 5% was reported in a recent review [5]. However, not all patients can be submitted to the procedure. Evaluating the extent and location of disease determines the operability (being diffuse and distal obstructions less resectable), as well as the pre-op hemodynamic parameters (mainly the PVR). PTE shall not be confounded with embolectomy, a considerably more simple procedure. PTE requires a referral center with experience in the perioperative management of PH and RV dysfunction including extracorporeal membrane oxygenation (ECMO) [5]. The most common post-op complication is reperfusion lung injury (RLI), being ECMO sometimes necessary to manage these patients. Persistent PH after PTE is common (16.7–35%), being medical support for symptomatic patients needed [5].

Other options of treatment are being recently considered and more studied. Balloon pulmonary angioplasty is a technique used to dilate stenotic segments of the pulmonary arteries, and it may offer several advantages in the treatment of inoperable CTEPH, but it is not currently recommended as an established treatment for CTEPH, because of the need for multiple procedures, significant IV contrast administration, lack of longer-term outcome data, and questions regarding optimal patient selection [5]. Also, it is not a permanent treatment like TPE, and the improvement of hemodynamic factors lasts about 2 years. Although, its methodology has substantially improved over the last years, decreasing the complications.

The medical therapy has also a role in CTEPH. Anticoagulation with warfarin is recommended for all patients (even after PTE and resolution of PH), as well as the symptomatic supportive therapy, especially oxygen therapy. Although, medications cannot reach the same results and replace TPE. For inoperable patients, prostacyclin analogs and phosphodiesterase-5 inhibitors are used for treatment, even without randomized clinical trials supporting it. The only drug that showed benefits in clinical trials is riociguat, a guanylate cyclase stimulator [5].

Concluding, in this case the patient took three and a half years until diagnosis, including a mediastinoscopy. On average these patients take up to 2 years for the correct diagnosis and several consultations before diagnosis [10]. With this, many patients may have important clinical worsening and lack of time until definitive treatment. The disease is often severe, but important advances in treatment options are being made in the last years: the surgeries are having better outcomes, with optimistic chances of cure; interventionist methods such as angioplasty have been introduced; and drugs for pre- and postoperative handling of pulmonary hypertension are being used.

References

1. Terra-Filho M, Ribeiro SCDC, Souza RD, Jatene FB. Tromboendarterectomia pulmonar em paciente com 80 anos de idade. J Bras Pneumol. 2004;30(5). Available at: https://doi.org/10.1590/s1806-37132004000500014.
2. Pengo V, Lensing AW, Prins MH, Marchiori A, Davidson BL, Tiozzo F, Albanese P, et al. Incidence of chronic thromboembolic pulmonary hypertension after pulmonary embolism. N Engl J Med. 2004;350(22):2257–64.
3. Dartavelle P, Fadel E, Mussot S, Chapelier A, Herve P, de Perrot M. Chronic thromboembolic pulmonary hypertension. Eur Respir J. 2004;22:637–48.
4. Tunariu N, Gibbs SJ, Win Z, Gin-Sing W, Graham A, Gishen P, Al-Nahhas A. Ventilation-perfusion scintigraphy is more sensitive than multidetector CTPA in detecting chronic

thromboembolic pulmonary disease as a treatable cause of pulmonary hypertension. J Nucl Med. 2007;48(5):680–4.
5. Robbins IM, Pugh ME, Hemnes AR. Update on chronic thromboembolic pulmonary hypertension. Trends Cardiovasc Med. 2016. Available at: https://doi.org/10.1016/j.tcm.2016.05.010.
6. Jamieson SW, Kapelanski DP, Sakakibara N, Manecke GR, Thistlethwaite PA, Kerr KM, Channick RN, et al. Pulmonary endarterectomy: experience and lessons learned in 1,500 cases. Ann Thorac Surg. 2003;76(5):1457–64.
7. Schölzel BE, Post MC, Bruaene AVD, Dymarkowski S, Wuyts W, Meyns B, Budts W, et al. Prediction of hemodynamic improvement after pulmonary endarterectomy in chronic thromboembolic pulmonary hypertension using non-invasive imaging. Int J Cardiovasc Imaging. 2014;31(1):143–50.
8. Rubens FD, Bourke M, Hynes M, Nicholson D, Kotrec M, Boodhwani M, Ruel M, et al. Surgery for chronic thromboembolic pulmonary hypertension—inclusive experience from a National Referral Center. Ann Thorac Surg. 2007;83(3):1075–81.
9. Jatene FB, Bernardo WB, Hueb AC, Aldunate JLCB, Terra-Filho M, Oliveira SA. Mortalidade pós-tromboendarterectomia pulmonar: é possível predizê-la? Rev Bras Cir Cardiovasc. 2004;19:196–220.
10. Cannon J, Pepke-Zaba J. Is distal chronic thromboembolic pulmonary hypertension treatable with PAH targeted drugs? Semin Respir Crit Care Med. 2013;34(05):620–6.

Intracardiac Embolization of Inferior Vena Cava Filter

Nágila Simon Ziebell, Augusto Emilio Hinterholz, Daniela Moraes, Fernanda Schuh Martins, and Francisco Coelho Lamachia

Clinical Presentation

MLC, male, 44 years old, former smoker, with history of diabetes mellitus, systemic arterial hypertension, and heart failure, comes to the hospital in September 2015 complaining about chest pain within the last 24 h, without any other symptom. The patient had a history of a grade III astrocytoma that was surgically removed 3 months before the day he was admitted in our hospital. After 1 month of this neurosurgery, the patient had another hospitalization due to a suspected cerebral abscess and acute dyspnea. During this hospitalization, a Doppler ultrasound of the legs diagnosed a deep vein thrombosis (DVT) and high-probability pulmonary embolism (PE). However, the recent brain surgery and cerebral abscess suspicion contraindicated the anticoagulation therapy. Therefore, the patient had undergone inferior vena cava filter (IVCF) insertion as the prophylaxis for PE, 2 months before looking for our service. After the procedure, the patient remained dyspneic for 2 more days and developed tachypnea, when a pulmonary angiotomography was taken, diagnosing a bilateral PE in main branches of the pulmonary

N. S. Ziebell (✉) · A. E. Hinterholz · D. Moraes · F. S. Martins
F. C. Lamachia
Santa Cruz do Sul University (UNISC),
Santa Cruz do Sul, RS, Brazil

R. M. S. Almeida, F. B. Jatene (eds.), *Cardiovascular Surgery*,
https://doi.org/10.1007/978-3-319-57084-6_34

arteries. The patient received anticoagulation therapy due to the high risk of mortality associated with the PE.

Diagnosis, Assessment, and Treatment

The patient was admitted to the hospital and an electrocardiogram (EKG) was made, which was normal. A serum troponin I level of 0.94 ng/mL (normal range <0.3 ng/mL) and CK-MB of 4 UI/L (normal range <24 U/L) were the laboratory findings. A transthoracic echocardiogram (Fig. 1) and a contrast-enhanced computed tomography (Fig. 2) were performed, diagnosing a foreign body inside the right ventricle. The patient underwent a cardiac catheterization that confirmed the diagnosis of the inferior vena cava filter inside the right ventricle (Figs. 3 and 4). After a few hours, the patient

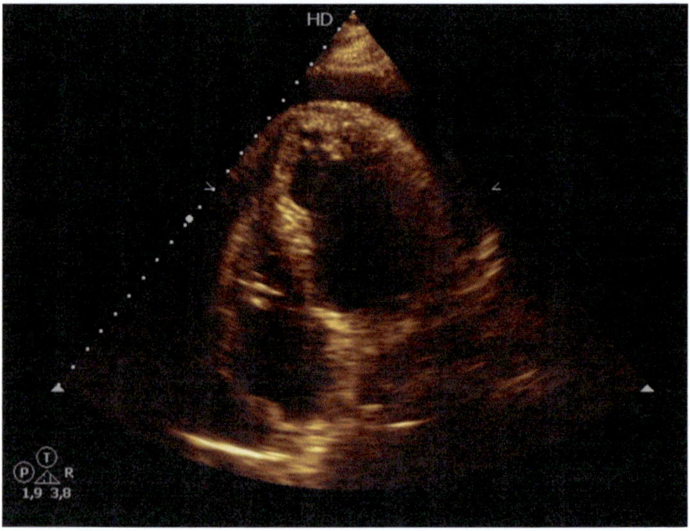

Figure 1 Transthoracic echocardiogram – modified four-chamber view. Visualization of the right atrium, right ventricle, and left ventricle. Abnormal echo-dense mass in the tricuspid valve. Evidence of pericardial effusion

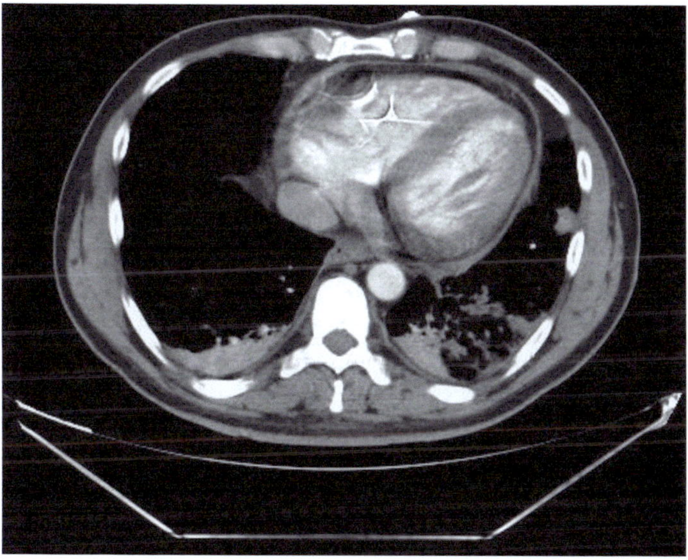

FIGURE 2 Contrast-enhanced computed tomography showing the ventricular chambers with a metal artifact inside the right ventricle. Evidence of a small pericardial effusion, pleural effusion, and bilateral pulmonary atelectasis

developed a cardiac tamponade and hemodynamic instability. He was submitted to a pericardiocentesis and admitted to the intensive care unit (ICU). He underwent a thoracotomy/open heart surgery, which on the filter was removed from the right ventricle, and a valvular lesion was repaired. He stayed in the ICU for 3 days and had no complications associated with the surgery.

Questions

1. What are the indications for inferior vena cava filter insertion?

The use of inferior vena cava filters (IVCFs) is increasing during the past few years. It is recommended for patients who

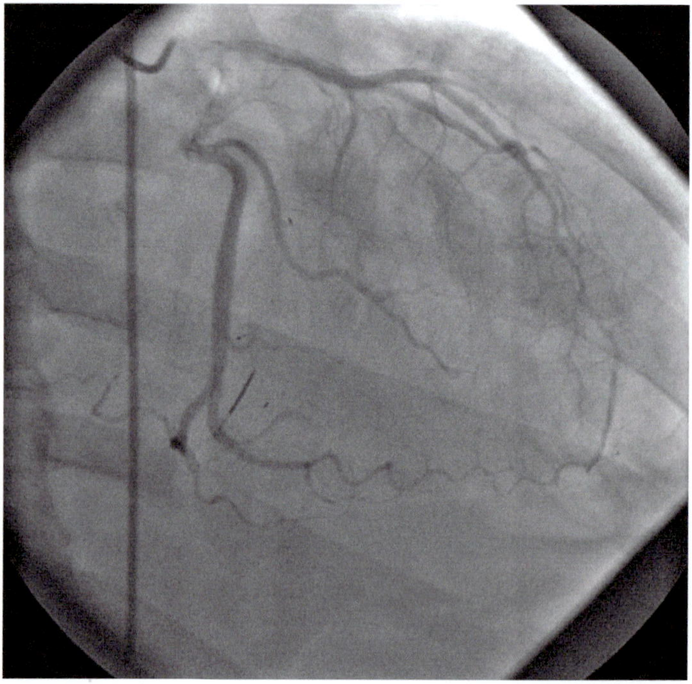

FIGURE 3 Cardiac catheterization – right oblique caudal view. JL catheter positioned inside the left coronary ostium. Radiopaque image in tricuspid position

developed deep vein thrombosis (DVT) or have another thromboembolic disease. The IVCF is used for secondary prophylaxis or pulmonary embolism (PE), especially in those patients with absolute or relative contraindications for anticoagulation or even in those who had developed PE recurrently despite adequate anticoagulation therapy. Contraindications (absolute or relative) for anticoagulation therapy are the most important indications for IVCF insertion. These are exemplified by the patient diagnosed with PE and active gastrointestinal bleeding, adverse effects of heparin (e.g., heparin-induced thrombocytopenia), thrombocytopenia (less than 50.000/mm^3), severe traumatic brain injury or

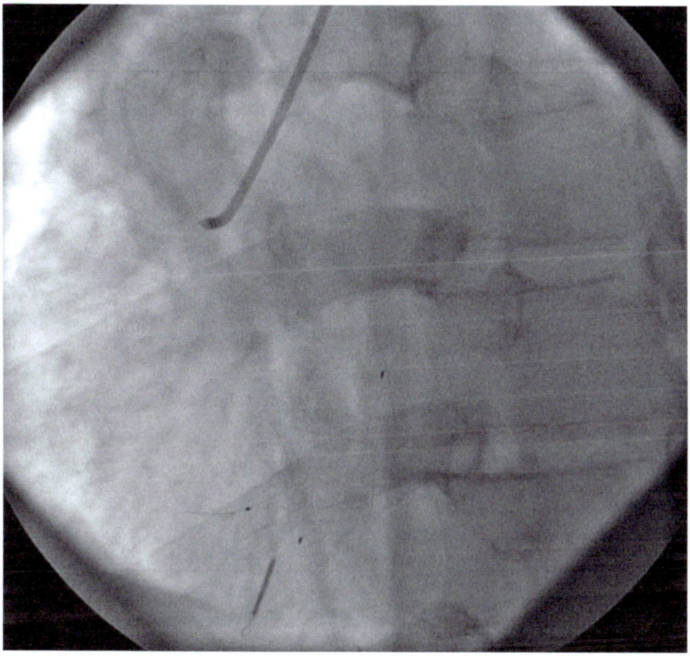

FIGURE 4 Cardiac catheterization – left oblique view. JR catheter positioned in the right coronary territory. Radiopaque image in tricuspid position

spinal cord trauma, central nervous system (CNS) bleeding on the past 6 months, CNS diseases (e.g., tumors), brain surgery, and active urinary tract bleeding on the past 6 months.

2. What are the most frequent complications related to the inferior vena cava filter?

Despite their effectiveness in preventing PE, IVCFs are associated with some complications inherent to their insertion or use. Therefore, the knowledge of those complications allows an early diagnosis and management, reducing the morbidity and mortality of these conditions. Inferior vena cava filter complications might be late or due to its insertion and even to its removal. The events that happen during the filter insertion are the most common complications and are exemplified by bleeding (the most frequent), hematomas (rarely large), inadvertent arterial puncture (mostly in obese patients and/or non-guided by ultrasound puncture), and wound infection. Misplacement of the device is another potential difficulty. More, defective filter deployment (in its expansion or with legs crossed) is a risk factor for migration and malfunctioning of the device.

Filter migration might be to another place in the inferior vena cava (IVC) or to the heart chambers. Some reports of right ventricle and even pulmonary trunk are described in literature.

Despite being used for PE prophylaxis, the IVCFs increase the risk for DVT, mainly in the inferior vena cava (IVC), and it is a complication in about 2.7–3.2% of the cases.

Inferior vena cava lesions, although frequent, are rarely associated with some clinical manifestation. However, there are some case reports about complete perforation of the IVC, causing aortic, ureteral, and intestinal penetration and, therefore, increased morbidity and mortality.

Device infection (mostly in retrieval filters, used in septic patients) and PE are some of the possible complications as well.

3. What is the incidence of intracardiac embolization of the inferior vena cava filter?

Inferior vena cava filter complications have incidence of about 3–12%. Among the most frequent are the hematomas, wound infection, and misplacement of the device. Filter embolization/complete migration is extremely rare, with reported rates of about 0.1–1.2% of the cases, associated mainly with misplacement of the filter, mechanical failure of the device, and IVC diameter less than 28 mm.

4. What are the complications associated with inferior vena cava filter intracardiac embolization?

Despite being rare, intracardiac embolization is a potentially serious condition that must be promptly managed. The main complications of this disorder is syncope, cardiac arrhythmia, dyspnea, cardiogenic shock, cardiac tamponade, myocardial infarction (MI), right ventricle free wall rupture, and even cardiac arrest.

5. What are the main differential diagnosis for inferior vena cava filter intracardiac embolization?

In the most of the cases of filter migration, no clinical manifestation is observed and the patient remains asymptomatic. However, when it migrates upward, mostly when related to the heart or great vessels, the patient might evolve with chest pain. In this perspective, every disease that presents with chest pain may enter the role of differential diagnosis. Knowing that patients who had undergone IVCF insertion are indeed at risk for thromboembolic events, diseases that share the same physiopathology should be listed as possible diagnosis. The most important causes of chest pain, in the presence of risk factors, are MI and PE. In the MI, typical angina associated with elevated cardiac biomarkers and abnormal electrocardiogram (EKG) confirms its diagnosis. Another differential diagnosis that must be excluded is PE, as the patient with the IVCF is, obviously, a patient with risk for this condition.

Pulmonary embolism and myocardial infarction (MI) must be the main differential diagnosis. Pulmonary embolism diagnosis is clinical and radiological (computed angiotomography or pulmonary angiography), but arterial gasometry, chest X-ray, EKG, and D-dimer (in low probability of PE) might be used.

Due to the vast possibilities of clinical manifestations of the IVCF intracardiac embolization, mainly when the patient presents with a cardiogenic or obstructive shock, conditions such as pneumothorax, constrictive pericarditis and cardiac tamponade set the range of differential diagnosis that must be investigated and excluded.

6. What are the exams that must be used to diagnose the inferior vena cava filter intracardiac embolization?

Patients with intracardiac embolization of the device are frequently symptomatic. However, other conditions must be excluded, and therefore, several exams may be used. Among others, the first diagnosing exam that should be performed is the transthoracic echocardiogram, due to its practicality and mainly when the patient is hemodynamically unstable. Even depending on the operator, it is not hard to visualize the foreign body inside the heart chambers by the echocardiogram.

Furthermore, ejection fraction, valvular lesions, as well as differential diagnosis and/or complications caused by the ectopic filter might be seen during the exam.

It is essential that PE and MI are excluded as soon as possible, and diagnostic tests related to those conditions must be used.

7. What are the treatment options for the inferior vena cava filter intracardiac embolization?

In the presence of intracardiac embolization of the IVCF, open heart surgery and endovascular approach are the treatment options. Weinberg, Kaufman, and Jaff [5] advocate that conservative management is a therapeutic option. However, there is no consensus of what is the best treatment method for the filter removal, nor if its removal is a good choice when the patient is hemodynamically stable. Due to the low incidence of this condition, there is no strong evidence to support one approach over the other, making the individualization of the case the basis for the best therapeutic option, allying clinical aspects and imaging exams to make the decision. Most authors suggest that the best approach would be the thoracotomy (open heart surgery), mainly when the patient is hemodynamically unstable.

8. What are the possible surgical complications of the removal of the filter?

Thoracotomy puts the patient at risk for MI, cardiac tamponade, vasoplegic syndrome, atrial fibrillation, and ventricular arrhythmias. Furthermore, when there are associated valvular lesions, its Plasty or rhaphy increases the risk for conduction abnormalities, atrioventricular block, and endocarditis. As well as described for other surgeries, complications related (or not) to procedure such as wound infection, bleeding, and atelectasis may happen.

Review About the Addressed Disease or Treatment

Cardiac tamponade can be classified as a cardiac emergency that requires immediate diagnosis and management. This condition is defined as an abnormal accumulation of fluid or gas in the pericardial sac, compromising the myocardial contractility, heart pumping flow, and systemic perfusion. It is one of the most common clinical presentations of penetrating chest trauma. The poor prognosis is directly proportional to delay on diagnosis. When classified as moderate to severe, it is not unusual that the patient develops severe dyspnea and chest pain, as shown in our report. Cardiac tamponade should be suspected in every patient who presents *pulsus paradoxus*/paradoxical pulse (a 10 mmHg decrease in the systolic blood pressure during the inspiration), Kussmaul sign (paradoxical elevation of the jugular venous distention/pressure during the inspiration), and/or the classical Beck's triad/acute compression triad, which is characterized by muffled heart sounds, jugular venous distention, and hypotension. The prompt diagnosis and management may prevent the development of an obstructive shock. Its usual treatment relies on performing a pericardiocentesis (acute treatment that allows the patient to remain hemodynamically stable) and posterior thoracotomy or median sternotomy (a definitive treatment, which repairs all the lesions that might be causing the cardiac tamponade). In our case, the patient developed a severe cardiac tamponade (secondary to the presence of an inferior vena cava filter inside the right ventricle) and was promptly managed.

Bibliography

1. Athanasoulis CA, et al. Inferior vena caval filters: review of a 26-year single-center clinical experience. Radiology. [Online]. 2000; 216:54–66. Available from: https://doi.org/10.1148/radiology.216.1.r00jl1254.
2. Caplin DM, et al. Quality improvement guidelines for performance of inferior vena cava filter placement for the prevention of pulmonary embolism. J Vasc Interv Radiol. [Online]. 2011;22(11):1499–506. Available from: https://doi.org/10.1016/j.jvir.2011.07.012.
3. Soeiro AM, et al. Intracardiac embolization of inferior vena cava filter associated with right atrium perforation and cardiac tam-

ponade. Rev Bras Cir Cardiovasc. [Online]. 2014;29(2):285–8. Available from: https://doi.org/10.5935/1678-9741.20140060.
4. Owens CA, et al. Endovascular retrieval of intracardiac inferior vena cava filters: a review of published techniques. J Vasc Interv Radiol. [Online]. 2009;20(11):1418–28. Available from: https://doi.org/10.1016/j.jvir.2009.08.001.
5. Weinberg I, Kaufman J, Jaff MR. Inferior vena cava filters. JACC Cardiol Interv. [Online]. 2013;6(6):539–47. Available from: https://doi.org/10.1016/j.jcin.2013.03.006.
6. Saeed I, Garcia M, McNicholas K. Right ventricular migration of a recovery IVC filter's fractured wire with subsequent pericardial tamponade. Cardiovasc Intervent Radiol. [Online]. 2006;29(4):685–6. Available from: https://doi.org/10.1007/s00270-005-0136-7.
7. Rossi P, et al. Fatal outcome in atrial migration of the tempofilter. Cardiovac Intervent Radiol. [Online]. 1999;22:227–31. Available from: https://doi.org/10.1007/s002709900372.
8. Nicholson W, et al. Prevalence of fracture and fragment embolization of Bard retrievable vena cava filters and clinical implications including cardiac perforation and tamponade. Arch Intern Med. [Online]. 2010;170(20):1827–31. Available from: https://doi.org/10.1001/archinternmed.2010.316.
9. Van Ha TG. Complications of inferior vena caval filters. Semin Intervent Radiol. [Online]. 2006;23:150–5. Available from: https://doi.org/10.1055/s-2006-941445.

Part XII
Valvular Heart Disease

Acute Mitral Valve Insufficiency Due to Multiple Trauma Accident

Vanessa Dias D'Avila Sperandio, Elisa Cao Bicalho, Priscilla Gomes Tosta, and Melchior Luiz Lima

Clinical Presentation

Female, 37 years old, was admitted to the intensive care unit (ICU) due to multiple trauma (car accident).

On admission, she presented posterior fracture of the 4th to the 10th left ribs with hemothorax, splenic injury grade III (according to the scale of organ damage of the American Association for the Surgery of Trauma – AAST), left renal laceration grade I (also according to the AAST), and peripancreatic hematoma. She underwent chest tube drainage due to left hemothorax, laparotomy with splenectomy, and raffia of the liver and drainage by pneumothorax due to puncture accident, in addition to antibiotic therapy with ceftriaxone and cefepime later on suspicion of lung infection. After stabilization of the patient, clinical history was taken, and physical examination was performed. The patient was in good general condition, with fever episodes. Sedation was performed with fentanyl and midazolam and mechanical ventilation via an endotrachcal tube. The ventilatory examination was tachydyspnea, with breath sounds reduced diffusely and saturation of 92%. After cardiovascular physical examination, she was

V. D. D' Avila Sperandio (✉) · E. C. Bicalho · P. G. Tosta · M. L. Lima
School of Sciences of Santa Casa de Misericórdia de Vitória (EMESCAM), Vitória, ES, Brazil

R. M. S. Almeida, F. B. Jatene (eds.), *Cardiovascular Surgery*,
https://doi.org/10.1007/978-3-319-57084-6_35

found with pulmonary hypertension (treated with sodium nitroprusside – Nipride) and high blood pressure (treated with losartan and atenolol).

Diagnosis, Assessment, and Treatment

After ninth day of admission, the patient developed acute respiratory failure following extubation attempt, being viewed foamy secretion in the endotracheal tube. Vasoactive drugs were then required, due to refractory hypotension. Transthoracic echocardiogram was perfomed was performed which showed an image in the posterior leaflet of the mitral valve, acute mitral regurgitation and acute heart failure. From then we started antibiotic therapy with daptomycin, and we requested assessment of cardiac surgery. On the same day, the patient was sent to the operating room for an emergency heart surgery. During the procedure envisioned is a laceration of the papillary muscle of the mitral valve, and native valve replacement with a bioprosthesis implant 29 mm is performed.

The patient recovered well from the standpoint of cardiac surgery but remained to show unexplained fever peaks. By doing physical assessment, an extensive pressure ulcer grade II was found, with fibrin tissue center and devitalized tissue stuck in the sacral region. Patient also developed grade II pressure ulcer in the right buttock.

Despite having the appropriate echocardiogram on the fifth day of treatment, without dysfunction of the bioprosthesis and with a left ventricle ejection fraction of 64%, the patient developed mediastinal abscess. So she was treated with debridement of the sternal wound washed with saline and drainage of serohematic fluid, with progressive improvement. After a long time of admission, the patient's cardiac condition improved and was discharged, following the guidelines, on the 14th day.

Questions

1. Which signs of the cardiological semiology made it possible to suspect a cardiac involvement in this patient?

The patient had a foamy secretion in the endotracheal tube, which may indicate an acute cardiogenic pulmonary edema. Moreover, he had tachydyspnea, decreased breath sounds, and hypoxemia, favoring the diagnosis of this entity.

2. What would be a plausible explanation for the clinical signs answered in the previous question?

Acute pulmonary edema of the patient's case (later confirmed by chest X-ray showing suggestive infiltrate) was probably caused by heart disease later confirmed by echocardiography, showing ruptured chordae tendineae with mitral valve insufficiency.

Cardiogenic shock is characterized by decreased myocardial contractility. This reduces cardiac output and blood pressure, which in turn causes a reduction in coronary perfusion leading to ischemia. The body uses several coping mechanisms to face this problem, among them is vasodilation plus increased left ventricular end-diastolic pressure, thereby causing acute edema.

3. What is the therapeutic approach to clinical signs answered in the first question?

The first step is to stabilize the patient. We should maintain mean arterial pressure greater than 60 mmHg; carry oxygen therapy with positive pressure ventilation, either by masks of O_2, nasal catheter, or endotracheal intubation; and still promote venodilation to increase venous return. The initial drug therapy aims to reduce the preload using diuretics, such as furosemide 1 mg/kg intravenously. Morphine is used at a dose of 2–4 mg/kg being a transitional venodilator and also decreases dyspnea and anxiety. If hypertension is detected, antihypertensives through parenteral route are employed, such as nitroglycerin, from 5 to 10 mcg/min, or sodium nitroprusside.

4. What are the main findings in cardiovascular physical examination that can be found in patients with mitral regurgitation?

The main findings are the displacement of the apex (beat stroke down and to the left), hypophonic first heart sound, and holosystolic apical murmur that often radiates toward the axilla. Moreover, one may develop pulmonary hypertension and right heart failure, as in the following.

5. What is the etiology of mitral regurgitation in the clinical case exposed? Besides this, what are other causes for this condition?

Laceration of the papillary muscle of the mitral valve. Other causes are myocardial papillary muscle infarction, annular calcification, endocarditis, myxomatous degeneration, collagen vascular diseases, and rheumatic heart disease.

6. What happens to the blood flow within the heart in the presence of mitral regurgitation? What is the ideal exam for evaluation of the flow?

In mitral insufficiency, the valve prolapses into the left atrium and may occur regurgitation of blood. In this condition, part of the blood that passes through mitral valve performs the anterograde and retrograde path, leading to the left chambers overload. The test that better evaluates the blood flow is transthoracic echocardiography with Doppler.

7. What is the main cause of mediastinal abscess? What are the main risk factors for its development?

The median sternotomy, esophageal perforation, and deep neck infections are the leading causes of mediastinal abscess. Rare causes are pleural empyema, vertebral or costal osteomyelitis, and retroperitoneal or subphrenic abscesses. The most significant risk factors are the use of internal thoracic artery graft, diabetes mellitus, emergency operations, external cardiac massage (resuscitation), obesity, postoperative shock, multiple blood transfusions, prolonged cardiopulmonary bypass or operation, reoperation, sternal dehiscence, and technical factors (electrocautery abuse, bone wax, or parasternal access). Such factors are likely synergistic.

8. What are the main etiological agents of postsurgical acute mediastinitis and your best treatment?

Most cases (70–80%) of postsurgical acute mediastinitis indicate infection caused by gram-positive cocci, usually by *Staphylococcus aureus* or *Staphylococcus epidermidis*. Associated infections by gram-positive and negative occur in about 40% of cases and gram-negative isolation are rare.

You must use specific treatment for the etiologic agent after culture results guided by its sensitivity. Piperacillin-tazobactam and vancomycin can be used as empiric treatment. Patients allergic to penicillin can receive quinolones and clindamycin.

Review About the Addressed Disease or Treatment

Rupture of chordae tendineae is the most common cause of acute mitral regurgitation. Most of these patients present congestive heart failure (CHF) and rapidly progressive increase in pulmonary capillary wedge pressure, requiring surgical treatment. Performed with extracorporeal circulation and general anesthesia, the procedure is the removal of the native valve and replacement with a prosthesis which can be mechanical or biological. The indications for selecting the type of prosthesis depend on the individual patient. Mechanical prosthesis is implanted in new patients whose life expectancy is over 25 years, with necessity of anticoagulant therapy for the rest of their lives. Bioprosthesis has the great advantage of not needing anticoagulation but lasts approximately about 20 years. The patient's surgery lasted 4 h and 30 min, with 65 min of cardiopulmonary bypass and 135 min of perfusion. The surgery complications were severe hypotension due to anesthesia and complete atrioventricular block, requiring ventricular pacemaker.

The prognosis of patients with severe regurgitation is poor, and median survival is around 33% – in 8 years without surgery – with a mortality rate of about 5% per year in the most severe cases; most deaths are related to heart failure or ventricular arrhythmias.

Other complications associated with mitral regurgitation include atrial fibrillation, cerebrovascular accident, transient ischemic events, and predisposition to develop endocarditis. Patients with mitral regurgitation due to rheumatic fever usually have associated mitral stenosis, which associates worse prognosis. The atrial dilatation influences the prognosis in patients primarily associated with atrial fibrillation. Patients with ischemic dysfunction of papillary muscles also have worse prognostic and require urgent intervention.

In cases of dilated cardiomyopathy, on which occurs annular dilatation and mitral regurgitation, are observed left ventricle geometrical changes and systolic dysfunction, leading to bad prognosis.

Bibliography

1. Goldman L, et al. Goldman cecil medicine. 24ª ed. Brazil: Elsevier; 2014.
2. Long DL, et al. Harrison Treaty internal medicine. 18° ed. Mexico: The McGraw-Hill Companies; 2013.
3. Jiménez MF, Macri P, Novoa N, Varela, GA. Descriptive of a series of patients diagnosed with acute mediastinitis [Online], 39 (2003). Available: http://www.archbronconeumol.org/en/linkresolver/analisis-descriptivo-una-serie-casos/S0300289603754192/.

Endocarditis: The Precipitation of a Mitral Insufficiency

Anna Luiza Amâncio Vidal, Lucas Alves Bessa Cardoso, Eduardo Teles de Lima Lopes, and Rodolpho Poeys Lima

Clinical Presentation

D.S.B.G., 18 years old, female, scholar, born in Teixeiras, Minas Gerais, Brazil, comes to the appointment complaining: "I'm feeling very tired and my hair is falling down." During the patient interview, she reports a progressive fatigue that started 3 months ago, associated with lack of appetite (she could only eat tomatoes and drink water) and a 10-kilo weight loss. After a month having the disease, she began to notice hair loss associated with fever, which was not measured. Two months later, little purplish spots appeared in her hands and feet, lasting a week, which soon disappeared and reappeared elsewhere. Currently, she is reporting fatigue on minimal efforts, fever, and purple spots.

Previously healthy, she reports that she went to several doctor appointments, who prescribed only symptomatic treatments. In the past medical reports: tooth extraction 1 month before the opening frame and tooth root canal surgery 6 years before. No family disease reported.

A. L. A. Vidal (✉) · L. A. B. Cardoso · E. T. de Lima Lopes
R. P. Lima
Federal University of Viçosa (UFV), Viçosa, MG, Brazil

R. M. S. Almeida, F. B. Jatene (eds.), *Cardiovascular Surgery*,
https://doi.org/10.1007/978-3-319-57084-6_36

At physical examination

No fever, tachycardia, pale 3+/4+, anemic 2+/4+, hydrated, acyanosis, eupneic. Regular heart rhythm, with presence of S3 and holosystolic murmur 3+/6+, irradiating to the left axilla. Nails with purple spots compatible with Janeway lesions. Blood pressure of 100/60 mmHg, heart rate 130 bpm.

Diagnosis, Assessment, and Treatment

The fatigue on minimal efforts – that got better when she was resting – drew attention to possible dysfunction of the cardiovascular system; the suspicion was confirmed, with important murmur auscultation during the physical examination. A fever with slurred evolution led to think about a subacute bacterial infection or perhaps atypical bacteria. As there was bacteremia caused by the dental procedure, the etiology for the main symptoms may be common, which led the hypothesis of bacterial endocarditis, which was reinforced with injuries consistent with Janeway spots. As bacterial endocarditis is rare in patients with no previous valve damage, a better knowing of her medical past was necessary. She denied known cardiac defects, both at birth or acquired, but reported history of multiple sore throats in childhood and adolescence, most of which were untreated. Taking in consideration the high prevalence of rheumatic fever in Brazil, it was assumed that the cause for initial valve deformity was a rheumatic fever episode caused by an untreated bacterial tonsillitis.

With the suspicion of infectious endocarditis (IE), the patient was admitted after consultation and evaluated for the referred disease with complete blood count (CBC) application, blood culture, electrocardiography (ECG), and transesophageal echocardiography and went through an empiric treatment with gentamicin and ampicillin. The CBC showed anemia and leukocytosis with a left shift, suggestive of bacterial infection, and ECG showed left ventricular hypertrophy, later confirmed by echocardiography, and also vegetation

(8 mm). Culture showed infection by *Streptococcus viridans*. With these results, there were two major criteria for IE (Duke criteria); thus the disease could be diagnosed. The first treatment option was valvuloplasty surgery, but after discussion between the surgical team and the patient, the approach chosen was a valve replacement, with the use of a biological one, to allow future pregnancy.

Questions

1. What is the pathophysiology of infectious endocarditis?

The characteristic lesion of infectious endocarditis is vegetation which is composed of platelets, fibrin, microorganisms, and inflammatory cells. Pathogenic bacteria are concentrated in the core of the vegetation, being covered with fibrin layers, thus impairing the action on neutrophils agents.

Symptoms reflect the existing infectious process, the mechanical changes resulting from local growth of vegetation, septic embolization, and circulating immune complexes.

The origin of the vegetation takes place in the presence of endothelial injury, which is derived from any abnormal heart chamber (e.g., ventricular septal defect, valvular insufficiency and stenosis, presence of prostheses, or installed catheters) and/or the state of presence of hypercoagulability (this factor is less commonly found in autopsy findings). The first step to form the vegetation is called Non-Bacterial Thrombocytopenic Endocarditis (NBTE), being fostered by: (1) the impact of high-speed jet *with the damaged wall of the chamber*, (2) the flow between chambers with a high pressure gradient (3) flow through a narrowed orifice on high speed. An inflammatory process damages the endothelium, which *releases cytokines and recruits and activates a fibrin coagulation cascade*, progressively increasing the thrombus.

The vegetation is formed facing the chamber with lower pressure, because of that, atrioventricular lesions form in the atrium and injuries of semilunar valves are formed in the respective ventricles.

With NBTE, the pathogenic microorganism may *aggregate* itself to the already formed thrombus, initiating the process of infective endocarditis. The origin of this germ is undetermined, usually originating from a damage to the mucosa that carries bacteria into the circulation (in this context, damages to the oral mucosa have great relevance). For the aggregation of the microorganism, it needs to be resistant to the bactericidal activity mediated by a complement of the immune system. The mechanism of aggregation of microorganisms is dependent on adhesion molecules called adhesins. The adhesins act on fibronectin, a glycoprotein produced by the endothelium, in response to the damage, making the connection between the fibrinogen and the endothelial collagen. Thus, when the germs bind to fibronectin, they adhere to both the fibrinogen and the endothelial collagen, remaining stable within the vegetation.

Once joined, the virulent organisms can be internalized to the endothelial cells, promoting their proliferation, which *lyses* the host cells, thereby increasing the agent population and stimulating new fibrin deposition and plaque stretching at the site of lysed cells, creating a feedback where more fibrin deposit facilitates more cell infections, and those, when *lysed*, create more fibrin. With the rapid growth plate associated with hyperproliferation of pathogens, there is the possibility of fragmentation and gelatinous or septic embolization of the thrombus, resulting in infarction and/or infection.

Intracardiac consequences *range from vegetation without tissue damage associated with leaflet lesions to chordae rupture, which narrows the valve opening, not all patients with chordae rupture generates a congestive heart failure.* It is also possible that the local spread of infection can create abscesses, which disrupt the cardiac conduction system, leading to arrhythmias and electrocardiogram changes and the possibility of purulent pericarditis.

2. What are the risk factors for infectious endocarditis?

Since the 1950s, a major shift in the paradigms related to microbiology and risk factors of the disease has occurred; however, the overall incidence of IE keeps around 3–9 per

100,000 individuals, with a mortality of about 25%. The use of prosthetic valves, both natural and mechanical, is the greatest risk factor for the disease. It can be distinguished in two groups: *natural valve endocarditis* and *prosthetic valves.*

Urban populations are more affected than rural ones, which may reflect certain socioeconomic factors, such as injecting drug use and higher rates of hospitalization (with consequent nosocomial infection). Endocarditis in natural valves is more prevalent in men at a ratio of 1.7:1. Regarding the average age, the last decades quite changed the scenario of the disease: in the early 1940s, the average age of those affected was 35 years old, and only 10% were over 60 years old. Today, the average age is 55 years old, and 50% of the patients are older than 60 years old. This change can be attributed to:

Reduction in the incidence of rheumatic heart disease in childhood with the use of treatment of streptococcal infections

Longevity of patients with heart disease and rheumatic injury due to surgical technology advances

Increase of degenerative heart diseases, especially in elderly patients

Use of invasive therapeutic interventions (e.g., catheters, pacemakers, and hemodialysis) that affect older patients, increasing the risk of nosocomial infection

Valve prostheses, which usually appear in older patients

Preexisting heart conditions are high-risk indicators for IE (because they represent the endothelial damage which is the basis of the pathogenesis of the disease). The American Heart Association (AHA) proposes the following classification:

High risk: presence of prosthetic valve, previous endocarditis, congenital cyanotic heart disease and pulmonary systemic shunts surgically performed

Moderate risk: cardiac birth defects, acquired valvular dysfunction (including rheumatic ones), hypertrophic cardiomyopathy, and mitral valve prolapse

The prosthetic valve endocarditis (PVE) is the most severe form, which affects from 1% to 6% of patients who underwent the exchange, with no predilection for mechanical or biological prostheses. Nosocomial infections are responsible for 37% of cases of PVE.

3. What are the surgical indications to infectious endocarditis? (Table 1)

The indication for surgical procedure in asymptomatic patients remains controversial, even with large vegetation or other comorbidities. So, in these cases, the need and time for surgery are a surgeon's criteria. On the other hand, with severe impairment of the valve, or symptomatic patients, surgical approach is considered the only curative one.

In some occasions, the intervention has to be immediate, as with an infection by *Staphylococcus aureus* or by fungus. In cases of fungal infection associated with mycotic aneurysm, causing hemorrhagic stroke, the surgery has to be delayed for 4 weeks to lower the risks of intracranial hemorrhage.

During the surgery, after exposure, the infected tissue is debrided to remove all the infection, and based on the left

Table 1 Surgical indications for native endocarditis and prosthetic valve endocarditis

1 Severe mitral regurgitation, with or without symptoms of congestive heart failure
2 Uncontrolled sepsis despite proper antibiotic therapy
3 Presence of an antibiotic-resistant organism
4 Fungal endocarditis or endocarditis caused by *S. aureus* or gram-negative bacteria
5 Presence of mitral annular abscess, extension of infection to intervalvular fibrous body, or formation of intracardiac fistulas
6 Onset of a new conduction disturbance
7 Large vegetations (>1cm), particularly those that are mobile and located on the anterior leaflet and thus at high risk for embolic complications
8 Multiple emboli despite appropriate antibiotic therapy

Table adapted from Cohn [3]

tissue, the reconstruction technique is chosen. During the debridement, abscesses, fistulas, and fibrosis of intervalvular tissue have to be observed, and all the infected tissue has to be removed. After the debridement, if the reconstruction of the valve is possible without tension on the tissue, repair should be made; otherwise replacement is indicated.

If the repair is possible, the technique depends on the extension of leaflet affected. In the anterior repair, the autologous tissue from pericardium is used, but the posterior repair is made by quadrangular resection of the middle scallop (Figs. 1 and 2).

4. In rheumatic mitral disease, how is the surgical approach?

The rheumatic mitral valve repair aims to restore the valve mobility and keep its function, reducing the regurgitation in several cases.

The procedure consists in debriding calcifications and scars, in papillary muscle and chordae.

The annuloplasty is indicated when the regurgitation compromises the daily activities (patients classified as II, III, and IV by New York Heart Association). And valvular replacement is indicated when the mitral valve area is 1 cm^2 or less,

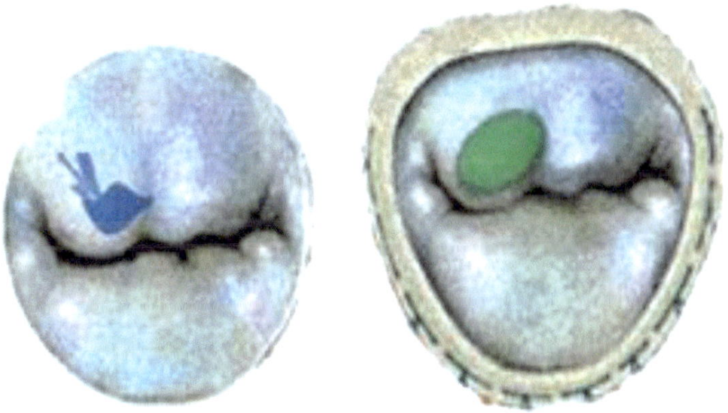

FIGURE 1 Anterior leaflet (autologous pericardium) and posterior annuloplasty

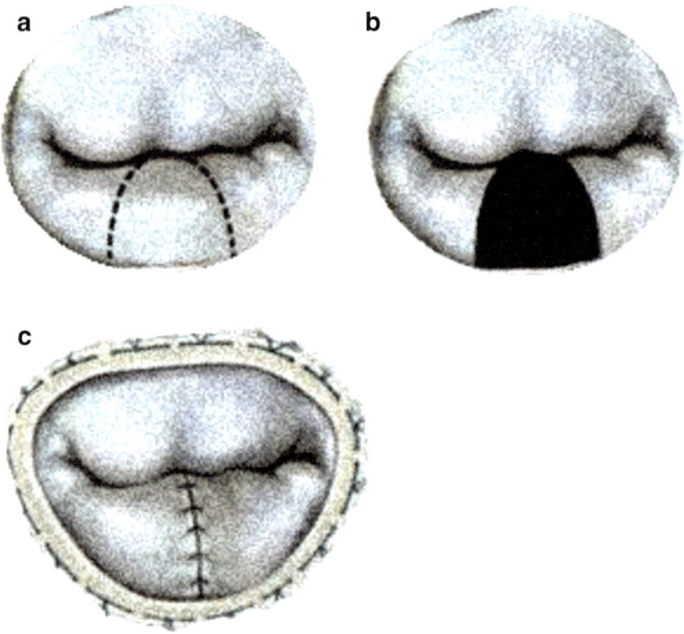

FIGURE 2 Repair of posterior mitral leaflet by quadrangular resection. (**a**) Resection of infected tissue. (**b**) A portion on both sides of the resected part of the annulus is detached, and (**c**) the remaining parts of the leaflet are sutured to the annulus and posteriorly are reapproximated

but in case of mixed lesion (stenosis + regurgitation), this indication is not used, once the patient can be symptomatic with less commitment.

As stated above, the choice of annuloplasty, or replacement, is multifactorial, but if the repair is possible, it should be done because it usually has better results.

5. The patient has been under a valve replacement. Was the replacement result better than the plastic? Why?

The choice is made based on the abnormality of the apparatus, clinical repercussion, surgeon's ability, and other factors. Nonetheless, the valve plastic is preferred over the replacement, because of better results.

Some patients in which the replacement was done had left ventricular function deteriorated, contributing to increased mortality and morbidity, i.e., cases with the discontinued valve-chordae-myocardium, where deformities and impaired left ventricle ejection are not rare. In addition, there are risks inherent to surgical intervention, such as endocarditis, use of anticoagulants in mechanical valves, and thromboembolism in biological valves.

The patient had a severe mixed lesion (stenosis + regurgitation) and was symptomatic, so the plastic one was not chosen.

6. Why the biological valve was indicated for the patient?

When the valve replacement is indicated, bioprosthetic or mechanical valves can be used. The mechanical valves last longer and usually do not need changes, and biological valves periodically need replacement. The changing time of the prosthetic valve depends on the age of the patient: in younger patients, the replacement is earlier.

The bioprosthetic valves can be porcine or pericardial; both have the same duration, but the pericardial valve has better hemodynamic results. The bioprosthetic valves are recommended in patients who have to avoid anticoagulation therapy, such as patients with gastrointestinal bleeding, pregnant women, and in renal chronic failure and hypercalcemia caused by hyperthyroidism.

The patient of the case manifested the desire of being pregnant in the future. So, considering possible future pregnancy complications, bioprosthetic valve was used, although it requires new future replacements in young patients due to valve degeneration.

7.What are the complications of the mitral valve replacement?

Multiple complications are possible in mitral valve replacement: valve calcifications are not rare, as myocardial infarction, arrhythmias, endocarditis, and low cardiac debit and shock can happen during or after this cardiac procedure.

Other systems frequently affected are nervous, respiratory, and renal ones.

8. What is the prophylaxis for endocarditis in the entail procedures?

The AHA and the American College of Cardiology (ACC) point dental procedures as high risk for the formation of endocarditis in patients already susceptible to IE. These organizations recommend the use of penicillin prophylaxis in procedures that handle gingival tissue or periapical region of the teeth or perforation of the oral mucosa, due to the fact that mucosa houses a large number of bacterial pathogens that, when released into the circulation, have high potential for bacterial aggregation in an injured cardiac site. Procedures in the lung and at genitourinary and gastrointestinal sites are considered of lesser importance and not always in need of prophylaxis.

With age profile changes in the population and expansion of risk factors to the disease, the profile of the main germs had great change involvement. The are about 50 germs that can cause IE but, *Streptococcus* viridans was the main identified agent (about 80% of cases), in association with major infection of injured natural valves (for rheumatic or congenital heart lesion) in young patients.

Considering the higher rate of treatment for streptococcal infections and increased longevity of the population, which is subjected to more invasive risk procedures (prosthetic valve replacement, catheterization, dialysis, dental procedures, etc.) and intravenous drug use, *Staphylococcus aureus* has gained greater importance in the IE scenario. It is currently primarily responsible for the framework of the training (30% of community cases and 46% of hospital). This change profile, negative coagulase *Staphylococcus*, also gained a lot of space in the pathogenesis of the disease, mainly in tangent to hospital invasive procedures (catheter and parenteral nutrition).

Review About the Addressed Disease or Treatment

Valve regurgitation (or insufficiency) is defined as abnormal reversal of blood through an incompetent valve. In theory, any valve can be affected; however, those affecting the left heart (aortic and mitral valves) are more common.

In the mitral regurgitation (MR), which was observed in the patient, the symptomatology depends on the patient's atrial complacency. In decreased or normal complacency (usually in acute cases of MR), the atrium does not have time to adjust to the regurgitant volume, thus, increasing its pressure rapidly to a relatively small volume, causing symptoms of heart failure. On the other hand, the increased complacency (more common in chronic cases) causes a greater accommodation of blood on the left side, and it dilates the left heart, usually leading to symptoms of low cardiac output. It is worth mentioning that most patients have combinations of both situations.

The treatment of MR dependents on the functional class of New York Heart Association and presence of ventricular dysfunction. The surgical treatment is indicated in any symptomatic patient (classes II to IV) or in the asymptomatic patients with alterations of left ventricular function or dimensions. The clinical treatment is usually used in patients who cannot undergo surgery or await on it, with purpose of improving symptoms.

Valve regurgitation has several etiologies; all have a degree of involvement with structures of the valve apparatus (leaflets, annulus, chordae tendineae, and papillary muscles). Those alterations can be caused by a large spectrum of diseases, i.e., Marfan syndrome, valve prolapse, rheumatic fever, and endocarditis. In developed countries, such as the USA, the most common cause of MR is mitral valve prolapse, while in Brazil, it is rheumatic fever. This knowledge is important because the recognition of MR can lead to the diagnosis of other diseases.

In rheumatic fever, the valve damage is caused by molecular mimicry by pathogens, usually bacteria found in the mouth or in the superior airway. Therefore, it is recommended the use of penicillin prophylaxis in dental procedures and the correct treatment of bacterial tonsillitis. The diagnosis of rheumatic fever is given by Jones criteria. Because of the lesion in the valve apparatus, rheumatic fever is an important risk factor for the development of IE.

IE is very rare in patients without prior valve lesion, so as soon as it is diagnosed, a more detailed investigation of the patient's past is necessary. The installation of endocarditis leads to the destruction of the valve apparatus due to bacterial growth, besides the possible embolization that will affect other organs and systems. It can worsen the already damaged heart and/or create other symptoms. Duke criteria are used for your diagnosis.

Bibliography

1. ACC/AHA 2006 guidelines for the management of patients with valvular heart disease: executive summary: a report of the American College of Cardiology/American Heart Association Task Force on practice guidelines (Writing Committee to revise the 1998 guidelines for the management of patients with Valvular heart disease): developed in collaboration with the Society of Cardiovascular Anesthesiologists: endorsed by the Society for Cardiovascular Angiography and Interventions and the Society of Thoracic Surgeons. Circulation. 2006;114(5):450–527.
2. Braunwald E, Bonow R. Braunwald's heart disease. 1st ed. Philadelphia: Saunders; 2012.
3. Cohn L. Cardiac surgery in the adult. 1st ed. New York: McGraw-Hill Medical; 2008. p. 1072.
4. Little A. Complications in cardiothoracic surgery. 1st ed. Elmsford: Blackwell Futura; 2004.
5. Sandoe J. Guidelines for the diagnosis and antibiotic treatment of endocarditis in adults: a report of the Working Party of the British Society for antimicrobial chemotherapy–author's response. J Antimicrob Chemother. 2012;67(12):3017.

Valvular Commitment in Hunter Syndrome

Manuela Xavier Cajado Sampaio, Pedro Guimarães Silva, Eugênio Antônio Mascarenhas Colonnezy, Roque Aras Júnior, and André Maurício Souza Fernandes

Clinical Presentation

A 30-year-old white patient with a history of rheumatic fever during his teenage years was admitted at the hospital after being referred by his general practitioner. He had a 6-month story of dyspnea on exertion, which at first occurred during his regular activities, but had been recently presenting on minimal efforts. The patient reported that he has been having such episodes of "fatigue" for almost 10 years, which were more pronounced during periods of great exertion and were accompanied by pallor and lipothymia. At the occasion, it was detected that both aortic and mitral valves were committed by lesions that suggested a valvulopathy of probable rheumatic origin. He was then oriented to undergo a surgery for the replacement of both mitral and aortic valves. Nevertheless, the patient refused to submit to surgical treatment at first, maintaining only his clinical vigilance at the referred hospital. He started taking up monthly doses of benzathine penicillin as a prophylaxis for rheumatic heart disease since the time of diagnosis, but did not undergo any other sort

M. X. C. Sampaio (✉)
Salvador University (UNIFACS), Salvador, BA, Brazil

P. G. Silva · E. A. M. Colonnezy · R. A. Júnior · A. M. S. Fernandes
Federal University of Bahia (UFBA), Salvador, BA, Brazil

R. M. S. Almeida, F. B. Jatene (eds.), *Cardiovascular Surgery*,
https://doi.org/10.1007/978-3-319-57084-6_37

of treatment. A previous transthoracic echocardiogram (TTE) and a recent transesophageal echocardiography (TEE) performed with an interval of 6 years showed an important progression of the preestablished valvular lesions, which were compatible with the development of the symptoms referred by the patient. He also complained about a severe diffuse arthralgia, with an important limitation of articular movements, from which he has been suffering for as long as he could remember. As far as his medical history is concerned, the patient presented a series of deformities that trace back to the time of his infancy, such as thoracic-wall dysmorphism (pectus excavatum), bilateral reduction of visual acuity, abnormal gait, and multiple permanent osteoarticular deformities. In the past, he was evaluated by a neurologist, who tried to perform a genetic investigation of his malady, but did not go on. Both the patient and the family reported no cognitive deficit or developmental delay when compared to people of the same age and locality. There was no report of another known case of genetic disease in the family.

At the physical examination, the patient presented good general aspect, with preserved orientation of time/space; eupneic, with pink/red and hydrated mucosae; afebrile, anicteric; and acyanotic. Anthropometric data was normal, and vital signs were stable. At inspection, several dysmorphisms could be perceived: large-bridged nose with a saddlelike morphology, rude facial expressions, deformed dental arcade with short and protruding teeth, asymmetrical pectus excavatum, kyphoscoliosis with a right-sided deflection, long superior and inferior limbs with articular misalignment, rigidity, thick fingers, and a "claw-like" disposition of both hands.

During cardiovascular assessment, he presented a moving precordium, with a palpable ictus at the encounter of the 6th intercostal space and the anterior axillary line, second heart sound split, and hyperphonetic pulmonary component. At the aortic auscultation site, it was perceived a diamond-shaped mid-systolic murmur (4+/6+), associated with palpable fremitus, radiating to the neck. No jugular distention was detected. The abdomen presented prominent and tender hepatomegaly (2 cm off the costal border) and splenomegaly (dullness on percussion of Traube's area) along with a non-tender indirect inguinal herniation on the right side. Both lower and upper extremities presented no signs of edema nor hypoperfusion.

Diagnosis, Assessment, and Treatment

During follow-up, the patient eventually accepted a surgical approach to his heart disease and then was submitted to a cardiac surgery for the replacement of his compromised aortic valve by a metallic prosthesis.

The performed X-ray images obtained corroborated with abnormal osteoarticular deformities (1–2), along with the suspected presence of an enlarged left ventricle (Figs. 1, 2, and 3), which was confirmed by a 12-lead ECG (Fig. 4).

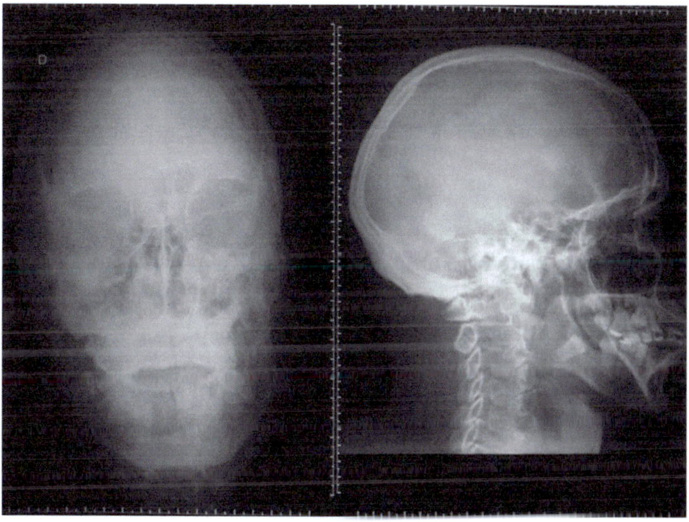

FIGURE 1 X-ray imaging of the patient's skull and cervical spine. Notice the areas of altered bone density in the superior dental arcade

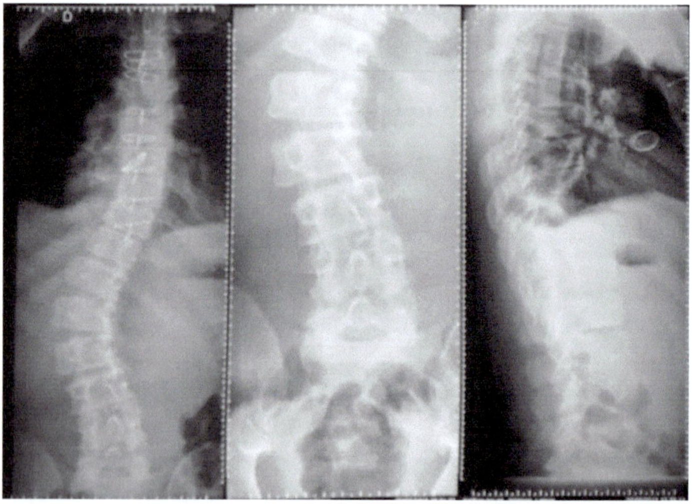

FIGURE 2 X-ray images of the patient's thoracic and lumbar vertebrae, confirming the finding during physical examination

Questions

1. What kind of valvular commitment is most related to rheumatic heart disease, and what is its most common clinical presentation?

The valves most affected by rheumatic fever, in order, are the mitral, aortic, tricuspid, and pulmonary. In most cases, the mitral valve is involved with one or more from the other three. In acute disease, small thrombi form along the lines of valve closure. In chronic disease, there are thickening and fibrosis of the valve resulting in stenosis or, less commonly, regurgitation [7].

2. What is the pathophysiology related to rheumatic heart disease?

Rheumatic fever is a late inflammatory and nonsuppurative complication of pharyngitis caused by group A-hemolytic streptococci. Rheumatic fever results from humoral- and

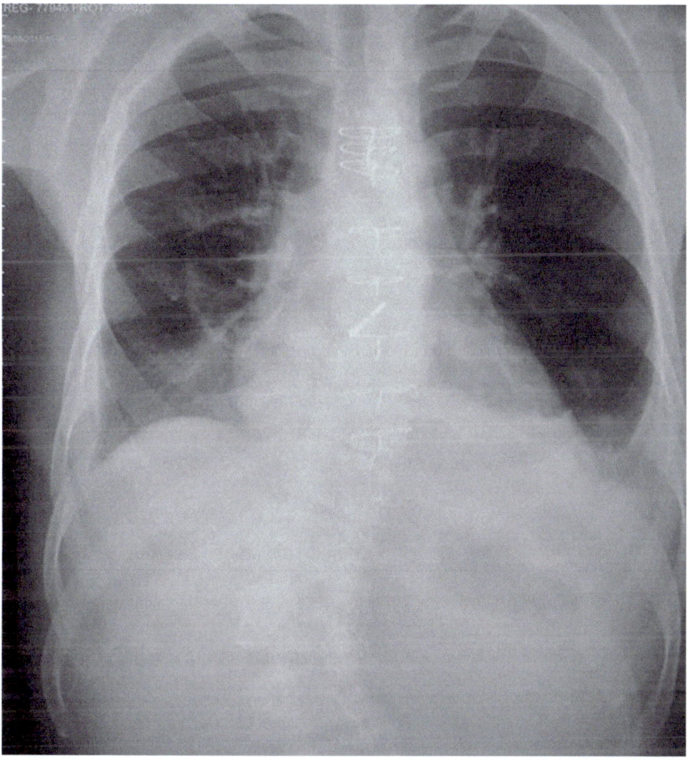

FIGURE 3 An X-ray of the patient's chest, in which it is immediately perceived as an enlarged mediastinum, a cardiac figure, and a congestive pattern of the pulmonary vessels

cellular-mediated immune responses occurring 1–3 weeks after the onset of streptococcal pharyngitis. Streptococcal proteins display molecular mimicry recognized by the immune system, especially bacterial M-proteins and human cardiac antigens such as myosin and valvular endothelium. Antimyosin antibody recognizes laminin, an extracellular matrix alpha-helix coiled protein, which is part of the valve basement membrane structure [1].

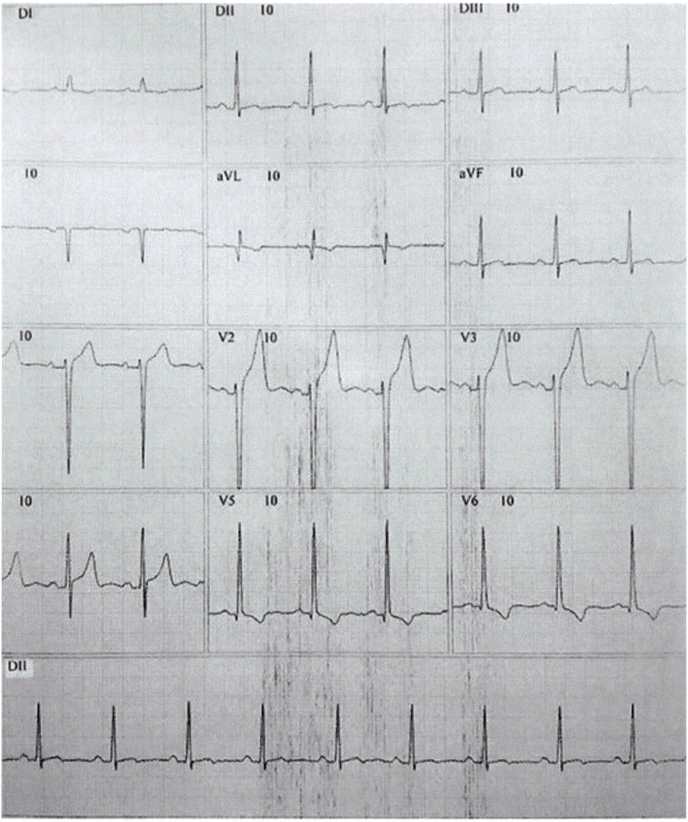

FIGURE 4 An ECG in which there is a clear pattern of left ventricular hypertrophy (notice the presence of the "strain pattern" in leads V5 and V6, along with the high R waves and the deep S waves in V1 to V3)

3. How would you manage a patient whom you suspect that suffers from a rheumatic valvulopathy?

The diagnosis of rheumatic fever is clinical and there is no specific exam. The Jones's criteria is the gold standard, for the diagnosis of the first outbreak/manifestation of the RF. They are divided on major and minor diagnostic criteria, and the diagnosis is made with two major or one major and two minor criteria, which are:

- Major diagnostic criteria: carditis, polyarthritis, chorea, erythema marginatum, subcutaneous nodules
- Minor diagnostic criteria: fever, arthralgia, previous rheumatic fever or rheumatic heart disease, acute phase reactions, erythrocyte sedimentation rate/C-reactive protein/leukocytosis, prolonged PR interval

An electrocardiogram (ECG) and a chest X-ray are usually carried out in conjunction with a clinical examination. TTE (transthoracic echocardiogram) is recommended in the initial evaluation of patients with known or suspected valvulopathy to confirm the diagnosis, establish etiology, determine severity, assess hemodynamic consequences, determine prognosis, and evaluate for timing of intervention [9].

Despite the absence of a randomized comparison between the results of valve replacement and repair, it is widely accepted that, when feasible, valve repair is the optimal surgical treatment in patients with severe lesion.

The management of symptomatic patients depends on the left ventricular dysfunction; if ejection fraction (EF) ≤30%, the surgery is recommended (repair whenever possible); if EF >30% and is refractory to medical therapy, the valve repair should be considered; if EF >30% and it is not refractory to medical therapy, the treatment of heart failure is extended. The management of asymptomatic patients is controversial; however, surgery can be proposed if the valvular damage is severe.

The indication for antibiotic prophylaxis has been significantly reduced in the recent European Society of Cardiology guidelines [10].

4. What kind of genetic disease could be responsible for the abovementioned physical deformities?

Marfan syndrome, Hunter syndrome (mucopolysaccharidosis type 2), Rubinstein-Taybi syndrome

5. Is any single genetic disease a possible diagnosis for the totality of this patient's health problems?

Yes, it could be a case of Hunter syndrome.

6. What is the pathophysiology of the mucopolysaccharidosis, and what type is more related to this patient's clinical framework?

The mucopolysaccharidoses (MPSs) are inherited metabolic disorders caused by genetic defects that result in the absence or severe deficiency of one of the lysosomal hydrolases responsible for the degradation of glycosaminoglycans (GAGs). MPSs are part of the group of lysosomal storage disorders (LSDs) which are all autosomal-recessive, with the exception of Hunter syndrome, or MPS II, which is an X-linked recessive disease [3].

Hunter syndrome is caused by a deficiency of iduronate 2-sulfatase (I2S, EC 3.1.6.13), which normally cleaves a sulfate group from the GAGs, heparan and dermatan sulfate. A shortage of I2S leads to an accumulation of undegraded GAGs within the lysosomes of various organs and tissues, including the central nervous system (CNS) [3].

7. What further tests or exams would you perform in order to obtain a diagnosis for this patient genetic disease?

Diagnosis is based on screening urinary glycosaminoglycans and confirmation by measuring I2S activity and analyzing I2S gene mutations.

8. What was the most probable cause of this patient cardiac problem: his genetic disease or a rheumatic valvulopathy?

Because of the rarity of MPS, cardiac studies involving large numbers of individuals with a particular type are uncommon. Nevertheless, the prevalence and severity of cardiovascular disease in individuals with MPS (especially MPS I, II, and VI) is strikingly high, occurring in 60–100% of those studied [4–6]. Cardiac valve involvement appears more common in those syndromes in which dermatan sulfate catabolism is deranged (MPS I, II, and VI but not MPS III and IV) [4–6].

Bibliography

1. Cunningham M. T cell mimicry in inflammatory heart disease. Mol Immunol Feb. 2004;40(14–15):1121–7.
2. Remenyi B, et al. Valvular aspects of rheumatic heart disease. Lancet. 2016;387(10025):1335–46.

3. Neufeld E, Muenzer J. The mucopolysaccharidoses. In: Scriver CR, Beaudet AL, Sly WS, Valle D, editors. The metabolic and molecular bases of inherited disease. 8th ed. New York: McGraw- Hill; 2001. p. 3421–52.
4. Chen MR, Lin SP, Hwang HK, Yu CH. Cardiovascular changes in mucopolysaccharidoses in Taiwan. Acta Cardiol. 2005;60:51–3.
5. Dangel JH. Cardiovascular changes in children with mucopolysaccharide storage diseases and related disorders: clinical and echocardiographic findings in 64 patients. Eur J Pediatr. 1998;157:534.
6. Leal GN, de Paula AC, Leone C, Kim C. Echocardiographic study of paediatric patients with mucopolysaccharidosis. Cardiol Young. 2010;20:254–61.
7. Burke AP. Pathology of Rheumatic Heart Disease; 2015. Available: http://emedicine.medscape.com/article/1962779-overview#a1. Upload: 15 Oct 2015.
8. Braunlin EA, Harmatz PR, Scarpa M, Furlanetto B, Kampmann C, Loehr JP, Ponder KP, Roberts WC, Rosenfeld HM, Giugliani R. Cardiac disease in patients with mucopolysaccharidosis: presentation, diagnosis and management. J Inherit Metab Dis. 2011;34:1183–97.
9. Special Writing Group of the Committee on Rheumatic Fever, Endocarditis, and Kawasaki Disease of the Council on Cardiovascular Disease in the Young of the American Heart Association. Guidelines for the diagnosis of rheumatic fever. Jones Criteria, 1992 update. JAMA. 1992;268(15):2069–73. Erratum in: JAMA 1993 Jan 27;269(4):476.
10. Vahanian A, Alfieri O, Andreotti F. ESC/EACTS guidelines on the management of valvular heart disease. Eur Heart J. 2012. https://doi.org/10.1093/eurheartj/ehs109 & Eur J Cardiothorac Surg. https://doi.org/10.1093/ejcts/ezs455.

Rheumatic Mitral Valve Stenosis: A Surgical Case

Vitor Abaurre Amaral, Lissa Canedo Rocha, Gabriel Donato Amorim, and Melchior Luiz Lima

Clinical Presentation

A 61-year-old woman came to a cardiology checkup consultation. She was asymptomatic at the time. Her blood pressure was 122/67 mmHg, and the auscultation revealed an opening snap associated with a diastolic murmur at the mitral area.

Diagnosis, Assessment, and Treatment

An electrocardiogram (ECG) was performed, and a first-degree atrioventricular block (AVB) was found, without signs of left ventricular overload. The patient had a history of rheumatic disease, which suggested, along with the ECG and auscultation findings, a possible rheumatic mitral valve stenosis.

A series of tests were made including urinalysis, lipid profile, glycemic profile, and complete blood count. Also, considering the high possibility of mitral valve disease, an echocardiogram

V. A. Amaral (✉) · L. C. Rocha · G. D. Amorim · M. L. Lima
School of Sciences of Santa Casa de Misericórdia de Vitória (EMESCAM), Vitória, ES, Brazil

R. M. S. Almeida, F. B. Jatene (eds.), *Cardiovascular Surgery*,
https://doi.org/10.1007/978-3-319-57084-6_38

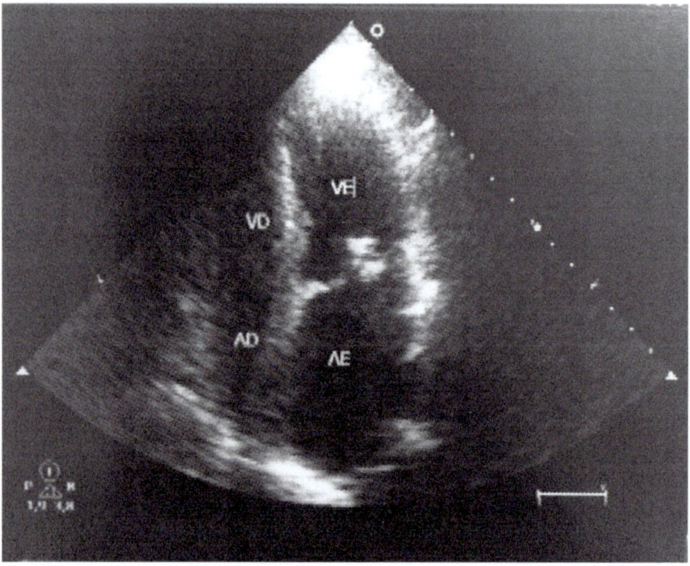

FIGURE 1 Echocardiography photo of the four cardiac chambers displaying severe mitral valve calcification

with Doppler (Figs. 1, 2, and 3) was performed, with the following results.

Structural Parameters

Aorta, 20 mm; left atrium, 52 mm; right ventricular diameter, 24 mm; final diastolic diameter of the left ventricle, 40 mm; diastolic septal thickness, 9 mm; diastolic thickness of the left ventricle posterior wall, 8 mm; mitral valve area of 0.88 cm2

Left atrium/aorta relation, 2.60; ejection fraction (Teichholz), 71%; ejection fraction (65%); left ventricular mass, 102 g; mass index of the left ventricle, 68.08 g/m2; percent encurt cavidade, 40%; septum/pulmonary pressure of the left ventricle relation, 1.13; final diastolic volume of the left ventricle, 70 ml; final diastolic volume index, 47 ml; systolic volume of the left ventricle, 50 ml; volume/mass relation, 0.63 ml/g; final systolic volume, 20 ml

Left atrium volume index, 65; E/A relation, 0.94; E/e' relation, 36; deceleration time, 745 ms

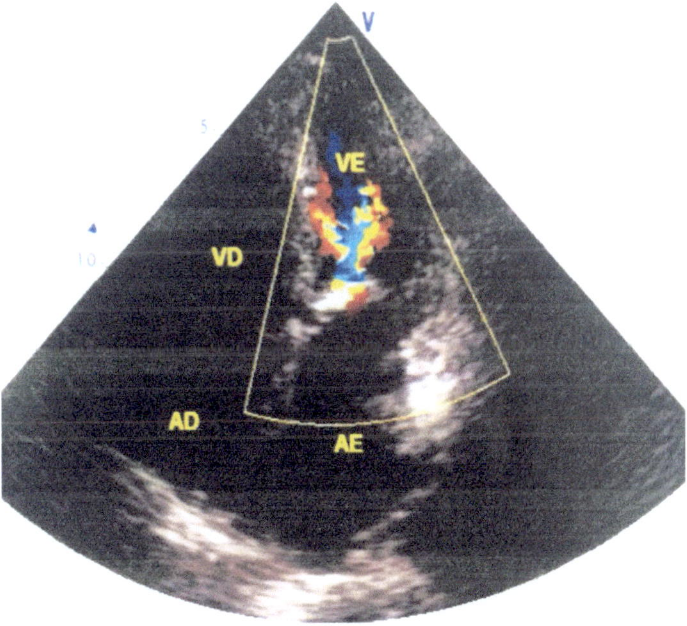

FIGURE 2 Echocardiography photo of the four cardiac chambers showing turbulent flow at the left ventricle due to severe mitral stenosis

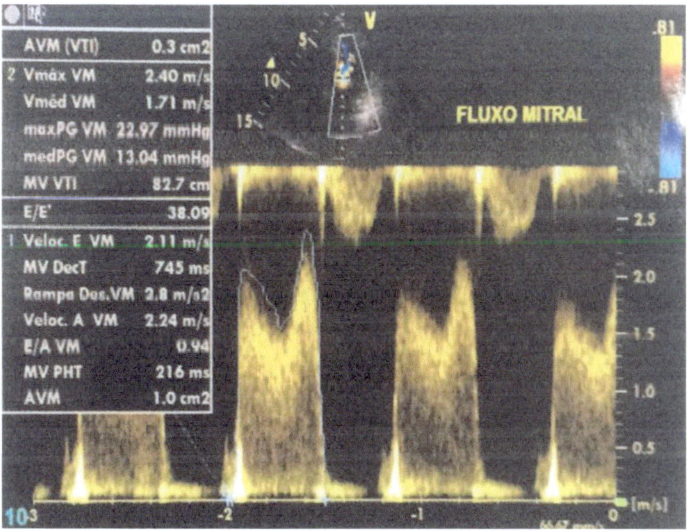

FIGURE 3 Pathologic mitral valve flow displaying important stenosis

Severe increase of the left ventricle, normal myocardial contractility at rest, severe mitral stenosis, minimum aortic and mitral regurgitation, discreet pulmonary hypertension

Conclusions

Severe mitral stenosis, severe increase of the left atrium, preserved biventricular systolic function, discreet pulmonary arterial hypertension

The echocardiogram with Doppler, as seen from Figs. 1, 2, and 3, confirmed the hypothesis of severe mitral stenosis, with intense calcification and area of 0.88 cm^2. At the time of this evaluation, the patient was referring important dyspnea, even at rest (leading to a NYHA IV classification of heart failure).

How to proceed?

For a best intervention indication, the symptomatic mitral stenosis NYHA functional class III–IV fluxogram (Fig. 4) was followed. Considering the valve area of 0.88 cm2 and non-favorable valve morphology for PMBV (percutaneous mitral balloon valvuloplasty) and also that the patient was not a high-risk surgical candidate, mitral valve replacement was indicated. Favoring surgical intervention, the echocardiogram examiner concluded in his report 12-point Wilkins score (Table 2). The types of valve prosthesis were explained to the patient, and the surgical decision for a bioprosthesis was made considering her will.

With surgery indicated, some preoperative exams were requested (Figs. 5, 6, and 7), with the following results.

Cineangiocoronariography

Coronary arteries without obstructive lesions

Blood Count

Surgery description

The patient was received in the operating room awake and well. The anesthetist explained how the anesthesia would be performed. Electrodes were placed in her back, followed by

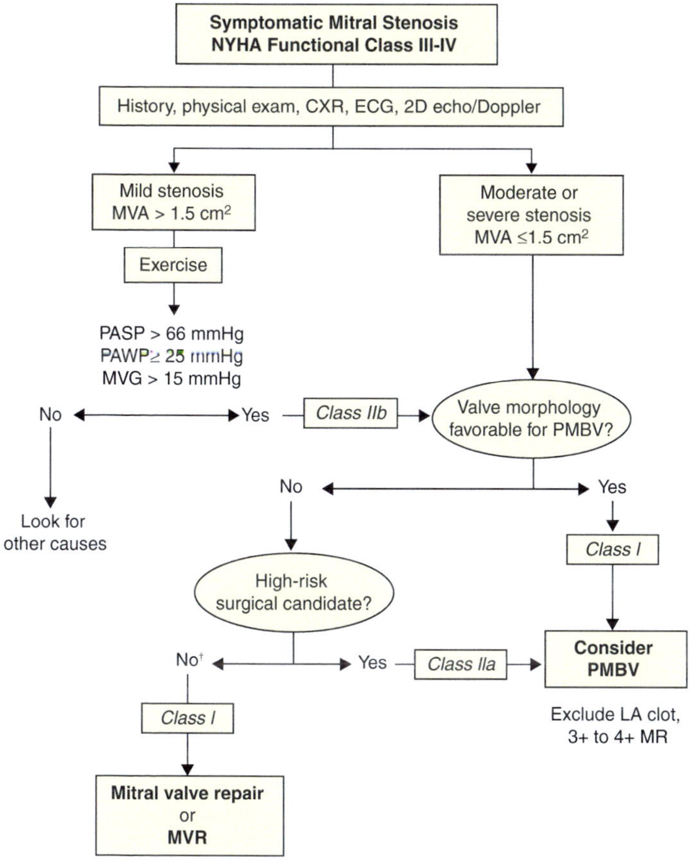

FIGURE 4 (Kirklin/Barratt-Boyes Cardiac Surgery, fourth edition)

peripheral venous catheterization with a Jelco 14 catheter and radial artery catheterization for median blood pressure.

Anesthesia was induced with fentany 15 mcg/kg (using 15mcg/kg during the whole procedure), propofol 2 mg/kg (followed by orotrachcal intubation for mechanical ventilation), and rocuronium for neuromuscular blockade with 0.6 mg/kg (plus 0.6mk/kg with the extracorporeal circulation). General anesthesia was kept with both venous and gas (sevoflurane) anesthetics.

Bladder catheterization was performed with an 18 Foley catheter. Then, her internal jugular vein was also catheterized

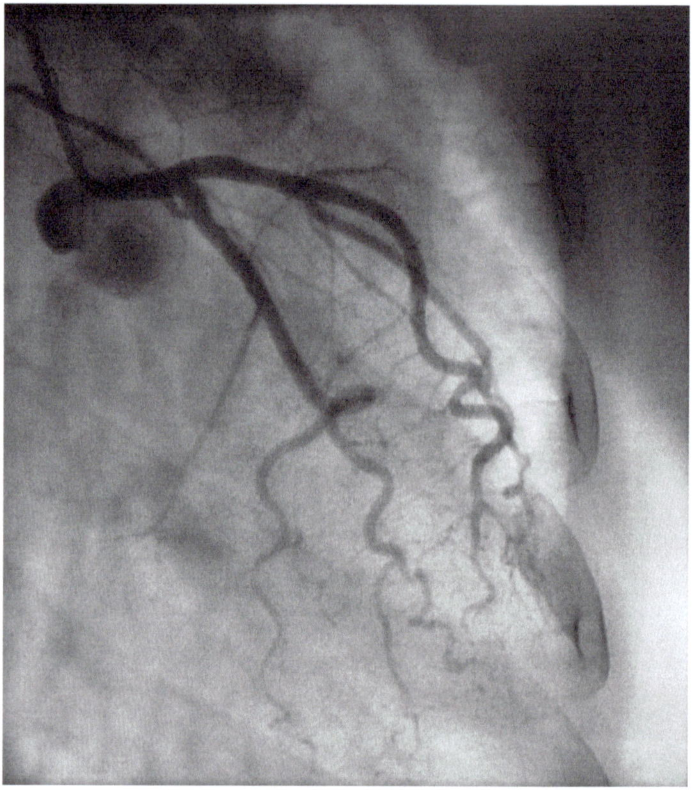

Figure 5 Left coronary artery cineangiocoronariography showing no significant obstructive lesions

using Seldinger's technique to insert a triple-lumen catheter for drug injection (e.g., sodium nitroprusside or norepinephrine). Asepsis and antisepsis were made and the surgical field was assembled.

For this surgery, median sternotomy was performed, followed by pericardiotomy and exposure of the heart. Purse string sutures were made for superior and inferior vena cava (simple purse string suture) and aorta (double purse string suture) cannulation. For the aorta, a cannula number 22 was used and for the venae cavae, cannulas number 3/8 were

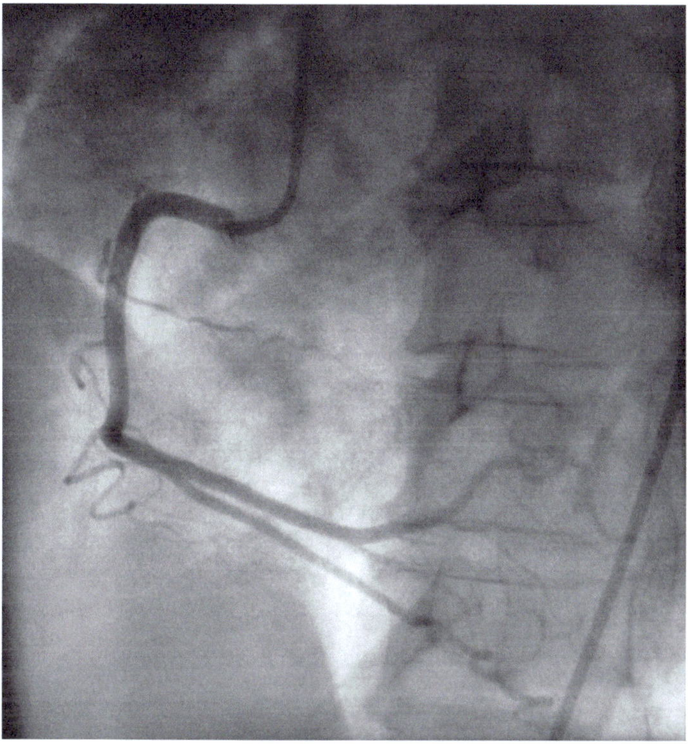

FIGURE 6 Right coronary artery cineangiocoronariography showing no significant obstructive lesions

inserted. The patient was heparinized (230 mg of heparin), and extracorporeal circulation was initiated.

Priming hypothermia was not necessary. The priming had the operation room's temperature (about 23 degrees Celsius). Antegrade hypothermic (15 degrees Celsius) hyperkalemic cardioplegia was used through the ascending aorta. An aortic clamp was placed and the cardiac chambers were all drained.

To approach the mitral valve, left atriotomy was made, and, for better exposure of the sick valve, a Cooley's retractor was used. First, the left auricle was inspected looking for blood thrombus. After that, the surgical inspection of the

Blood count:
Eritrogram

Red blood cells.. 4.85mm^3
Hemoglobin.. 14.9 g/dL
Hematocrit... 44.1%
MCV... 90.9 u3
MHC... 30.7 Pg
MCHC... 33.8%
RDW... 13.1%

Leucogram

Leukocytes..10170mm^3
Segmented neutrophils................................. 55.5% ... 5644mm^3
Lymphocytes... 30.8% ... 3132mm^3
Monocytes... 10.6 % ... 1078 mm^3
Eosinophils.. 2.5% ... 25mm^3
Platelets.. 271,000mm^3
Prothrombin Time....................................15.2 ... INR 1.14
Activated Partial Thromboplastin Time............ 22.5
Glucose... 85 mg/dL
Total Cholesterol.................................... 226 mg/dL
HDL Cholesterol..................................... 52 mg/dL
Triglycerides... 119 mg/dL
Urea.. 48 mg/dL
Creatinine.. 0.80 mg/dL
Uric acid.. 5.2 mg/dL
Calcium... 10.3 mg/dL
Magnesium.. 1.9 mg/dL
Aspartate transaminase........................ 32 U/L
Pyruvic transaminase........................... 30 U/L
Total bilirubin...................................... 0.5 mg/dL
Direct bilirubin.................................... 0.1 mg/dL
Indirect bilirubin.................................. 0.4 mg/dL

FIGURE 7 Blood count and urinalysis

Urinalysis: volume of 45ml, density of 1020, pH 6,0, coloration: light yellow, clear, no others abnormalities.

Anti HBS.. reagent
Anti HCV.. non reagent
Anti HBC IgG.................................... non reagent
Anti HBC IgM.................................... non reagent
HIV 1 and 2....................................... non reagent

Blood.. AB negative
Coagulation time.............................. 5.40
Bleeding time (DUKE)......................... 1.10 minutes

Sodium.. 140 mmol/L
Potassium.. 4.5 mmol/L
Fibrinogen.. 300.7 mg/dL

FIGURE 7 (continued)

mitral valve showed severe calcification on the anterior leaflet and commissures, leading to an intraoperative diagnosis compatible with the echocardiographic one.

The anterior leaflet and commissures were removed and all the calcium lumps carefully withdraw. Part of the posterior leaflet was preserved, as well as the secondary chordae to protect the posterior wall from disruption. As figured, the disease was in a very advanced stage and the patient was at imminent death risk.

Figure 8 (Cooley's retractor)

Following the removal of the valve (Fig. 8), a biological prosthetic valve size 29 was implanted with the interrupted suture technique (Fig. 9), and the final result can be seen in Fig. 10.

After checking for the correct prosthetic valve's position, the left atrium was sutured; cavitary air was removed as well as the aortic clamp. Normothermic myocardial reperfusion was initiated.

With the heartbeatings recovered, extracorporeal circulation was interrupted. The cannulas were removed from the

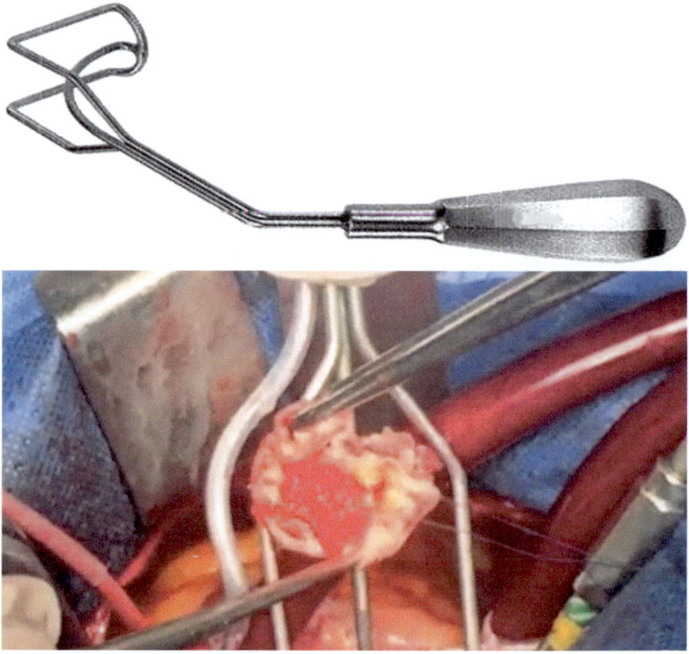

Figure 8 Photography of the removed mitral valve anterior leaflet. Severe calcification and thickness are displayed

aorta, superior vena cava, and inferior vena cava, and protamine was injected to antagonize the effects of heparin.

Medium mediastinal drainage was installed, along with an epicardial pacemaker. Hemostasis was checked and, after suturing all planes, the procedure was over.

Surgery's Stats

- Patient's age: 61 years old
- Patient's stature: 147 cm
- Patient's weight: 57,5 kg
- Corporal surface: 1500 m^2
- Extracorporeal circulation time: 85 min

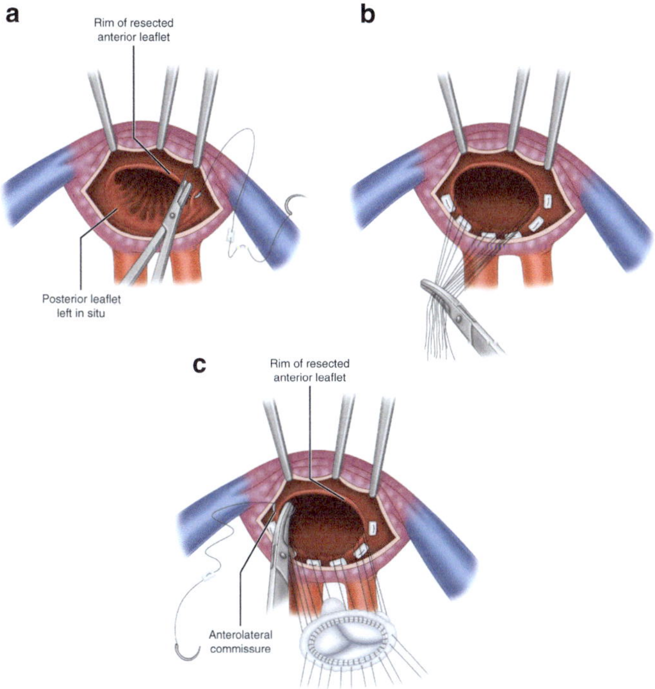

FIGURE 9 (Kirklin/Barratt-Boyes Cardiac Surgery, fourth edition)

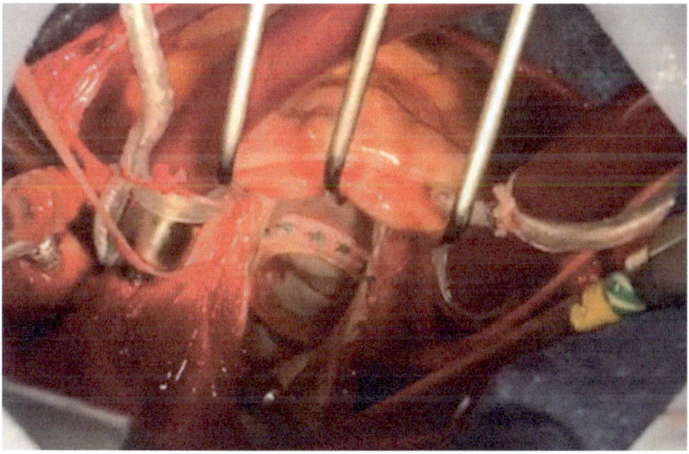

FIGURE 10 Implanted mitral valve bioprosthesis

- Aortic cross clamp time: 75 min
- No perioperative complications
- Post-extracorporeal circulation blood balance: -23 ml

She had a good recovery and was sent home after 1 week and 2 days.

Questions

1. When surgery should be indicated in a patient with mitral stenosis?

Surgery is indicated for symptomatic patients (NYHA functional class III–IV) with any of the following contraindications to percutaneous mitral balloon valvuloplasty: unfavorable valve anatomy (Wilkins score greater than 8 associated with calcification and insufficiency of the subvalvular apparatus), presence of mitral lesion with moderate to important insufficiency, concomitant tricuspid or aortic significant valve disease, and persistent left atrial thrombus (without resolution after adequate oral anticoagulation).

Surgery also benefits patients with moderate to important mitral stenosis associated with important embolic events, despite adequate anticoagulation therapy and those with CF I or II, with severe pulmonary hypertension and without favorable anatomy for percutaneous mitral balloon valvuloplasty. Patients with atrial fibrillation (AF) who will undergo valve surgery may benefit from concomitant surgical treatment of AF (as maze surgery or radiofrequency ablation).

2. What is the Wilkins score?

The Wilkins score (Table 1), described in 1988, consists in echocardiographic assessment of the mitral valve with an emphasis on the description of structural aspects. Four parameters are considered: mobility of the leaflets, valvular thickening, calcification degree, and involvement of the subvalvular apparatus. A degree of four points for each item results in a score, which can range from 4 to 16 points. Patients with lower Wilkins score or equal to 8 are candidates for

TABLE 1 Wilkins score

Grade	Mobility	Subvalvular thickening	Thickening	Calcification
1	Highly mobile valve with only leaflet tips restricted	Minimal thickening just below the mitral leaflets	Leaflets near normal in thickness (4–5 mm)	A single area of increased echo brightness
2	Leaflet mid- and base portions have normal mobility	Thickening of chordal structures extending up to one third of the chordal length	Mid-leaflets normal, considerable thickening of margins (5–8 mm)	Scattered areas of brightness
3	Valve continues to move forward in diastole, mainly from the base	Thickening extending to the distal third of the cords	Thickening extending though the entire leaflet (5–8 mm)	Brightness extending into the midportion of the leaflets
4	No or minimal forward movement of the leaflets in diastole	Extensive thickening and shortening of all chordal structures extending down to the papillary muscles	Considerable thickening of all leaflet tissue (>8–10 mm)	Extensive brightness through much of the leaflet tissue

The total echocardiographic score was derived from an analysis of mitral leaflet mobility, valvar and subvalvular thickening, and calcification which were graded from 0 to 4 according to the above criteria. This gave a total score of 0–16

percutaneous mitral valvuloplasty, in the absence of other contraindications.

3. What types of prosthetic heart valves are available in the treatment of mitral stenosis? How to choose which type should be used?

There are two types of prostheses: the mechanical and biological.

Mechanical valve prostheses are formed by metal rings that support the discs, or balls cages, which could be of Silastic®, metal, or pyrolytic carbon. They are subdivided into prosthetic valve ball cage, double hemi-disc prosthesis, and single-disc prosthesis.

The biological valve prostheses emerged as an alternative to mechanical valves due to complications of permanent anticoagulation and high thrombogenic risk. They can be heterologous, such as porcine prosthesis and bovine pericardium, or homologous, which are subdivided into heterografts, when removed from human cadaver tissues, and autografts, when the non-valvular tissue is obtained from the patient.

The first stage of choice is the decision between a mechanical and biological prosthesis, and the risks/benefits should be taken into account. Factors that favor the use of the mechanical one include patient desire, other anticoagulation indications, risk of rapid deterioration valve, and age <65 years, with high life expectancy; bioprosthesis is favored with patient's desire, when optimized anticoagulant therapy is not possible, age over 65 years and low life expectancy, and women of childbearing age.

After defining the type of prosthesis, the doctor needs to assess which of the mechanical has less thromboembolic risk or which bioprosthesis has more durability. It is also important to observe the hemodynamic performance and transprosthetic gradient.

4. How is rheumatic fever diagnosed?

The diagnosis of the rheumatic fever is clinical, with no pathognomonic signal or specific exam. The laboratorial exams, although nonspecific, support the diagnosis of the inflammatory process and the streptococcal infection. The

TABLE 2 Guidelines for the diagnosis of an initial attack of rheumatic fever (1992)

Major manifestations	Minor manifestations	Supporting evidence of antecedent group A streptococcal infection
Carditis	Clinical findings: Arthralgia Fever	Positive throat or rapid streptococcal antigen test, OR Elevated or rising streptococcal antibody titer
Polyarthritis Sydenham chorea Erythema marginatum	Laboratory findings: Elevated acute phase reactants Erythrocyte sedimentation rate C-reactive protein	
Subcutaneous nodules	Prolonged P-R interval	

If supported by evidence of preceding group A streptococcal infection, the presence of two major manifestations or of one major and two minor manifestations indicates a high probability of acute rheumatic fever

criteria of Jones, established in 1944, had its last modification in 1992 and keeps being considered the "gold standard" for the diagnosis of the first outbreak of rheumatic fever (Table 2). The division of the criteria in major and minor is based on the specificity and not in the frequency of the manifestation. The probability of the rheumatic fever is high when there is evidence of previous streptococcal infection, determined by the elevation of antistreptolysin O titer, beyond the presence of at least two major criteria or one major criterion and two minor.

5. What are the main comorbidities resulting from rheumatic heart disease?

Carditis is the most severe manifestation of rheumatic fever, because it is the only one that can have long-term sequels and result in death. The cardiac involvement is characterized by pancarditis; however, the valve lesions are responsible for the clinic condition and prognostic. The pericardial involvement is not usual, does not occur in isolation, and does not result in constriction. The involvement of the endocardium (endocarditis/valvulitis) which is the diagnostic hallmark of carditis involves more often the mitral and aortic valves. In the acute phase, the most frequent lesion is the mitral regurgitation, and in second place comes the aortic regurgitation. On the other hand, the valvular stenosis occurs lately, in the chronic phase.

6. Is there prevention for rheumatic fever?

Rheumatic fever comes as a result of a non-treated pharyngotonsillitis caused by the group A beta hemolytic *Streptococcus pyogenes.* Thus, prevention for the rheumatic disease is an effective treatment of the pharyngotonsillitis, with benzathine penicillin or erythromycin. With the correct clinical treatment, the patient will not develop the fever and its complications.

7. Which complications are related to valve surgery?

After mitral valve repair, the anterior systolic movement can influence negatively on the left ventricular fraction of ejection, and, in general, the incidence of thromboembolism is low. About the surgery, the mortality is higher in procedures of resuscitation, especially in reoperations. The most important causes of morbidity and mortality are related with the chronic myocardial dysfunction, thromboembolism, endocarditis, bleeding by anticoagulants, and coronary artery diseases.

8. Are there any other forms of treatment for mitral stenosis?

Beyond the surgery, there are other options of treatment, as the pharmacological and the percutaneous mitral balloon valvuloplasty (PMBV). The drug therapy could just relieve symptoms, without any direct effects on the fixed obstruction. In case of mild mitral stenosis, with the patient asymptomatic and in sinus rhythm, there is no need of specific pharmacological intervention. In patients with moderate to important mitral stenosis, pharmacological treatment could be displayed while the patient waits for interventionist procedure, aiming the improvement of the symptoms or controlling the complications (e.g., atrial fibrillation).

The PMBV has a high rate of success, which swings between 80% and 95%. However, the obtainment of those results requires an experienced and trained hemodynamic team. The main contraindications to this technique are the previous existence of moderate to important mitral insufficiency, left atrium thrombus, unfavorable Wilkins score (above 8 points), presence of other concomitant valvulopathies that require surgery treatment, and coronary artery disease with indication of revascularization surgery associated.

Bibliography

1. Kouchoukos N, Kirklin J. Kirklin/Barratt-Boyes cardiac surgery. 1st ed. Philadelphia: Elsevier/Saunders; 2013. p. 473–540.
2. Who.int. WHO | Rheumatic fever and rheumatic heart disease. [online]. 2017. Available at: http://www.who.int/cardiovascular_diseases/publications/trs923/en/. Accessed 1 Oct 2016.
3. Mota CCC, et al. Rheumatic fever prevention program: long-term evolution and outcomes. Front Pediatr N.p. 2015. Web. 1 Oct 2016.
4. TARASOUTCHI F, et al. Diretriz Brasileira de Valvopatias – SBC 2011/ I Diretriz Interamericana de Valvopatias – SIAC 2011. Arquivos brasileiros de cardiologia, São Paulo. 2011;97(5, supl. 1):1–67.
5. Barbosa PJB, Müller RE, Latado AL, Achutti AC, Ramos AIO, Weksler C, et al. Diretrizes Brasileiras para Diagnóstico, Tratamento e Prevenção da Febre Reumática da Sociedade Brasileira de Cardiologia, da Sociedade Brasileira de Pediatria e da Sociedade Brasileira de Reumatologia. Arquivos brasileiros de cardiologia., São Paulo. 2009;93(3, supl. 4):3–18.
6. Rajamannan NM, Antonini-Canterin F, Moura L, Zamorano JL, Rosenhek RA, Best PJ, Lloyd MA, Rocha-Goncalves F, Chandra S, Alfieri O, Lancellotti P, Tornos P, Baliga RR, Wang A, Bashore T, Ramakrishnan S, Spargias K, Shuvy M, Beeri R, Lotan C, Suwaidi JA, Bahl V, Pierard LA, Maurer G, Nicolosi GL, Rahimtoola SH,

Chopra K, Pandian NG. Medical therapy for rheumatic heart disease: is it time to be proactive rather than reactive? Indian Heart J. 2009;61(1):14–23.
7. Liguori GR, Barros LN, Tenório DF, Jatene FB, Almeida RMS. Manual Acadêmico de Cirurgia Cardiovascular, São Paulo; 2014. p. 199–211.

Sutureless Aortic Prosthesis Implantation: The First Brazilian Experience with Perceval Device

Rodrigo Petersen Saadi, Marina Petersen Saadi, João Carlos Guaragna, and Eduardo Keller Saadi

Clinical Presentation

A 63-year-old physically active man diagnosed with aortic stenosis 2 years ago started with dyspnea NYHA class II. The physical examination showed a systolic murmur. His current echocardiography showed severe aortic stenosis with a heavily calcified tricuspid aortic valve (peak and mean gradient, 129/75 mmHg, respectively; peak velocity, 4.5 m/s; and valve area, 0.9 cm^2).

Diagnosis, Assessment, and Treatment

This was a low-risk surgical patient with a mean Society of Thoracic Surgeons (STS) score of 0.97. Signs, symptoms, and echocardiography findings confirmed severe aortic stenosis. Because of the severe symptomatic aortic stenosis, surgery was indicated. Open surgery was chosen because of the low operation risk. Rapid deployment technique was preferred

R. P. Saadi (✉) · M. P. Saadi · J. C. Guaragna · E. K. Saadi
Pontifical Catholic University of Rio Grande do Sul (PUC- RS), Porto Alegre, RS, Brazil
e-mail: rodrigosaadi@terra.com.br

R. M. S. Almeida, F. B. Jatene (eds.), *Cardiovascular Surgery*,
https://doi.org/10.1007/978-3-319-57084-6_39

mainly because of the lower gradient with this prosthesis. The surgery was performed in May 2016 at the Hospital de Clínicas de Porto Alegre, Brazil, according to Dedeilias technique description [4]. After a median full sternotomy, a routine cannulation to the extracorporeal circulation was carried out with aortic cannula at the distal part of the ascending aorta and a two-stage venous cannula at the right atrium. The cross clamp was applied as distal as possible in the ascending aorta, and a transverse aortotomy was performed 1 cm distal to the sinotubular junction (approximately 3.5 cm above the valve ring), followed by direct cannulation of the coronary ostium and delivering of cold hyperkalemic cardioplegia solution (St. Thomas). After the calcified native aortic valve leaflets were removed and the aortic annulus decalcified and measured, three guiding sutures were positioned 2 mm below the nadir of the native leaflet insertion line of each valve sinus. These sutures were passed through the corresponding eyelets in the prosthetic inflow ring, as a reference for alignment of the inflow section of the prosthesis with the insertion plane of the native leaflets. The device is selected at the time of operation with dedicated sizers, and the annulus diameter should be more than 19 mm and less than 27 mm.

The prosthetic valve was released in two phases, first, the inflow section of the valve, followed by the opening of the outflow part (Fig. 1), and then a post-implant dilatation was done with a balloon catheter at pressures of 4 atm for 30 s (Fig. 2). Once the prosthesis was completely deployed, the guiding sutures were removed.

Three-dimensional transesophageal echocardiography performed by experienced echocardiographer was available during all the procedure.

In order to allow expansion and anchorage of the device and reduce migration risk, the ratio between the sinotubular junction diameter and the aortic valve annulus couldn't exceed 1.3.

The procedure was performed with participation of a doctor of the University of Graz in Austria. The cardiopulmonary bypass time was 38 min and the cross-clamping time was

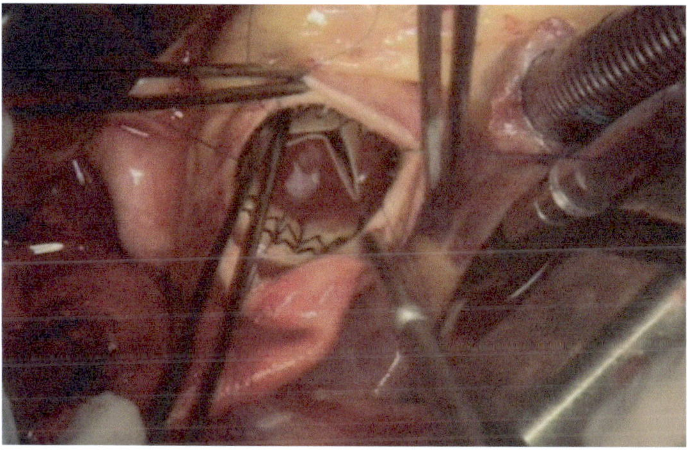

FIGURE 1 Sutureless valve after deployment

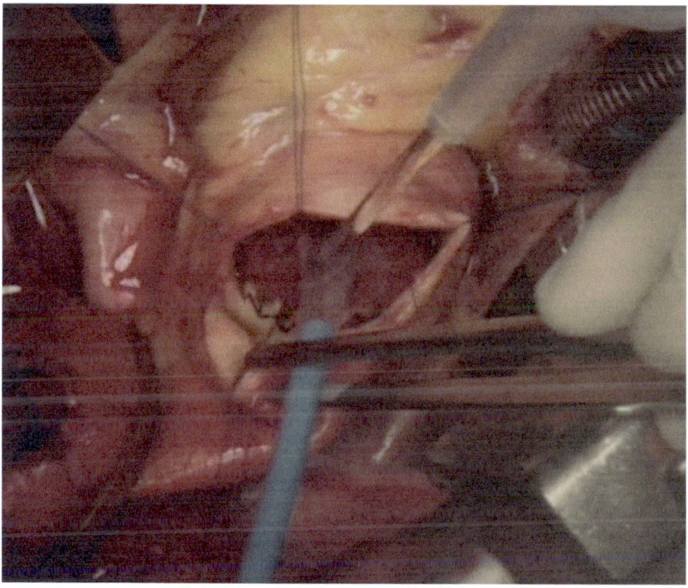

FIGURE 2 Balloon accommodation of the sutureless valve with warm saline

30 min. Mechanical ventilation weaning, postoperative bleeding control, and intensive care unit stay were carried out according to the routine of the cardiovascular surgery postoperative care (48 h in ICU and 3 more days on the ward).

Postoperative echocardiography showed mean gradient 8 mmHg and there was no paravalvular leak.

The patient had favorable postoperative clinical course. There was no major complication or atrioventricular block determining need of pacemaker implant. He was discharged on the 5th postoperative day.

Questions

1. What is a sutureless valve?

It is a self-expandable valve that does not suture to the aortic annulus and consists of a nitinol cage and bovine pericardium leaflets. It is collapsed into a delivery system at the time of operation and is a rapid deployment device inserted through an aortotomy.

2. What are the potential clinical indications?

It is indicated in low-risk physically active patients with severe aortic stenosis, because of the low gradient during exercise than the conventional prosthesis patients. It has been shown to be beneficial in intermediate-risk patients in a gray zone between conventional surgery and transcatheter aortic valve implantation.

3. For what valve position it can be used?

So far, just for aortic position.

4. What are the potential advantages comparing to conventional surgical valves?

Reducing the duration of the operation, length of hospitalization, less blood transfusion which is ideal for combined operation (double valve or valve and myocardial revascularization). It is also very good for elderly people with a small annulus due to excellent hemodynamic performance with lower residual gradients.

5. Are there contraindications?

Pure aortic insufficiency and a ratio >1,3 between the diameter of the sinotubular junction and the annulus diameter. This is measured by the preoperative transthoracic echocardiography. When the ascending aorta is dilated above this ratio, there is a risk of device migration, and its use is contraindicated. When the annulus is less than 19 mm or more than 27 mm, the valve should not be used.

6. Should the native valve be removed before implanting this device?

Yes. After opening the aorta, the calcified leaflets of the aortic valve are removed and the calcium carefully removed.

7. How is the size selected?

After leaflet removal and decalcification, the device size is chosen with dedicated sizers during the operation. There are four valve sizes (small, medium, large, and extra large).

8. Are there studies on midterm durability?

There is a study, which was published in [7] with follow-up up to 5 years showing that there is no structural valve deterioration.

Review About the Addressed Disease or Treatment

The constant search for less invasive surgery techniques is extremely relevant for modern cardiovascular surgery. Once the aortic stenosis is the most frequent valvular disease, keeping pace with advances in its surgical treatment maintains a surgery group competitive and provides an opportunity for patients to have access to the best treatments available.

Even though worldwide several prospective studies and systematic reviews have demonstrated safety and excellent hemodynamic results with the Perceval sutureless bioprosthesis, this device had not been used in Brazil yet. It's a self-expanding bovine bioprosthesis valve mounted in a nitinol stent and designed to preserve aortic sinuses and sinotubular junction.

When we compare the aortic valve replacement using sutureless prosthesis with the conventional technique, we realize not only significantly shorter aortic cross-clamping, cardiopulmonary bypass, and surgery times but also less blood transfusion required, lower intubation time, shorter intensive care unit stay and hospital stay, and lower incidence of postoperative atrial fibrillation and respiratory insufficiency. This lower rate of postoperative complications resulted in reduced resource consumption in the sutureless group with a total cost saving of approximately 25% [5].

It is worth mentioning that Brazil already has experimental studies in animal models in order to develop a similar device but balloon expandable (Inovare Alpha prosthesis-Braile Biomédica). The results were published in 2015 by Gomes and demonstrated excellent clamping time (mean of 7 min, ranging from 6 to 10 min) and no paravalvular leak [6] after the prosthesis implant. It is now ongoing in Brazil a trial comparing Alpha (Braile biomedical sutureless device) with conventional aortic valve replacement (AVR) in patients with combined procedures. There is another sutureless valve (INTUITY/EDWARDS) that has just been approved some months ago for clinical use in Brazil. This device needs three sutures to be tight at the nadir of each cusp.

Bibliography

1. Horstkotte D, Loogen F. The natural history of aortic valve stenosis. Eur Heart J. 1988;9(Suppl E):57–64.
2. Canadian Agency for Drugs and Technologies in Health. Transcatheter aortic valve replacement in severe aortic stenosis: a review of comparative durability and clinical effectiveness beyond 12 months, vol. 2. Ottawa: CADTH Technology Overviews; 2013.
3. Leon MB, Smith CR, Mack MJ, Makkar RR, Svensson LG, et al. PARTNER 2 investigators. Transcatheter or surgical aortic-

valve replacement in intermediate-risk patients. N Engl J Med. 2016;374(17):1609–20.
4. Dedeilias P, Baikoussis NG, Prappa E, Asvestas D, Argiriou M, Charitos C. Aortic valve replacement in elderly with small aortic root and low body surface area; the Perceval S valve and its impact in effective orifice area. J Cardiothorac Surg. 2016;11(1):54.
5. Pollari F, Santarpino G, Dell'Aquila AM, Gazdag L, Alnahas H, et al. Better short-term outcome by using sutureless valves: a propensity-matched score analysis. Ann Thorac Surg. 2014;98(2):611–6.
6. Gomes WJ, Leal JC, Jatene FB, Hossne NA Jr, Gabaldi R, et al. Experimental study and early clinical application of a Sutureless aortic bioprosthesis. Braz J Cardiovasc Surg. 2015;30(5):515–9.
7. Meuris B, Flameng WJ, Laborde F, et al. Five-year results of the pilot trial of a sutureless valve. J Thorac Cardiovasc Surg. 2015;150:84–8.

Thrombosis of a Mechanical Mitral Valve Prosthesis

Gilberto Loiola De Vasconcelos, Saulo Victor Benevides Nunes, Joaquim David Carneiro Neto, and Camila Lopes do Amaral

Clinical Presentation

Patient A.N.S.H., 43 years old, female, married, brown, born and raised in the North-CE region. Previous medical history includes hypertension, rheumatic fever, and a mechanical mitral valve prosthesis for 7 years. Since the prosthesis, she performs a continuous oral anticoagulation therapy, having been asymptomatic during the clinical follow-up that she has performed since the postoperative.

Recently, the patient started to present hypermenorrhea and then she decided to look for her gynecologist. After that, she was diagnosed with a uterine myoma, with a hysterectomy indication. Shortly after, she was admitted in the local hospital for performing the gynecological surgery, when she was advised to discontinue oral anticoagulation for 5 days, due to the procedure.

On the 4th day of anticoagulant suspension, however, it evolved to orthopnea, chest pain, and dyspnea on medium efforts (being characterized as a functional class III, according to NYHA criteria).

G. L. De Vasconcelos (✉) · S. V. B. Nunes · J. D. C. Neto
C. L. do Amaral
Federal University of Ceará (UFC), Sobral, CE, Brazil

R. M. S. Almeida, F. B. Jatene (eds.), *Cardiovascular Surgery*,
https://doi.org/10.1007/978-3-319-57084-6_40

On the 5th day of hospitalization and drug discontinuation, she showed worsening of symptoms and was referred to the emergency department of cardiological service because of her hemodynamic instability, with an episode of nausea and vomiting, as well as intensification of chest pain and respiratory distress (already considered functional class IV, according to the NYHA criteria).

On admission, the patient was with 90 × 60 mmHg of blood pressure, heart rate of 85 bpm, symmetrical and full pulses, axillary temperature 36 °C, respiratory rate 25 cycles/min, and O_2 saturation 92%. In ectoscopy, the patient was acyanotic, afebrile, anicteric, pallor, sweaty, hydrated, and dyspneic, with atypical facies and poor general condition, but was conscious, oriented, and active (Glasgow 15).

During the examination of the cardiovascular system, she showed significant jugular venous distension and an auscultation with irregular heart rhythm, two times, with an important systolic mitral murmur (3+/6+) and the absence of mitral metallic click, without pericardial noises.

On examination of the respiratory system, the patient showed an atypical chest and tachypnea, and the pulmonary auscultation revealed vesicular murmur universally distributed with bibasilar crackles (suggesting pulmonary edema).

During abdominal evaluation, she presented flaccid abdomen, painless to palpation, with fluid sounds. Presented extremities were well perfused, heated, and without edema.

Diagnosis, Assessment, and Treatment

Laboratory tests were ordered, which showed the following results:

Hemogram [Hb, 10.4 g/dl; Ht, 33.6%; the presence of anisocytosis, anisochromia, hypochromia, and microcytosis]

Leukogram [leukocyte = 19.400/mm^3; basophils = 0; eosinophils = 0; metamyelocytes = 0; Bats = 1/mm^3; targeted = 85/mm^3]

Thromboram [336.000 platelets/mm^3]
Creatinine = 1.5 mg/dl; GLUCOSE = 114 mg/dl; UREA = 80 mg/dl;
Potassium = 4.7 mEq/l; SODIUM = 132 mEq/l
Urine [dark yellow color, cloudy, with a pH = 5, and the presence of sediment with mucus filaments and hyaline cylinders]
Coagulogram [prothrombin time = 28,1 s; prothrombin activity = 49%; international normalized ratio (I.N.R.) = 2.46; part-time thromboplastin active = 39,8 s]

The patient was hospitalized in the intensive care unit, where initiated a therapy with heparin in continuous infusion pump. A colorful Doppler echocardiography was ordered, performed 11 h after admission, which indicated the presence of metallic prosthesis in the mitral position with significant dysfunction and greatly reduced mobility of their brochures, with maximum systolic transvalvular gradient of 38 mmHg and an average of 27 mmHg, indicating thrombosis prosthesis.

Besides, a tricuspid valve with severe regurgitation, thickened and failed in the coaptation of its leaflets, was found, with a maximum gradient of 10 mmHg and an average of 4 mmHg. Systolic pulmonary artery pressure was equal to 60 mmHg and right ventricle with preserved function. The mitral valve area by PHT (pressure half-time's method or Hatle's method) was measured at 0,5cm^2.

It was indicated, within an urgency character, a surgery for replacement of the thrombosed mechanical prosthesis, which was started 17 h after the arrival of the patient. A preoperative electrocardiogram was performed, showing sinus rhythm, cardiac frequency of 63 bpm, normal electrical axis, normal AV and IV conduction, and some alterations of the ventricular repolarization (Fig. 1).

The surgery started with heparinization (4 mg/kg), establishing of an extracorporeal circulation, replacing of the mechanical prosthesis by a bioprosthesis number 25 St Jude (Fig. 2).

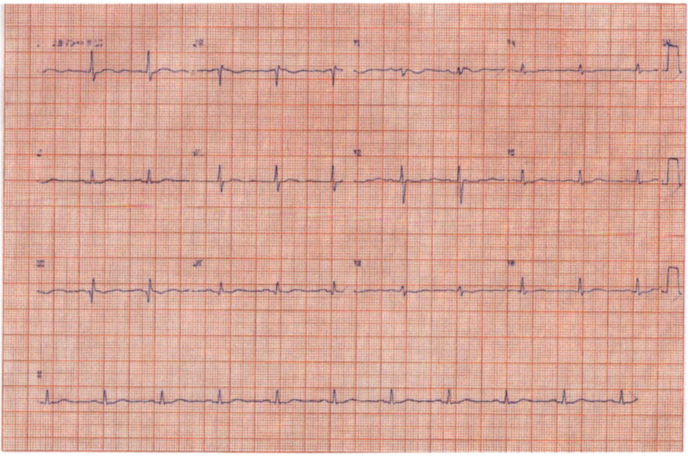

FIGURE 1 Preoperative electrocardiogram

The analysis of the surgical piece demonstrated a mechanical prosthesis waged by thrombi in both rocker switch of the leaflets regions (as visible in Figs. 3 and 4).

The entrance laboratory tests were performed again, presenting without changes. The patient was released from the ICU on the 12th postoperative day and from the ward on the next day, being driven on outpatient periodic control for clinical evaluation.

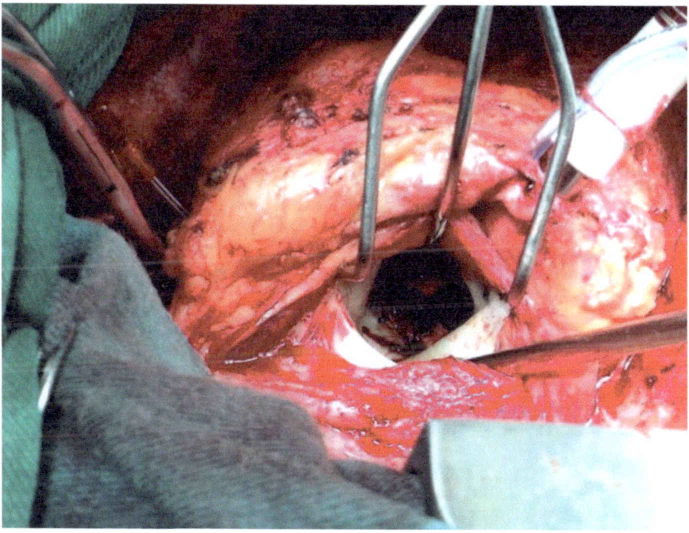

FIGURE 2 Prosthesis view during surgery

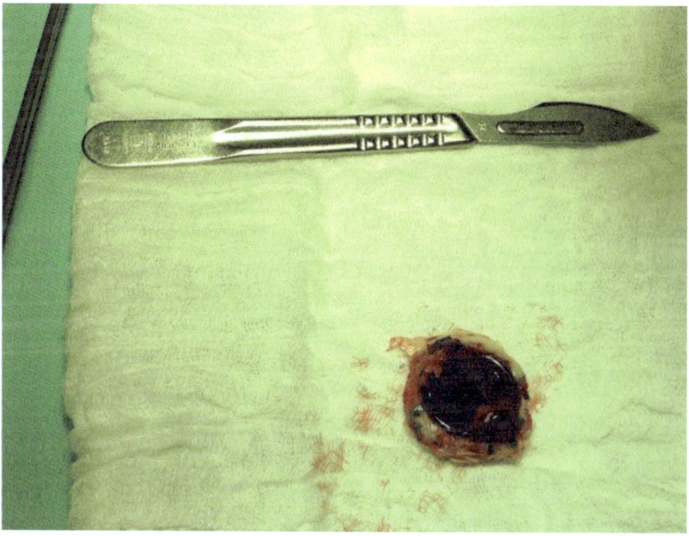

FIGURE 3 Mechanical prosthesis after excision

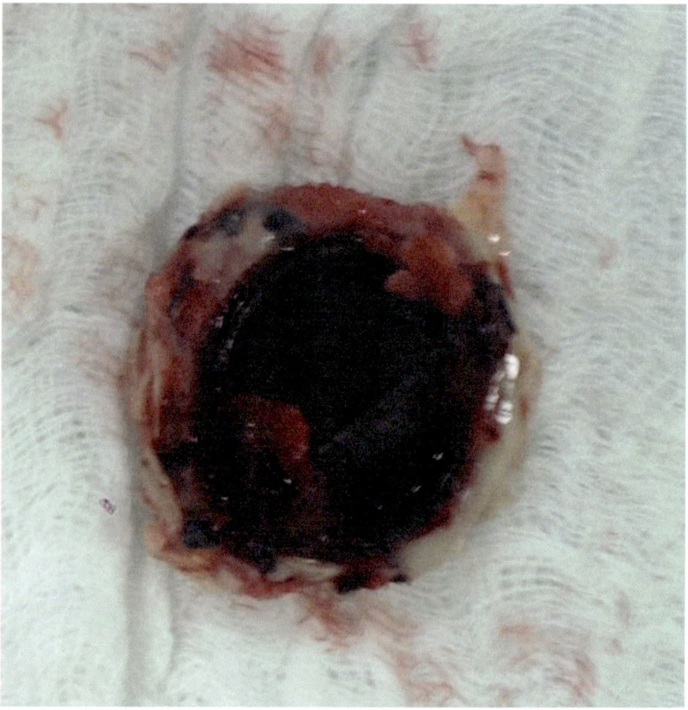

FIGURE 4 Mechanical prosthesis with evident thrombosis areas

Questions

1. What is the major etiology of the prosthetic valve thrombosis?

The main cause of prosthesis thrombosis is an improper anticoagulation or an inadvertent discontinuation of medication, which can be found in up to 82% of cases. Traditionally, we indicate the surgical valve replacement, but the morbidity and mortality rates are high. Currently, the use of fibrinolytic agents has become a therapeutic option especially for cases that affect the right cardiac chambers.

2. Is there any epidemiology defined for this pathology? Is there any relation between the pathology development and the type of prosthesis implanted in the patient's first procedure?

The incidence of thrombosis varies based on the effectiveness of anticoagulation, with the type and location of the implanted prosthesis and the presence of atrial fibrillation. In a meta-analysis published in 1994, with 13.000 carriers of prosthetic heart valves, the annual incidence of thrombosis was 0.2%, with thromboembolic events occurred in 1.8% per year. This incidence was higher in patients that received only antiplatelet agents, occurring in 1.6% to 8.2% for thrombosis and thromboembolism. Studies show that patients with mitral prosthesis had double risk for thrombosis when compared to patients with aortic prosthesis, and metal prosthesis in the tricuspid position had greater thrombogenicity. The "cage" metal prosthesis was the most thrombogenic. Other studies revealed that the cases of obstruction of the prosthesis are more frequent at 1 year after surgery.

3. Which are the main indications, relative contraindications, and absolute contraindications of the anticoagulant therapy?

The main indications are:

1. Thrombosis of tricuspid prostheses: first choice of treatment
2. Multiple valve surgeries or high surgical risk
3. Hemodynamically stable patients with double-disc prosthesis or recent onset of suggestive symptoms of prosthesis thrombosis
4. Patients with inadequate anticoagulation due to special situations (pregnancy, preparation for noncardiac surgery)

The absolute contraindications are:

1. A history of hemorrhagic stroke or diabetic retinopathy
2. BP > 200 × 120 mmHg
3. Presence of active internal bleeding
4. Active infective endocarditis
5. Recent head trauma

The relative contraindications are:

1. Gastrointestinal bleeding in the last 10 days
2. Recent ischemic stroke (within previous 2 months)
3. Large thrombus in the left atrium or in the prosthesis
4. Prior exposure to thrombolytic therapy (within 1 year)
5. Pregnancy

4. In special cases, like pregnant patients, is there any specific and more appropriate therapeutic scheme?

In all cases, we have to evaluate the risk benefit of using anticoagulant medication. In pregnant women, for example, there is controversy about the best anticoagulation scheme. There are no guidelines in order to define the best single or combined treatment option face to the potential risks of thrombosis, because no evidence is available for the effectiveness maternal side of fetal protection. The current recommendation has been for the replacement of warfarin in the first trimester of pregnancy by heparin or low-molecular-weight heparin (LMWH) until the 12th week of pregnancy. After this gestational age, warfarin is reintroduced until the 36th week of gestation, and later it is again replaced by LMWH 24 h before parturition. Literature data warns about the inefficiency in the use of unfractionated heparin (UFH) subcutaneously in preventing metal prosthetic valve thrombosis during pregnancy, due to difficulties in obtaining effective anticoagulation, its control, and the adherence of the patient to the drug. In other cases, we should assess the potency and half-life of the drug of choice and its related adverse effects.

5. Which are the most dangerous complications of this disease and what is the prognosis of these patients?

The existence of the thrombus, in itself, constitutes a serious impairment that requires immediate intervention. However, the complications related to prosthesis thrombosis include systemic embolization, especially to the brain. The risk is higher in mechanical prostheses in relation to biological, mitral valve to the aortic, and early (less than 3 months after surgery) in relation to late. The risk is increased by concomitant risk factors for thromboembolism, such as atrial fibrillation, ventricular dysfunction, left atrial dilatation, prior thromboembolism, and hypercoagulable conditions. The outcome is favorable when intervention is immediate.

6. What is the overall clinical picture presented by a patient with prosthetic valve thrombosis?

The clinical presentation is variable. The patient may manifest asymptomatically or even with extreme cases of cardiogenic shock. Clinical assessment by history and cardiac auscultation is the first step on the diagnosis of prosthesis thrombosis. The most obvious clinical finding is the change of pattern from opening-closing prosthesis click. There may also be the appearance of a new systolic or diastolic murmur. Most patients experience dyspnea in NYHA functional classes III and IV, which can develop into acute pulmonary edema; other presenting symptoms can occur such as systemic embolism, dizziness, and angina pectoris. Systemic embolism and acute pulmonary edema may be the first manifestation of the patient. At physical examination we can observe new murmurs or change of the old murmur pattern. Generally, the most common clinical manifestations are progressive exertional, dyspnea, and syncope.

7. Which are the diagnostic tools for prosthetic valve thrombosis?

Before the introduction of Doppler echocardiography, fluoroscopy was considered the fastest and most accurate method in the evaluation of mechanical prostheses. The exam shows the mobility of the disc and the calculation of the opening angle. It is performed in multiple projections, and the projection measurement is made using the maximum opening and closing of the single-leaflet prosthesis. The Doppler echocardiography is a key part in the diagnosis of prosthesis obstruction. During this exam, in cases of mitral valve prosthesis obstruction, the prosthesis becomes rounded, and a change of the "E" opening point is one of the most important signs. In the two-dimensional echocardiography, the mobility of the mitral and tricuspid prostheses can be well assessed in the apical four-chamber view. Generally, we observe in the thrombotic occlusion an increased density on echoes on the prosthesis region. When found obstruction, gradient is usually increased by the Doppler. In some special cases, we can better confirm by transesophageal echocardiography. Nowadays, there is consensus that cardiac catheterization is no longer necessary to establish the diagnosis of thrombosis of the prosthesis and is still a bleeding risk if used combined with thrombolytic treatment.

8. What is the appropriate conduct for this disease and which are the therapy success criteria?

Prosthesis thrombosis allows clinical treatment with thrombolytic or surgical therapy. It will be up to the medical therapeutic decision. When thrombosis involves the tricuspid valve or, much more rarely, the pulmonary valve, thrombolysis is the therapy of choice. Studies show low complications in this group of patients, regardless of clinical presentation (asymptomatic, mildly, or complete heart failure). When thrombosis involves left valves (mitral and aortic), some considerations must be made for choosing the best treatment. All patients should undergo transesophageal echocardiography before the definitive treatment, and the characteristics of the thrombus should be evaluated. Thrombus <0.8 cm^2 predicts successful thrombolysis. Therefore, for patients in these conditions, regardless of functional class, i.e., from asymptomatic to cardiogenic shock, and no matter what time of thrombosis settlement, thrombolytic therapy can be considered as first choice. This consideration is not valid if the patient has a history of stroke or present atrial fibrillation, because the risk of complications is higher. When the patient has a thrombus >0.8 cm^2, surgery should be considered as the first choice, unless the clinical conditions are unfavorable, as in cardiogenic shock (which has a high surgical risk), making thrombolysis, although potentially complicated, justified for the patient. Also in cases where they do not have heart surgery, thrombolysis may be an option, especially if there is extreme clinical severity. The reoperation in these cases increases the risk, with mortality rates ranging from 10% to 15% in some series. This surgical risk may be increased when the patient is in unfavorable conditions, such as hemodynamic instability.

9. Which are the criteria of choosing a metal or biological prosthetic valves? According to these criteria, could we consider the patient's first replacement (with a mechanical valve) adequate? And now, was the new replacement (changing the prosthesis from mechanical to biological) an appropriate conduct?

The first step in this decision-making process is to choose between a mechanical and a bioprosthetic valve. The most important factors that should be considered in this first step are the patient's age, life expectancy, preference, indication/contraindication for warfarin therapy, and comorbidities. From the recent American College of Cardiology/American Heart Association and European guidelines, the importance given to patient age has been reduced, whereas much greater importance is now given to the patient's preference.

The criteria in favor of using a mechanical valve include the following:

1. The informed patient wants a mechanical valve and has no contraindication for long-term anticoagulation.
2. The patient is already on anticoagulation (mechanical prosthesis in another position or at high risk for thromboembolism);
3. The patient is at risk of accelerated bioprosthesis structural deterioration (young age, hyperparathyroidism, renal insufficiency).
4. The patients is <65 years of age and has a long life expectancy.

On the other hand, a bioprosthesis may be preferred in the following situations:

1. The informed patient wants a bioprosthesis.
2. Good-quality anticoagulation is unavailable (contraindication or high risk, compliance problems, lifestyle).
3. The patient is ≥65 years of age and/or has limited life expectancy.
4. The patient is a woman of childbearing age.

Bioprostheses degenerate more rapidly in young patients and during pregnancy. Hence, a woman in her late 30s or early 40s who has completed her family should probably be advised to have a mechanical valve.

As we see, the patient in our case was correctly recommended for the mechanic valve in her first procedure. However, in front of her disease (the thrombosis), looking at her age and coagulation disturb, the current indication of biological prosthesis should be considered correct to reduce the actual risks of the patient.

Bibliography

1. Pibarot P, Dumesnil JG. Prosthetic heart valves: selection of the optimal prosthesis and long-term management. Circulation. 2009;119(7):1034–48.
2. Baron TH, Kamath PS, McBane RD. Management of antithrombotic therapy in patients undergoing invasive procedures. N Engl J Med. 2013;368:2113–24.
3. Katz M, Tarasoutchi F, Grinberg M. Thrombolytic therapy in prosthetic valve thrombosis. In: Arquivos Brasileiros de Cardiologia, vol. 85. 1st ed; 2005. p. 76–8.
4. Roudat R, Serri K, Lafitte S. Thrombosis of prosthetic heart valves: diagnosis and therapeutic considerations. Heart. 2007;93:137–42.
5. Cáceres-Loriga FM, Perez-Lopez H, Santos-Garcia J, Morlans-Hernandez K. Prosthetic heart valve thrombosis: pathogenesis diagnosis and management. Int J Cardiol. 2006;110:1–6.
6. Garcez JDS, Rosa VEE, Lopes ASSA, Accorsi TAD, Fernandes JRC, Pomerantzeff PM, Avila WS, Tarasoutchi F. Patient management with metallic valve prosthesis during pregnancy and postpartum period. Arq Bras Cardiol. 2015;105:426–9.
7. Lengyel M, Fuster V, Keltai M, Roudaut R, Schulte HD, Seward JB, Chesebro JH, Turpie AGG. Guidelines for management of left-sided prosthetic valve thrombosis: a role for thrombolytic therapy. J Am Coll Cardiol. 1997;30:1521–6.
8. Nishimura RA, Otto CM, Bonow RO, Carabello BA, Erwin JP, Guyton RA, O'Gara PT, Ruiz CE, Skubas NJ, Sorajja P, Sundt TM, Thomas JD. 2014 AHA/ACC guideline for the management of patients with valvular heart disease: executive summary. J Am Coll Cardiol. 2014;63:2438–88.

9. Vahanian A, Baumgartner H, Bax J, Butchart E, Dion R, Filippatos G, Flachskampf F, Hall R, Iung B, Kasprzak J, Nataf P, Tornos P, Torracca L, Wenink A, Priori SG, Blanc JJ, Budaj A, Camm J, Dean V, Deckers J, Dickstein K, Lekakis J, McGregor K, Metra M, Morais J, Osterspey A, Tamargo J, Zamorano JL, Angelini A, Antunes M, Fernandez MAG, Gohlke-Baerwolf C, Habib G, McMurray J, Otto C, Pierard L, Pomar JL, Prendergast B, Rosenhek R, Uva MS, Tamargo J. Guidelines on the management of valvular heart disease. Eur Heart J. 2007;28(2):230–68.

Correction to: Unusual Mechanism of Myocardial Infarction in Prosthetic Valve Endocarditis

Armindo Jreige Júnior, Felipe Bezerra Martins de Oliveira, Larissa Lucas Schloicka, Fernando Antibas Atik, and Claudio Ribeiro da Cunha

Correction to: R. M. S. Almeida, F. B. Jatene (eds.), *Cardiovascular Surgery*, https://doi.org/10.1007/978-3-319-57084-6_16

This chapter was inadvertently published with incorrect order of Given name and Family name for the author "Armindo Jreige Júnior" and the name has been updated to correct order –
Given Name: Armindo
Family Name: Jreige Júnior

The updated version of this chapter can be found at https://doi.org/10.1007/978-3-319-57084-6_16

R. M. S. Almeida, F. B. Jatene (eds.), *Cardiovascular Surgery*, https://doi.org/10.1007/978-3-319-57084-6_41

Index

R. M. S. Almeida, F. B. Jatene (eds.), *Cardiovascular Surgery*,
https://doi.org/10.1007/978-3-319-57084-6

MIX
Papier aus verantwortungsvollen Quellen
Paper from responsible sources
FSC® C105338

If you have any concerns about our products,
you can contact us on
ProductSafety@springernature.com

In case Publisher is established outside the EU,
the EU authorized representative is:
Springer Nature Customer Service Center GmbH
Europaplatz 3, 69115 Heidelberg, Germany

Printed by Libri Plureos GmbH
in Hamburg, Germany